PATHOLOGIE

C000254616

THE WELLCOME INSTITUTE SERIES IN THE HISTORY OF MEDICINE

Forthcoming Titles

Dangerous Liaisons:
A Social History of Venereal Disease
in Twentieth-Century Scotland
Roger Davidson

From Lesion to Metaphor:
Chronic Pain In British, French and
German Medical Writings: 1800–1914
Dr Andrew Hodgkiss MD MRCPsych

Academic enquiries regarding the series should be addressed
to the editors C. J. Lawrence, V. Nutton and Roy Porter at
the Wellcome Institute for the History of Medicine,
183 Euston Road, London NW1 2BE, UK

PATHOLOGIES OF TRAVEL

edited by
Richard Wrigley and George Revill

Amsterdam – Atlanta, GA 2000

First published in 2000
by Editions Rodopi B. V., Amsterdam – Atlanta, GA 2000.

© 2000 Wrigley, Richard and Revill, George

Design and Typesetting by Alex Mayor, the Wellcome Trust.
Printed and bound in The Netherlands by Editions Rodopi B. V.,
Amsterdam – Atlanta, GA 2000.

All rights reserved. No part of this book may be reprinted or reproduced or utilized in any form or by any electronic, mechanical, or
other means, now known or hereafter invented, including photo-
copying and recording, or in any information storage or retrieval
system, without permission in writing from the
Wellcome Institute for the History of Medicine.

British Library Cataloguing in Publication Data
A catalogue record for this book is available from the British
Library
ISBN 90-420-0598-X (Paper)
ISBN 90-420-0608-0 (Bound)

Wrigley, Richard and Revill, George
Pathologies of Travel –
Amsterdam – Atlanta, GA:
Rodopi. – ill.
(Clio Medica 56 / ISSN 0045-7183;
The Wellcome Institute Series in the History of Medicine)

Front cover:
Albrecht Dürer: illustration to Sebastian Brandt,
The Ship of Fools (1494), woodcut

© Editions Rodopi B. V. Amsterdam – Atlanta, GA 2000

Printed in The Netherlands

All titles in the Clio Medica series (from 1999 onwards) are available to
download from the CatchWord website: http://www.catchword.co.uk

Contents

Acknowledgements   i

Notes on Contributors   iii

Introduction
George Revill and Richard Wrigley   1

Letting Madness Range:
travel and mental disorder c.1700-1900
Jonathan Andrews   25

The Continental Journeys of Andrew Duncan Junior:
a physician's education and the international culture of
eighteenth-century medicine
Malcolm Nicolson   89

Richard Jago's *Edge-Hill* Revisited:
a traveller's prospect of the health and disease of
a succession of national landscapes
Matthew Craske   121

'The Rime of the Ancient Mariner':
a ballad of the scurvy
Jonathan Lamb   157

Lassitude and Revival in the Warm South:
relaxing and exciting travel (1750-1830)
Chloe Chard   175

Pathological Topographies and Cultural Itineraries:
mapping 'mal'aria' in eighteenth- and nineteenth-century Rome
Richard Wrigley   203

The Railway Journey and the Neuroses of Modernity
Ralph Harrington   229

Mobility, Syphilis, and Democracy:
pathologizing the mobile body
Tim Cresswell   261

The Politics of Medical Topography:
seeking healthiness at the Cape during the nineteenth century
Harriet Deacon   279

10 Sleepers Wake:
    André Gide and disease in *Travels in the Congo*
    Russell West 299

    Index   317

Acknowledgements

This volume originated in a conference held at the Humanities Research Centre, Oxford Brookes University in 1996. We would like to thank all those who helped to organise the conference, as well as the participants. It was the success of the conference which encouraged us to take on the business of preparing a volume of related texts. We are extremely grateful to Roy Porter and Alex Mayor at the Wellcome Institute, for their efficiency, and amicable collaboration. Finally we would like to thank all the collaborators for their hard work and exemplary punctuality, which have helped to bring to fruition what we believe to be a worthwhile project – hopefully readers will share this view.

Notes on Contributors

Jonathan Andrews is Wellcome Trust Research Lecturer in the History of Medicine at Oxford Brookes University. He is the author of *"They're in the trade ... of lunacy They 'cannot interfere' - they say'" The Scottish Lunacy Commissioners and Lunacy Reform in Nineteenth-Century Scotland* (London: Wellcome History of Medicine, Occasional Publications No. 4, 1998). He is the co-author of *The History of Bethlem* (Routledge, 1997), with Asa Briggs, Roy Porter, Penny Tucker, and Keir Waddington. He co-edited with Anne Digby *Perspectives on Class and Gender in the History of Psychiatry* (forthcoming). He has written widely on the history and historiography of forensic psychiatry and criminal insanity.

Chloe Chard is a literary historian who works on travel writing and imaginative geography; her recent publications include a book, *Pleasure and Guilt on the Grand Tour* (Manchester University Press, 1999), and the co-editing with Helen Langdon of a collecton of essays, *Transports: travel, pleasure, and imaginative geography, 1600-1830* (Yale University Press, 1996). She has recently been a Visiting Fellow at the Centre for Cross-Cultural Research, Australian National University, Canberra, and a Visiting Scholar at the University of Tasmania, Hobart.

Matthew Craske is Henry Moore Research Fellow at Oxford Brookes University. He is the author of *Art in Europe 1700-1830* (Oxford University Press, 1997), a forthcoming study of Joseph Wright, and *Death and Decorum* (Yale University Press), on British funerary sculpture from the seventeenth to the nineteenth centuries.

Tim Cresswell is a Lecturer at the Institute of Geography and Earth Sciences, University of Wales, Aberystwyth. He is the author of *In Place / Out of Place: geography, ideology, and transgression* (University of Minnesota Press, 1996), and *Making up the Tramp* (Reaktion Boks, forthcoming).

Harriet Deacon is currently Research Co-ordinator at the Robben Island Musuem in Cape Town, South Africa. She has published in a number of African History and Medical History journals, and has edited a book on the history of Robben Island.

Ralph Harrington is a Lecturer in the History Department, University of York, and is Transport History Research Trust Lecturer in the History of Urban Transport in the Institute of Railway Studies. He also holds an Honorary Curatorship at the National Railway Museum. He has written on attitudes to 'railway spine' in Victorian Britain; train accidents, trauma and technological crisis in nineteenth-century Britain; and fast trains and modernity from the later nineteenth to the mid twentieth centuries.

Jonathan Lamb teaches English at Princeton University. He is the author of *Sterne's Fiction and the Double Principle* (Cambridge, 1989), and *The Rhetoric of Suffering* (Oxford, 1995). His latest book, *Preserving the Self in the South Seas*, is to be published by Chicago University Press, together with an anthology of Pacific writing co-edited with Nicholas Thomas and Vanessa Smith, *Exploration and Exchange*.

Malcolm Nicolson is Senior Lecturer and Wellcome University Award Holder at the Wellcome Unit for the History of Medicine, University of Glasgow. He is also an honorary member of the Department of Science Dynamics, University of Amsterdam. His principal interests are now in the history of diagnostic practice, in the nineteenth and twentieth centuries.

George Revill is senior lecturer in cultural geography at Oxford Brookes University. His research interests are in music landscape and national identity and in the historical meanings of railway work. He is co-editor of *The Place of Music* (Guilford/Routledge), Landscapes of Defence (Longman) and co-author (with John Gold) of *Representing the Environment* (Routledge).

Russell West is Professor of British and American Studies at the Fachschule/University of Applied Sciences in Magdeburg. He is the author of *Conrad and Gide: translation, transference, and intertextuality* (1996), *Figures de la maladie chez André Gide* (1997), the co-editor of *Marginal Voices: diaries in European literaure and history* (1999, forthcoming)

Richard Wrigley is Principal Lecturer in History of Art, Oxford Brookes University. His publications include *The Origins of French Art Criticism: from the Ancien Regime to the Restoration* (Oxford University Press, 1993), and numerous articles on the politics of visual culture in revolutionary France. He is currently preparing *The Politics of Appearances: the symbolism and representation of dress in revolutionary France.*

Introduction

Travel has been represented as improving and wasteful, as a blessing and a curse. The speed and ease of modern travel have created undreamt of opportunities for many; at the same time, the burgeoning transport infrastructure has brought forth the worst excesses of environmental degradation and exploitation. Travel both demonstrates the health and strength of western technological and social organisation, and symbolises its deepest malaise. To view travel as evidence of a pathology is not, however, novel. Travel has long been associated with both personal and social ailments and also with their remedies. The act of pilgrimage has carried the curative power of personal and national salvation across cultures and time. Exploration has sought scientific, medical, and economic remedies for the social and technological ills of the western world. Travel has been a metaphor for regeneration that is at once personal, psychological and aesthetic. This collection of essays contributes to the growing literature on and around the subject by exploring a range of symbolic and practical aspects of travel, health and illness from the eighteenth to the twentieth centuries.

In recent years metaphors of travel have come to dominate large areas of the humanities and social sciences. Such concepts as mobility, displacement, diaspora, frontier, transience, dislocation and permeability have become central for thinking about the nature of subjectivity, the formation of identity, and the elusive co-ordinates of belonging in the world of late modernity.[1] Relationships between the journey and the narrative take on particular importance in a theoretical context which interprets the world as text.[2] Metaphors of travel assume a politically charged resonance in a world of mass mobility and forced migration, generating a need to search for origins, authenticity and community.[3] The contradictions inherent in trajectories of exploration and discovery acquire a particular significance in light of the preconceptions and prejudices which shape the production of knowledge.[4] In contemporary theory, travel constitutes the direct route to many key areas of current social, cultural and historical investigation: imperialism, postcolonialism, the formation of scientific knowledge, the clinical

1

and social definition of the modern subject. To this extent it has become very difficult to think through these historical issues outside this conceptual framework.

Yet there is an everpresent danger that a critical vocabulary whose terms seductively emphasis the transitory and fluid nature of the world themselves congeal and coalesce into a new orthodoxy, forgetting its origins in contingency and mobility. It is at this point that we need to remember the historical specificity of the language and vocabulary of travel. This implies not merely that travel means different things at different times to different people, but that the words and concepts deployed in contemporary theoretical contexts have a history, the recognition of which will undermine any tendency towards the solidity of convention. James Clifford recognises this in his essay 'Traveling Cultures', in which he calls for cross-cultural, historically and geographically sensitive studies of travel.[5] He argues that the term 'travel' is inextricably bound up with a history of European, literary, male, bourgeois, scientific, heroic, recreational meanings and practices.[6] A complex set of problems are raised, he suggests, when 'travel' is used as a metaphor for the experience of, for example, immigrant and migrant workers, whose stories of mobility are substantially governed by the forces of necessity and coercion. Yet he says:

> I hang on to 'travel' as a term of cultural comparison, precisely because of its historical taintedness, its associations with gendered, racial bodies, class privilege, specific means of conveyance, beaten paths, agents, frontiers, documents, and the like.[7]

For Clifford, 'travel' is a 'translation term', 'a word of apparently general application used for comparison in a strategic and contingent way'. For him, and for us also, the value of a term such as travel lies in the difference between travel as an historically situated practice and any subsequent claims to universalise the experience of travel. There is a substantial and growing literature on the culture of travel, which explores the meanings of travel in specific contexts and is both theoretically and historically sensitive. This collection of essays aims to make a contribution to this corpus, and to acknowledge the centrality of travel in the history of modernity and the modern subject, whilst at the same time focusing on the meanings of travel within specific historical circumstances. By adopting the term 'pathology' as an organising theme, this volume recognises that the association of travel with theories of the subject, of the body, of organism and social organisation, has a long and richly ambiguous history worthy of investigation.

It is not intended that this introduction or the contributions gathered here should exhaustively define the term pathology. Rather, as the collection's title implies, the theme was chosen precisely because of the multiplicity of possible meanings arising out of the conjunction of pathology – or more accurately pathologies – with travel. The aim of the book is to keep these meanings open and trace the ways in which the term is defined and contested in particular historical contexts. In this sense, we adopt the term pathology in a similar spirit to that in which Clifford adopts the term travel. In today's parlance, and indeed in earlier parlance, the term pathology is at once specific – implying a causality that can be clinically determined – and also diffuse, carrying with it a marked social and moral charge. During the twentieth century, it has become current in popular and political as well as professional and technical discourses. The idea of pathology suggests at one and the same time something deepseated and fundamental and yet also clearly observable.[8] The fusion of hidden depth with visible objective evidence, and the conflation of scientific fact with social and moral prescription gives the notion of pathology a distinctive place within cultural politics. The medical associations of the term are important because they throw into question relationships between the individual and the social whole as a functional and organic entity, bringing into play metaphors of national health and the condition of the body politic. It is precisely the ways in which the 'scientific' is mapped on to the 'moral' and vice versa that gives the pathology of travel an important role in the cultural politics of the body. Through observation, description and classification, the material and metaphorical practices of travel produce a terrain which organises social and moral values in terms of a physical topography which give such values an authority vested in empirical fact. Because of this, the theme of pathology facilitates examination of the ways in which the material and metaphorical practices of travel negotiate the boundaries between culture and nature, individual and society, wilderness and civilisation, deviancy and conformity, health and sickness, producing moral geographies simultaneously in the mind, of the body, and on the ground.

The period embraced by the essays in this book saw three important cultural dynamics in the 'transport revolution': the rise of tourism from its origins in the Grand Tour, the mechanisation and democratisation of travel concomitant with the coming of the railways, and the increasing centrality of communications

3

technology in governance of the nation state and establishing the formal rule of Empire.[9] Increasing mobility of the 'lower orders', and the perceived fears of social mixing on the road and in railway stations acted as a counterpoint to the facility of mechanised travel and communication to integrate, order, and subdue. Containment of the poor by legal conditions of settlement, polite society's fear of massed 'rootless' labour represented by the gangs of navvies who built railways and canals, no less than the still familiar rounds of invective against the invasion of the countryside suggested, for example, by Wordsworth's sonnet *On the Projected Kendal and Windemere Railway* (1843) – all involve a conception of mobility as social pathology.[10] Modern authors who have engaged with these themes have adopted a variety of strategies which reflect the tension between representations of travel as a stabilising and destabilising force. Labour historians like Eric Hobsbawm pay homage to the 'tramping artisan'[11] as a model for ordered, respectable, self-help at the same time that celebrants of cultural modernity like Paul Virilio revel in the destabilising revolutionary implications of speed and movement:

> All through history there has been an unspoken, unrecognised revolutionary wandering, the organisation of a first mass transportation – which is nonetheless revolution itself.[12]

Most useful for our purpose are those studies which work with the tension between order and disorder in conceptions of travel. The discourses of tourism and anti-tourism in the mid-nineteenth century considered by James Buzard occupy this territory.[13] 'Travellers' as opposed to 'tourists' are represented as both travelling for a purpose and engaging with people and place in meaningful ways which cannot be predetermined. In contradistinction, tourist experiences are represented as predictable and repetitive, a combination of purposelessness and certainty which results in vulgarity and ignorance. Buzard characterises this in a recurrent association between the image of tourism and that of the *beaten track*.[14] Figured as a social other, a cultural stereotype from which society constructs a counter representation of itself, the image of the traveller is itself subject to a process of stabilisation. Crowther's study of the tramp in Victorian Britain highlights the diversity of vagrants, tinkers, sailors, beggars, gamblers, craft workers, Irish immigrants, seasonal agricultural workers, gipsies, travelling showmen and fairground people, family groups and lone males.[15] She shows how the idea of the tramp was stereotyped both in

4

popular romanticisation and governmental regulation disguising a complex set of social, economic and political relationships. She says:

> the vagrant aroused three powerful emotions, fear, pity and envy. These are not mutually exclusive, and each age constructs its own version. The sturdy beggar of Tudor times, the intimidating Victorian 'moucher' and the twentieth-century alcoholic provoked different kinds of fear, reflected in official policies.[16]

The pioneering application of ideas from psychoanalysis to the study of bourgeois culture by Stallybrass and White links the stabilising and destabilising effects of mobility with scientific and moral constructions of public health.[17] Their examination of the refiguring of the Victorian city looks at the ways in which the bourgeoisie came to terms with the phenomenon of industrial urbanism through techniques which increased knowledgability and heightened visibility through social scientific survey and report. They show how notions of cleanliness and confinement were used to classify, map and regularise people and place, connecting for example 'slums to sewage, sewage to disease, and disease to moral degradation'.[18] Their argument centres on the city as a body and its means of public circulation, its streets and sewers being the key to ordering and separating the masses, their products and effluvia into sound and manageable units subject to the civilising axioms of public health. They argue that the concepts of 'the slum, the sewer, the nomad, the savage, the rat' are just as important for remapping the body as they are in ordering the city, articulating notions of shame, embarrassment and disgust which reflect back to structure the bourgeois imaginary.[19] Such notions of otherness link darkest London to darkest Africa through the cultural oppositions which construct European bourgeois identity. By implication this marks out an important place for travel within the four symbolic domains – 'psychic forms, the human body, geographical space and the social order' – which they believe articulate bourgeois identity. For the period under consideration here, a number of authors have usefully explored the relationships between travel and pathology examining issues of travel for, and as generative of, health, and travel as itself a malady. Located at the intersection of issues concerning travel and health, each of these studies brings into focus various aspects of the four symbolic domains of bourgeois identity suggested by Stallybrass and White, indicating, as Clifford and others have argued, the key role of travel in the formation of bourgeois western subjectivity.

The symbolic domain of the human body is an essential site for this formation. In terms of physique, deportment, and behaviour, the human body has become a malleable and ultimately transformable location of self-realisation. Since the beginnings of Romantic tourism, travel has played an active role in this; it is a means both of secular emotional pilgrimage and personal bodily transformation. In *Walking, Literature and English Culture: the origins and uses of peripatetic in the nineteenth century* (Oxford, 1993), Anne Wallace discusses the way in which walking came to be interpreted as therapeutic in the later eighteenth and early nineteenth centuries. She traces this to changing attitudes to travel accompanying the transport revolution from the mid-eighteenth century onwards, when walking began to become an option rather than a necessity and therefore more acceptable to middle-class and aristocratic tastes. She demonstrates how walking became aesthetically representable in the work of William Wordsworth, through the literary device of the 'peripatetic'. This constitutes the conjunction of a Georgic sensibility which stressed agrarian values of cultivation, and a Romantic sensibility which valorised proximity to nature. Both cohere around a notion of walking as labour, grounding care for locality in both work and knowledge. Following the 'peripatetic' through the nineteenth century and finding clear traces in current ideas of psychic and physical health in the western world, she observes:

> Essays by William Hazlitt, Henry David Thoreau, John Burroughs, Robert Louis Stevenson, and Leslie Stephen, although differing in detail, all argue that the natural, primitive quality of the physical act of walking restores the natural proportions of our perceptions, reconnecting us with both the physical world and the moral order inherent in it, and enabling us to recollect both our personal past and our national and/or racial past – that is, human life before mechanization. As a result, the walker may expect an enhanced sense of self, clearer thinking, more acute moral apprehension, and higher powers of expression.[20]

The realm of psychic form suggests not only bourgeois notions of individuality and creativity, but also those of repression and the subconscious. The desire for the exotic within the West finds historically specific expression in eighteenth- and nineteenth-century travellers and collectors. At the same time, journeys into the subconscious begin to provide a technical means for revealing the inner conflicts associated with illicit passions. John Barrell, for example, builds his study of Thomas De Quincey (1785-1859), the essayist, critic, admirer of Coleridge and Wordsworth and self-confessed opium addict, around a metaphor of 'infection'.[21] The notion of mobility here operates at the level of an idiosyncratic imaginative geography. Barrell adopts this metaphor to address what he sees as twin recurring fears in De Quincey's work. For Barrell, De Quincey's pathology of travel conflates the guilt of empire with personal shame. These derive from an attempt both to envision the Orient and its place in the British empire, and reconcile what he perceived as a fear of class-conflict encapsulated in a concern with republicanism and sedition in Britain. These fears are manifest, for example, in dream-like sequences of topographical description in *Confessions of an English Opium-Eater* which provide a confusing kaleidoscope of Oriental imagery. Barrell demonstrates how 'The English Mail Coach' conflates the plebeian with the Oriental. An upstart 'democratic' rival to the Mail-coach is characterised as having 'as much writing and painting on its sprawling flanks as would have puzzled a decipherer from the tombs of Luxor';[22] a coachman riding alongside De Quincey on the lower-class outside of the coach is transfigured into the threatening spectre of an Egyptian crocodile.[23] Barrell adopts the concept of infection from Roland Barthes to explain these problematic invasions of a vivid irrationality:

> 'One immunizes the contents of the collective imagination by means of a small inoculation of acknowledged evil; one thus protects it against the risk of a generalised subversion' (Barthes). The apparently mixed metaphor here, which seems to identify political opposition and disease, is particularly appropriate to De Quincey's scheme, which figures the oriental as infection, and also as rebel, mutineer or subversive immigrant. De Quincey's life was terrorised by the fear of an unending and interlinked chain of infections from the East, which threatened to enter his system and to overthrow it, leaving him visibly and permanently 'compromised' and orientalised.[24]

For bourgeois society, the inherent instabilities of capitalist economic relations provide a deeply traumatised basis on which to build a symbolic domain of the social order. As itself a product of capitalism, the negotiation of this conflict is something bourgeois society cannot avoid in the figuration of its own sense of social stability.

In his study of the culture of railway travel in the nineteenth century, Wolfgang Schivelbusch examines the psychosocial consequences of capitalism's cyclical, crisis-ridden economic relations, and its drive for technological innovation. His concern is with the relationship between medical knowledge, the social practices of travel, and the creation of broader notions of socio-technical order and stability. He shows how the inception of new technologies of transport brought with them a complex of pathologised perceptions that operate on levels which conjoin the symbolic realms of the social and the psychological. In *The Railway Journey*, Schivelbusch examines the traumatic experience induced by the speed of railway travel and the danger of accident as indicative of the shock of modernity. The consequent coping strategies engendered by the new experience of risk are, he believes, a demonstration of the broader cultural responses to both capitalism and industrialisation. He sets this in the context of the new technological environment of industrialisation exemplified by the railway:

> the more civilized the schedule and the more efficient the technology, the more catastrophic its destruction when it collapses. There is an exact ratio between the level of the technology with which nature is controlled, and the degree of severity of its accidents...

The breaking of a coach axle in the eighteenth century merely interrupted a slow and exceedingly bumpy trip on the highway; the breaking of a locomotive axle between Paris and Versailles in 1842 led to the first railroad catastrophe that caused a panic in Europe.[25]

Schivelbusch reviews a range of coping strategies including upholstered and sprung coaches, reading whilst travelling, and 'panoramic perception'. These, he suggests form a new psychic layer, 'that obscures the old fears and lets them lapse into oblivion'.[26] He shows how the deleterious force of railroad disasters was manifest not only in the destruction of machinery and damage to life and limb, but also in symptoms of psychic and physical deterioration which occurred in victims only sometime after the event. He shows how the medical explanation of this phenomenon shifted from an early pathological explanation which depended on the physical shock transmitted to the central nervous system and called 'railway spine', to more psychopathological explanations which constituted a 'traumatic neurosis'. He examines Freud's engagement with nineteenth-century pathological theories and in particular his theory of the stimulus shield in his account of the relationship between anxiety and fright. In doing so he is able to relate the psychopathology of industrialised travel to the progressive trajectory

8

of western modernity more generally, such that:

> the 'civilising process' described by Norbert Elias can be understood
> as the formation of a stimulus shield, just as we have understood
> the process of travel by rail to be one.[27]

It can be argued that the symbolic domain of geographical space is key in terms of the authority claims of bourgeois society. Such claims are, of course, vested not simply in tradition, church or monarchy, but in that which is empirically verifiable. Geographical space plays a fundamental role in the production of such truth claims, mapping out causal links and demonstrating the spatial arrangement of physical facts. A notable product of the revolutions which punctuated the rise of bourgeois society is the increasing centrality of the nation state as both container and arbiter for economic, political, and social relations and transactions. Like the ordering of the city central to Stallybrass and White's argument, so in a broader geographical sense, the idea of the nation undermined by the challenge to traditional modes of authority itself required refiguring. Mobility derived from social change and the reformation of social hierarchies no less than industrialisation and transport technology, challenges the wholeness and coherence of the nation. This wholeness is at once both dependent on, and undermined by, such mobility. Here, the nation as a whole was pathologised: the material practices of travel are mapped on to metaphors of the body and together these have been used to diagnose its state of health. In his essay 'J.M.W. Turner and the Circulation of the State', Steve Daniels uses Turner's own mobility and pictoral concern with routeways, 'turnpikes, droveroads, railways, rivers, canals and sea lanes' to examine the idea of travel as a metaphor for national strength and wellbeing.[28] Daniels discusses Turner's extensive tours throughout Britain and Europe explaining how routeways often organize his compositions, he says: 'Routeways in Turner's art are not just lines of linkage, but arenas of bustling activity.' He concludes that: 'It was circulation rather than property which shaped Turner's landscape imagery, even in depictions of landed estates....'[29]

Discussing the painting *Leeds from Beeston Hill*, Daniels suggests that the view is more than just a record of Leeds as a place; rather, the picture documents the city's growth and its industrial activity. It tells an instructive story of worthwhile labour; from the distant mills and the factory workers returning from the night shift, to the man carrying a roll of cloth from the weaving sheds and the workers hanging out cloth to dry on the tenter frames adjacent to the road. Here Turner echoes John Dyer's patriotic poem *The Fleece*, a Georgic exposition which traces the process of cloth production – 'Britannia's fleece' – as it travels from hill to factory, to port, charting its influence in overseas trade. Turner imitates the patriotism of this poem in his own lines written on the flax industry of Bridport. Daniels relates this fusion of travel with the state of the nation to Turner's view of a train crossing Maidenhead viaduct, *Rain, Steam and Speed*, his view of the *Fighting Temeraire*, and a painting of *The Burning of the Houses of Parliament*. He argues that the presence of the River Thames, a thoroughfare at the heart of the nation whose scenery had long signified the nation's condition and power, is important to these works. Quoting some of Turner's own verse, Daniels considers his attitude towards London as national capital:

> It was the railway which most dramatically expressed this vision of London as an epicentre of energy, both explosive and implosive, creative and destructive, noble and base, and in *Rain, Steam and Speed*, Turner shows the exact place at Maidenhead Bridge where the capital's main arteries can be seen 'far stretching East and West', the 'concentrated focus' of 'hope', for Turner a driving but duplicitous force of history.[30]

Given the importance of the mobile sovereign individual to bourgeois subjectivity, it is perhaps not surprising that the body, health, and travel are represented together in the European imagination. This is not to suggest that health and travel are somehow inextricably connected, and constitute some form of master discourse, or give some form of singularly privileged access to social and cultural formation. The association between, for example, human health and the structures of capitalism prominent in our discussion of Schivelbusch, for instance, is hardly confined to travel as a metaphorical vehicle. Perhaps one may usefully cite Susan Sontag's study *Illness as Metaphor* here. For example, she argues that medical ideas about illnesses such as tuberculosis were informed by metaphors of reckless and non-productive expenditure closely associated with the conceptual world of early capitalist accumulation.[31] However, we do wish to suggest that the fortunes of people informed by the technologies of an increasingly medicalised body find some kind of expression within the material and metaphorical practices of travel. Mobility provides a vehicle with which to explore society's individualistic and liberatory possibilities at the same time as those of regulation and confinement. Transport provides the physical means to threaten social and corporeal stability and purity, yet also facilitates the re-establishment of a sense of order. At the same time, travel provides a means of gaining knowledge about self and world necessary to enforce such regimes. The experience of travel and the practice of medicine are, if not necessarily together, fundamental to the experience of the subject in the modern world. Yet when health and travel are conjoined, the ensuing cultural ramifications may be both extensive and complex.

A recent study which exemplifies the importance of such a perspective is Anne McClintock's *Imperial Leather: race, gender and sexuality in the colonial context*, which discusses the development of soap as a fetishised commodity for the bourgeois imperial household. This story of travel, trade colonialism and health draws on a wide spectrum of the Victorian imagination from the mundane to the exotic. She examines the relationships between domesticity, cleanliness, imperial exploration, conquest, control and trade. She argues that the economic systems of indigenous peoples were derided as irrational and fetishistic, typified by non-utilitarian exchange of trinkets, beads and baubles, and that this functioned to disguise and rationalise the rampant profiteering of westerners in the colonial economy. Yet, at the same time, British travellers, traders and explorers became dependent an equally fetishistic symbolic framework which reworked the trajectory of colonialism in terms of domesticity, racial purity, health and strength. In the case of soap, for example, she says it:

> offered the promise of spiritual salvation and regeneration through commodity consumption, a regime of domestic hygiene that could restore the threatened potency of the imperial body politic and the race.[32]

According to many accounts of European travellers and colonials, McClintock claims ENO's Fruit Salts as amongst the most 'potent' of fetishistic artifacts. If soap cleansed the outer body, ENO's guaranteed internal purity and ensured male potency in the arena of war. She describes an incident in Kenya when Joseph Thompson staged a mock ceremony in which he posed as a white medicine man by 'conjuring an elaborate ruse with a tin of ENO's'. At this ceremony, Thompson apparently wore gloves, brandished a sextant, and had an assistant fire a gun in an attempt to make the Masai believe in the power of Fruit Salts as an efficiacious remedy. She comments:

11

While amusing himself grandly at the imagined expense of the
Masai, Thompson reveals his own faith in the power of his fetishes
(gloves, as a fetish of class leisure, sextant, and a gun as a fetish of
scientific technology, and ENO's as a fetish of domestic purity).[33]

Thus, for McClintock the incident epitomises Western fears of travel
and conquest in terms of infection, purgative, and purity, at the same
time that it justified the imperial trajectory as a cleansing and
civilising mission. The story of cleanliness and empire claimed to be
liberatory and progressive, moving 'savage' peoples to a civilised and
rational world of consumer commodities and making the bounty of
empire available to purify and sanctify the European home. However,
this story of commodification merly traps the indigenous peoples in
highly iniquitous trading relationships and imprisons Western
women in the private sphere as guardians of the home.[34]

Brian Turner's discussion of agoraphobia ranges across isssues of
mobility and domesticity in a way which has similar implications for
the place of women in nineteenth-century society. He shows how
urbanism became viewed as a threat to the dominant culture of the
eighteenth-century elite. Urban life was increasingly problematised
as having a deleterious consequence on the morality of the
population. The moral anxieties of urban life were focused on
middle-class women who were seen as especially vulnerable to the
sexual dangers of urban space. As the regulation of cities reached a
point where women's travel within cities became safer, anxiety
increased. It was at this time that the first coherent medical
descriptions of agoraphobia started to appear. Shilling summarises
Turner's argument thus:

> Agoraphobia in wives expresses the anxiety of husbands over their
> control of the domestic household, but is also a manifestation of
> the wife's dependence on the security and status of the bourgeois
> family setting. Fear of urban areas and the market place became
> converted into a medical condition which legitimated the power of
> husbands over wives.[35]

The above studies by McClintock and Turner begin to indicate
some of the ways in which travel and the technologies of mobility
impinge on the medicalisation of the body through social,
economic, legal, and political structures operating across a range of
geographical spaces from the household to the empire. The
foregoing discussion may help to show that the culture of travel and
the history of the human subject in the eighteenth and nineteenth

centuries are more complexly related than they might at first sight appear. Historians have paid considerable attention to the social implications of the various scientific, economic and political 'revolutions' which have shaped many of the contours of the modern world since the seventeenth century. In the process they have considered numerous ways in which these have inscribed the limits and potential of human subjectivity. One may perhaps venture that the implications of the 'transport revolution' have yet to be fully explored in this regard and that the metaphor of travel as pathology may help us begin to traverse some of this territory.

Many of the studies cited above exemplify the way in which the study of travel and mobility almost seems to necessitate an approach which is sceptical of disciplinary boundaries. Equally, the social and scientific connotations of the term pathology make it an ideal touchstone for the pursuit of interdisciplinary history. Our decision to engage with the notion of travel as pathological corresponds to our desire to go against the established grain of expectations of travel as beneficial, pleasurable, educational, and improving. This applies most obviously to those contributions which relate to, but depart from, existing literature on 'the age of the Grand Tour', and associated forms of cultural and educative travel. Taken as a whole, the contributions to the volume offer valuable insights into the inter-relations that existed between a variety of medical ideas and practices and the literature of travel in its various forms. Between these two types of discursive territory we find a range of exchanges and overlaps. The notion of travel as pathological provides a bridge by means of which a linguistically complex two-way traffic can be shown to circulate.

The first two texts, those by Jonathan Andrews and Malcolm Nicolson, contextualise aspects of medical ideas and practices, and seek to map the interplay between the two in terms of their relevance for our understanding of the scientific and cultural significance of travel. Jonathan Andrews' paper considers the complex and contested issue of whether travel was likely to be more beneficial that harmful in the treatment of madness and its various related conditions, and shows the degree to which, in the eighteenth and nineteenth centuries, this was a vexed question, which generated conflicting recommendations. Proponents of travel in one sense constituted 'a threat to medical practitioners' claims to special expertise in the treatment of insanity'. While travel might be thought of as working beneficially both on the sick mind and the ailing body, it can also be recognised as having been exploited to deal with the problem by removing the patient out of sight. Andrews shows that travel and relocation of the afflicted was a key matter in thinking about the most effective ways of controlling the causes and alleviating the symptoms of madness. In its detailed exposition of case histories, institutional histories, and dominant types of thinking on the matter, Andrews clearly demonstrates the inherent ambiguities involved in conceptualizing the benefits and drawbacks of travel for patients, as it was respectively encouraged or forbidden. This analysis is contextualised within the ongoing debates between asylum-based and private practitioners, who each had conflicting types of vested interest in seeking to confine patients or encourage a more flexible approach to their management. However, the very wealth of literature produced around medical aspects of travel necessitates a significant degree of contextualising caution, such that specific contributions to this body of ideas are anchored within their professional, institutional, and ideological contexts. Andrews also underlines the extent to which 'the prescription of travel was dependent on patients' social circumstances (as well as their conditions)'. Class and wealth were important factors in determining different forms of medical attention, especially as this applied to its peripatetic possibilities.

A key aspect of the complexity of competing ideas surrounding the benefits aand disadvantages of travel which Andrews brings to our attention, is the way that the growth of travel in the nineteenth century – whether recreational, or associated with colonial and military enterprises – spawned a considerable literature produced as much by as for a non-specialist audience. The greater frequency and scope of travel, as well as the new types of transport which helped to make it possible, above all the train, brought with them concomitant new forms of indisposition and affliction, thus generating new problems for medical commentary. It should also be noted that notions of travel or mobility take on a profoundly different complexion when that experience applies to individuals who are subjects of medical prescription, abovd all in relation to those who were treated as mad or mentally incompetent.

Medical men on the move were a familiar sight in the eighteenth and nineteenth centuries. Indeed, Malcolm Nicolson argues that different forms of mobility were central to the business of eighteenth-century medicine, whether in the form of military and naval service, 'as tutors and bearleaders on the grand Tour, as attendants to explorers and ambassadors, or as tourists and explorers in their own right'. Nicolson's paper analyses the experience of a young Edinburgh doctor, Andrew Duncan junior, travelling in search of technical knowledge, and as a means of consolidating both his reputation and his worldliness. Although Duncan's main concern was foreign medical institutions and medics, he did not insulate himself from the pursuit of more conventional cultural activities. In the constructing of a career, such areas of social activity were integral to the acquisition of a knowledge of the varieties of professional conduct. Furthermore such mobility was a necessary form of self-advertisement, and a means of positioning himself within a network across which flowed practical and theoretical knowledge. Ultimately, it also served as a potential source of clientele, gained through successive recommendations and the increased degree of contact that travel brought.

Matthew Craske's analysis of Richard Jago's poem, *Edge-Hill, or the Rural Prospect Delineated and Moralised* (1767), shifts attention from the traveller as responding to the health-giving or otherwise effects of a specific location on to the notion of pathologising a landscape. This pathologisation is shown to be driven by a desire to see in the prospect of the British landscape an expression of the condition of the body-politic. Such ideological colouration led in Jago's case to the inscription of a pro-Stuart and covertly Jacobite reading on to the prospect he surveyed. On another level, celebrations of sites such as Edge Hill were emphatically conceived as patriotic alternatives to the propensity to seek cultural inspiration abroad, especially in Italy. In Jago's terms, if the British landscape sometimes fell short of its continental counterparts, then this was directly ascribable to political mismanagement and neglect – natural effects were an ineluctable register of any deepseated, pervasive 'disease' which might be afflicting the state.

Jonathan Lamb considers Coleridge's *The Rime of the Ancient Mariner* in relation to travel accounts of South Sea exploration and their recording of the disturbing effects of scurvy. Lamb shows that apparently literary effects within the poem should be understood as reworking descriptions of the altered states of mind and body produced by the physical depredations of the disease. European voyaging in the South Seas not only involved conflict with indigenous peoples, but the sickness that accompanied such travel was associated with extreme degress of destabilisation, which engendered heightened modes of perception (as well as proving fatal to a large proportion of the crews of these expeditions). The chronic debilitation suffered by travellers was accompanied by an appalled euphoria at the spectacle of their physical decay, and at their 'otherworldly' surroundings. Such a perspective profoundly shifts our reading of travel narratives of long-distance naval expeditions, and at one and the same time undermines and makes more complex our picture of such travel as being fundamentally a matter of economic or nautical expansion, or merely extremely hazardous. Lamb shows how *The Rime of the Ancient Mariner* inscribes a 'pathology of travel' whose chronic effects were as unmanageable as they were all but unavoidable, confusing horror and euphoria. In Coleridge's text, the language of medical diagnosis applied to scurvy was transposed into a poetic idiom which obscured its sources and translated its content into a 'powerfully ambivalent' moral register.

Both Chloe Chard and Richard Wrigley discuss the theme of travel and the pathological as it relates to the experience of Italy, normally unerstood to be the classic reference point for the phenomenon of European cultural travel. Chard traces the reliance of descriptions of destabilized states of mind and body on contemporaneous physiological models. She also notes the ambiguity inherent in crediting such extreme states of mind with being natural, and therefore essentially pleasurable, but also hazardous in so far as destabilisation could descend into a chronic, irrecoverable state. Indeed, so much was this liable to be the case that travel could itself be credited with being pathological. Prescriptions of travel as a beneficial solution to physical and psychological malaise therefore clearly carried with them a high risk factor. Reflection on the underlying mechanics of physical, and therefore psychological, disposition was a way of seeking to consolidate explanations regarding the therapeutic reliability of such of relocation and change of scene.

Richard Wrigley draws attention to the way that accounts of travel to Italy, especially the culturally privileged site of Rome, resolve the conflict between the inspiring prospect of the Eternal City's artistic riches, and the insalubrious atmosphere which threatened natives and travellers alike. Valetudinary travellers had to contend with conflicting advice, not only as to when and where to go, but also regarding the particular effects associated with the pursuit of cultural tourism. This might be encouraged for its therapeutic effects, but was also recognized to be potentially hazardous because of the way it involved exposure to the dangerous inconstancy of Rome's climate. Thus, the key note in discussions of the likely effects to be produced by a sojourn in Rome is at best a wary empiricism, at worst a traumatising uncertainty. Only as the nineteenth century progressed was medical knowledge more precisely attuned to the relative benefits and disadvantages of the Roman climate for different forms of ill health, disease, and types of constitution. In the case of the incidence of 'mal'aria', uncertainty remained until the end of the nineteenth century. In exploring attitudes to Rome as a 'health station', it is abundantly clear that such views relied on a mixture of documented observations and personal experience, which were informed both implicitly and explicitly by a deepseated belief in the special transhistorical qualities of the Roman environment. This impinged on both the growing tide of tourism and artistic and archaeological practice in various, often contradictory, ways.

Ralph Harrington examines responses to railway travel within nineteenth-century British society. He argues that the railway, with its speed, power, and danger, became a focal point for the experience of nervous and psychological disorders within an urbanising and modernising society. The sense of crowding on platforms and in carriages, the anticipation of social mixing no less than the prospect of catastrophic accident, combined with the velocity and vibration of the journey to produce a range of embodied symptoms ripe for medical interpretation. Following Schivelbusch, Harrington believes that the pathologies of railway travel bring into sharp focus the experiences of psycho-social shock which accompanied the development of a machine-dominated, urbanised, fast-moving industrial modernity. He suggests that the scale of railway development, its extensive impact on the landscape, as well as its widely-felt social ramifications, provided a commonality of experience unique to nineteenth-century technologies. He concludes: 'other aspects of industrial civilisation, from gas lights to steamships, were on occasion dangerous and destructive; but no other technological system required large numbers of ordinary people to surrender their security and safety to a vast, fast-moving machine driven by incomprehensibly powerful and barely controllable energies, nor did any do so as frequently, and on such a scale, as the railway.'

Tim Cresswell addresses not a specific location as such, but the rail network which made possible both commercial and passenger mobility, and also the communication of disease and social undesirables. As with eighteenth- and nineteenth-century Rome – where visitors and local inhabitants were treated to differentiated medical analysis – pathologisation was deeply marked by perceptions of class identity – in this case the socially marginal group known as hobos. Cresswell unravels the complex and highly charged levels of meaning which inform the definition of the hobo problem and its link to the transmission of syphilis within a picture of the impact of

17

the railway on the highly charged politics of mobility. 'Tramps ... not only suffered from particular pathologies but were also represented as pathologies themselves.' Cresswell's analysis provides a counterpoint to the notion of increased mobility as part of the celebratory mythology of the settling and consolidation of North America.

Harriet Deacon traces the complexities of the changing reputation of the Cape, and the re-evaluation of its temperate, health-giving environment on the edge of Empire. As she shows, the Cape's reputation shifted from being simply beneficial because distanced from less hospitable parts of the Empire (being on the sea route to India and Australasia), to that of a location endowed with specific medical therapeutic effects (notably against tuberculosis). The nature of Cape Town itself directly affected the tenor of the claims made for the location. As the city grew, so its claims as a health station declined, and this function was transferred on to the 'sylvan beauty' of the suburbs: 'These shifts were consistent with a search for new health resorts in established settlements which were safely inside the moving colonial frontier, but not yet sullied by the foulness of the city.' Salubrity of locale was not an objectively fixed phenomenon, but subject to contingent perceptions informed by the evolving status of the Cape within the climatic and moral geography of Empire.

The final contribution, by Russell West, offers a case study of an individual travel narrative, André Gide's *Voyage au Congo*, and the role within it of the dimension of the pathological, attending to the way that Gide's use of medical language shifts from the practicalities of prophylaxis, to a metaphoric evocation of the depredations of French colonialism in Africa. Gide's arrival at a recognition of the damage caused by the state which was also his sponsor and protector, through his gradual willingness to recognise its devastating human effects – most tellingly registered through his recording of Africans' illnesses – was forcefully and bitterly expressed by the intensification of this metaphorical register. Thus the very nature of Gide's reflection on the implications of his experience, and its relation to that of the Africans whose lives he witnessed, can be seen to be progressively more sharply focused by means of his utilization of different modes of literary expression – shifting away from the laconic brevity of journal entries, towards a more analytic, interrogative idiom, which inscribes his consciousness of the political contradictions of his situation. The presence of the pathological in Gide's text moves from the descriptive to the metaphorical as his insomnia dominates his experience of Africa.

His insomnia registers his troubled sense of identity, as he struggled to come to terms with his complicity in the destructive impact of the French imperial presence.

From eighteenth-century England and Scotland, to twentieth-century North America, the experience of travel, and the business of representing that experience involved an obligatory engagement with the disturbing perception that travel's pleasures were inextricable from its dangers and ennuis. Despite the confidence of some medical authorities in their recommendations of the therapeutic benefits to be derived from 'change of air' as a way of restoring a state of health, such opinions failed to establish a consensus, either amongst those who followed such peripatetic prescriptions, or within the medical professions in general. Mad doctors and climatologists alike were forced to adopt an essentially partisan stance in arguing their case for such recommendations, and were confronted by rival practitioners who could marshal counter-case histories which demonstrated diametrically opposed conclusions concerning the advisability of travel. To this extent, the history of travel and its pathologies is a particularly revealing instance of the way medical thinking was dependent on localised studies which might do more to challenge the universal applicability of generally accepted theories than they did to confirm their diagnostic reliability.

One central issue running through the volume is the way that different definitions of the pathological are created and secured by means of recourse to an eclectic variety of vocabularies and rhetorics. Papers such as Chard and Andrews address what may be called the primary meanings of the term as manifest in more or less technical vocabulary applied to abnormal physical and psychological conditions and their relation to the experience of travel, whether prescribed or freely undertaken. Other papers focus on a more expanded usage and invocation of the pathological, in which the term is applied to political and cultural matters, habitually relying on characteristically partisan metaphor and judgemental analogy. The assimilation and appropriation of the vocabulary of health and sickness is a theme which can be seen to inform writings on travel almost without exception. In the period covered by these papers, such appropriation was all the more possible given the striking degree of uncertainty and divergence within professional opinion on a wide range of diseases and their causes and treatment. To this extent, the historical ambivalence regarding the advisability and benefits of travel was emphatically reinforced by the complex and proliferating, if unresolved, range of medical views on the subject in its different manifestations. The essays collected here not only contribute to our understanding of the conception and application of a variety of medical ideas, showing how they depended on beliefs about climate, corporeal constitution as well as often inconsistent data or *récits* culled from travellers and geographically dispersed case histories, but also open up illuminatingly complex perspectives on the uncertainties and dangers of the phenomenon of modern travel.

George Revill & Richard Wrigley

Notes

1 See, for example, E. Soja, *Postmodern Geographies: the reassertion of space in critical social theory* (London: Verso, 1989); S. Lash, *Sociology of Postmodernism* (London: Routledge, 1990); S. Lash and J. Friedman (eds), *Modernity and Identity* (Oxford: Blackwell, 1992); G. Robertson *et al.* (eds), *Travellers' Tales: narratives of home and identity* (London: Routledge, 1994); I. Chambers, *Migrancy, Culture, Identity* (London: Routledge, 1994).

2 M. De Certeau, *The Practice of Everyday Life* (Berkeley: University of California Press, 1984); P. Carter, *Living in a New Country: history, travelling and language* (London: Faber and Faber, 1992); S. Pile and N. Thrift, *Mapping the Subject: geographies of cultural transformation* (London: Routledge, 1995), 19-26.

3 See, for example, H. Bhabha (ed), *Nation and Narration* (London: Routledge, 1990); P. Gilroy, *The Black Atlantic: modernity and double consciousness* (London: Verso, 1993); P. Werbner and T. Modood (eds), *Debating Cultural Hybridity: multi-cultural identities and the politics of anti-racism* (London: Zed Books, 1997).

4 See, for example, E. Said, *Orientalism* (London: Faber and Faber, 1985); J. Clifford and G. Marcus (eds), *Writing Culture: the poetics and politics of ethnography* (Berkeley: University of California Press, 1986); R. Young, *White Mythologies : writing history and the West* (London: Routledge, 1990); D. Haraway, *Primate Visions: gender, race, and nature in the world of modern science* (London: Routledge, 1989); M.L. Pratt, *Imperial Eyes: travel writing and transculturation* (London: Routledge, 1992); D. Livingstone, *The Geographical Tradition* (Oxford: Blackwell, 1994); D. Gregory, *Geographical Imaginations* (Oxford: Blackwell, 1994).

5 J. Clifford, 'Traveling Cultures', in L. Grossberg, C. Nelson and Treichler (eds), *Cultural Studies* (New York: Routledge, 1992), 96-111.

6 *Ibid.*, 106-7.

7 *Ibid.*, 110.

8 R.C. Maulitz, *Morbid Appearances: the anatomy of pathology in the early nineteenth century* (Cambridge: Cambridge University Press).

9 P. Bagwell, *The Transport Revolution 1775-1985* (London: Routledge, 1988); J. Urry, *The Tourist Gaze* (London: Sage, 1990); B. Porter, *The Lion's Share: a short history of British imperialism* (London: Longman, 1996); S. Kern, *Culture of Time and Space 1880-1918* (Cambridge, Mass: Harvard University Press, 1983), esp. 92-3, 212-58.

10 I. Ousby, *The Englishman's England* (Cambridge: Cambridge University Press, 1990), 190-4; J. Urry, *Consuming Places* (London:

Routledge, 1995), 202-3; also, J. Simmons, *The Victorian Railway* (London: Thames and Hudson, 1991); D. Brooke, *The Railway Navvy: that despicable race of men* (Newton Abbott: David & Charles, 1983); C. Tilly and L. Tilly, *Class Conflict and Collective Action* (London: Sage, 1981); S. Daniels, *Trainspotting: images of the railway in art* (Castle Museum Nottingham, 1985); see also H. Jennings, *Pandaemonium 1680-1886: the coming of the machine as seen by contemporary observers* (London: Deutsch, 1985).

11 E. Hobsbawm, *Primitive Rebels: studies in archaic forms of social movements in the 19th and 20th centuries* (New York: Norton, 1965), and *Labouring Men: studies in the history of labour* (London: Weidenfeld, 1968).

12 P. Virilio, *Speed and Politics: an essay in dromology* (Andromedia: London, 1986), 5.

13 J. Buzzard, *The Beaten Track: European tourism, literature, and the ways to culture 1800-1918* (Oxford: Clarendon Press, 1993).

14 *Ibid.*, 4-5.

15 A. Crowther, 'The Tramp', in R. Porter (ed.), *Myths of the English Polity* (Cambridge: Polity, 1992).

16 *Ibid.*, 92.

17 P. Stallybrass and A. White, *The Politics and Poetics of Transgression* (London: Methuen, 1986).

18 *Ibid.*, 131.

19 *Ibid.*, 148.

20 A. Wallace, *Walking, Literature, and English Culture: the origins and uses of peripatetic in the nineteenth century* (Oxford: Clarendon Press, 1993), 13.

21 J. Barrell, *The Infection of Thomas de Quincey: the psychopathology of imperialism* (New Haven and London: Yale University Press, 1991).

22 *Ibid.*, 9.

23 *Ibid.*, 17.

24 *Ibid.*, 15.

25 W. Schivelbusch, *The Railway Journey: industrialisation and the perception of time and space in the nineteenth century* (Leamington Spa: Berg, 1986), 130.

26 *Ibid.*, 130.

27 *Ibid.*, 168.

28 S. Daniels, 'J.M.W. Turner and the Circulation of the State', in *Fields of Vision: landscape imagery in England and the United States* (Cambridge: Polity, 1993), 112-145.

29 *Ibid.*, 113.

30 *Ibid.*, 137.

31 S. Sontag, *Illness as Metaphor* (Harmondsworth: Penguin, 1983); see also C. Shilling, *The Body and Social Theory* (London: Sage, 1993), 48.

32 A. McClintock, *Imperial Leather: race, gender, and sexuality in the colonial context* (London: Routledge, 1995), 211.

33 *Ibid.*, 229.

34 See also D. Arnold, *Imperial Medicine and Indigenous Societies* (Manchester: Manchester University Press, 1988), and R. Hyam, *Empire and Sexuality: the British experience* (Manchester: Manchester University Press, 1991).

35 B.S. Turner, *The Body and Society* (Oxford: Blackwell, 1984), 107-8; Shilling, *op. cit.*, 91. On the ideological strands that intersect in ideas on agoraphobia see also E. da Costa Meyer, 'La donna e mobile', *Assemblage*, 28 (1996), 6-15.

1

Letting Madness Range:
Travel and Mental Disorder, c1700-1900

Jonathan Andrews

Introduction (i): Travel as Banishing the Pathological

Hamlet: Ay, marry, why was he sent into England?
1 Clown: Why, because a' was mad: a' shall recover his wits there, or if
        a' do not, 'tis no great matter there.
Hamlet: Why?
1 Clown: 'Twill not be seen in him there, there the men are as mad as he.[1]

The clown's joke that Hamlet's madness would not be noticed in England because everyone was mad there conveys a serious point about the importance of context in the definition of madness. But it also alludes to a practice common in early modern Britain, and even more common in the nineteenth century, of sending the mentally affected on a journey, of placing them at a distance – both for reasons of therapy, and for reasons of outcast. On the one hand, it was believed, travel could provide distraction for the distracted mind, a new perspective, or distancing from present morbid preoccupations and fixed objects of concern.

King: Haply the seas, and countries different,
        With variable objects, shall expell
        This something-settled matter in his heart,
        Whereon his brains still beating puts him thus
        From fashion of himself.[2]

On the other hand, sending the deranged away might also be a way of disposing of the dangers they posed; of better ensuring the safety and peace of mind of those around them; or, for more selfish reasons, of safeguarding the interests, person and reputation of oneself and one's family.

King: I like him not, nor stands it safe with us

> To let his madness range. Therefore
> … he to England shall along with you.[3]

In the Greco-Roman world banishment was a standard punishment for crime, although, when committed in a state of madness, limits might be recommended for the term – Plato's *Laws* stipulating a year's ostracism in 'another land and country' for an insane homicide.[4] The so-called 'Ship of Fools' of medieval times appears to have been a literary and artistic trope, rather than a reality.[5] Yet outcast remained an important aspect of contemporaries' motivations for sending away the nervous, deranged and unbalanced. Such motivations continued to be significant throughout the period 1700-1900. For many patients and their families it was hoped that the expedient of sending patients away, whether to asylums or to distant relatives, whether into the country, to the seaside or abroad, might save their reputations and sensibilities from the prying eyes and gossip of their neighbours and of the general city *hoi polloi*. Recent historiography has confirmed that the appeal of travel and change of scene in this period was acutely felt by the well-to-do, who not only 'possessed the financial wherewithal to employ relays of private attendants to cope with lunatics' eccentricities and disruptions', but who moreover had the motivation 'to send those who threatened to embarrass the family name abroad' or to country retreats.[6] John Monro, Physician to Bethlem Hospital, England's archetypal madhouse, alluded to such factors even when talking about confinement for the insane, which he stressed:

> is more likely to be of service abroad, than at home; and the country
> is preferable to the town for the opportunities it affords of using
> exercise, without the danger of being exposed.[7]

By the end of the next century, critics of the use of travel in treating mental disorders, like George Henry Savage, the former Superintendent at Bethlem, were putting particular emphasis on such motivations. Savage saw extirpation, getting 'rid' of the mentally disordered and placing them 'out of sight', as one of the primary reasons for sending patients abroad, stressing 'the irksomeness of looking after [such] persons', and especially those 'suffering from the slighter forms of mental disorder'.[8] He alleged that contemporaries were often 'willing to send the sufferer away anyhow' to avoid the 'social stigma … of their having an insane relative'. Furthermore, such inducements were not confined to the laity, argued Savage, 'but the family doctor' too is often driven to desperation by the neurotic friends, and feels that if the invalid remains he will run the risk of becoming a nervous patient himself.[9]

Quite apart from this, patients might also be 'sent away to avoid certification' and confinement in an asylum. Indeed, Savage and many other contemporaries believed that English lunacy law encouraged such avoidance by its wrapping up of the process of certification in bureaucracy and legal technicalities, arguing that the 'weakest feature' of the new 1890 Act had been 'magisterial interference'. Without doubt, because informed by a deeper anxiety about false confinement, English law lacked the flexibility of the Scotch statutes which permitted temporary non-certificated treatment of the insane on notification to the Lunacy Board.

Nevertheless, some historians, who have contended that genteel contemporaries were anxious, 'at almost all costs, to avoid gossip and publicity about the existence of the object of their shame', may have exaggerated the extremity of such concerns, as well as contemporaries' ability to satisfy them.[10] The presence of a substantial and growing number of private patients at many asylums as the period wore on suggests that asylums sustained a significant, if limited, appeal for certain sectors of the moneyed classes. Removal to the country was no guarantee of avoiding scandal. The country was still a highly public place, with established nobility and gentry (or what Horace Walpole called 'the gentlemen of the country')[11] abounding in their country seats. Some eccentric individuals managed to maintain a relatively free rein whilst there. When, in the 1770s, Walpole's mad nephew, Lord Orford 'resumed the entire dominion of himself … is gone into the country, and intends to command the militia', Walpole exclaimed 'what a humiliation, to know he is thus exposing himself'.[12] Even the continent was no safe haven from society gossip when half the gentry was there during the summer.

Introduction (ii): Travel as Therapy for the Pathological

Primarily, moreover, from the earliest times, mentally deranged individuals seem to have left, or been removed from, their domiciles for the sake of their health. It was less for reasons of outcast than of therapy that the Hippocratic and Galenic corpus sometimes prescribed removing the insane to distant parts. During the Middle Ages, the mentally afflicted were occasionally amongst those sick persons who embarked on pilgrimages, and were transported to the thaumaturgical realms of holy shrines and places.[13] By the 1600s, travel was recommended most commonly of all by contemporary authorities as a cure for melancholy. Recycling a wide range of classical advice on the benefits of travel, Robert Burton, in his Anatomy of Melancholy (1621), offered perhaps the firmest medical endorsement of travel for the melancholic. There was, said Burton, 'no better physick for a melancholy man than change of aire and variety of places, to travel abroad and see fashions'.[14] Travel and change of scene have continued to be embarked upon by mentally troubled and ill individuals, and to be recommended for mental and nervous afflictions well into the twentieth century. Whether as a symptomatic response to mental unrest and trauma of the type now sometimes understood by psychiatrists under the umbrella term 'fugue';[15] a sign of disorientation or manic hyperactivity; or a means of working out trauma and of pursuing, or accidentally arriving at, self-knowledge, wandering and journeying have long had an association with mental unrest. Culturally, travel has meant and still means radically different things to different societies, be it the dreamtime walkabouts of aboriginals, the many-faceted routes taken in American road movies, or the mental journeys pursued during certain forms of meditation. Yet many of these modes of travel have had aspects of mental healing at their very centres.

In the period under consideration here, travel was recommended in mental cases for a variety of reasons: traditionally, simply because it took sufferers away from the place, people and surroundings with which their mental afflictions were held to be associated, and because of its metaphysical virtues of diverting sufferers' minds from current troubles. Burton cited sources which stressed the virtues of travel in offering, on the one hand, simple 'variety', whether 'of actions, objects, aire, places' or company. (In general, claimed Burton, 'peregrination charmes our senses with … unspeakeable and sweet variety').[16] On the other hand, travel might present new, diverting and uplifting 'prospects' to the melancholy mind.[17] Travel thus afforded a pageant of pleasing spectacle: it offered healthy sustenance and release to the senses, and through them to the mind. According to the Burtonian view, it was not only the actual survey of new countries, towns, cities and rivers, but the very anticipation or expectation of such sights that might affect the mind positively. Travel was perceived as a particularly good antidote for love melancholy. For, far from making the heart grow fonder, absence and time might 'wear away pain and grief'. Travel put the loved one out of sight and mind, while providing new distractions to aid the process of forgetting and change.[18]

During early modern times, these prescriptions, which dated back to antiquity, were fortified and elaborated by sensationalist or associative models of mental pathology, which tended to stress the origins (and manifestations) of insanity in intellectual processes. According to such models, mental disorder was in part the result of mistaken sense impressions, or misassociation of ideas (e.g. Locke, Battie).[19] In essence this meant that, whether through mental shock, strain, or other stimuli; through physiological imbalances, blockages or superfluities in the body's fluids and vessels; or through tensions and laxities in its nerves or fibres, the senses were providing distorted impressions of the objects and associations for the mind or judgement. Such interpretations highlight the centrality of both misconceptions and fixed ideas (or what the French later termed *idées fixes*) in definitions of mental disorder. And such definitions have clear links with the nineteenth-century concept of monomania, and twentieth-century notions of paranoid psychoses and also of obsessive disorders.[20] The pathogenesis and perpetuation of these misassociated or fixed ideas were often themselves seen as the result of remaining too long in one place, or too long in the place where some calamity or trauma had occurred, of the mind settling and forming its patterns of thought upon the same unchanging and unhealthy objects and associations. The principle of diversion, or interruption of a set pattern of thought, was therefore the bedrock of doctors' advice to their patients to travel.

Coexistent and sometimes competing with this model, however, were other models of mental pathology which, for example, saw madness as in essence vitiated judgement (e.g. Robinson, Monro, Cullen).[21] Proponents of this model argued that, rather than in the sense impressions or imagination, the fundamental problem resided in the judgement, as affected by the same physiological imbalances as mentioned above, which were inhibiting and distorting patients' powers of judgement. While these models were essentially mutually exclusive, nevertheless, associative psychological and physiological interpretations of madness were common to both and tended to be espoused concurrently. Often medical men adopted and adapted portions of both interpretations. The Edinburgh specialist on nerves, William Cullen, for example, while seeing madness as 'false judgement', stressed how there was concurrently 'false association', but how ultimately both 'produced', depended upon, or were caused by 'an increased excitement of the brain', or 'a morbid organic affection ... in some part of the brain'.[22] Richard Mead accepted that madness could be caused by 'an excessive intention of the mind, and

29

the thoughts long fixed on any one object', or by 'continually present' images or objects giving 'a wrong turn to' the mind. Fundamentally, nevertheless, he believed madness to have its seat in 'the inward parts of the animal body', and 'chiefly in the nervous fluid, commonly called animal spirits'.[23]

Partly because of their psychological content, primarily organic models like the latter did not seriously undermine the putative healthiness of removing patients from their customary surroundings. Anyway, those surroundings could be just as implicated in the bodily causes of nervous disorders as in their more psychological ones. Throughout the eighteenth century, travel tended to be recommended to mental cases as much because it might afford an occupation and an environment with a healthier impact on patients' physiological system, as because of its potential psychological benefits. The effect of 'diversions' were themselves often understood in physiological terms, whether in that the exercise they could afford might help to enliven the animal spirits, invigorate the blood and jolt the patient's physiology out of its torpor, or because *vice versa* the relaxation travel and other diversions could provide might ease the tension in the body's nervous integuments.

The title of this chapter is something of a misnomer, for travel was rarely seen as advisable, helpful or practicable in full-blown cases of madness. The disincentives and practical problems in advocating travel for the acutely or violently mentally disordered seem obvious and need little elaboration here. In such cases confinement and restraint were the general rule, strategies that were emphasised as paramount by almost every medical specialist on insanity during the period.[24] Specialists whose practices were largely restricted to asylums, might even claim to have little experience of trying travel and change of scene for patients. Partly as a result, many of them said very little about travel in their publications on insanity. The manuscript casebook (1766) of John Monro, Physician to Bethlem, mentions change of scene being prescribed for only two or three out of 100 private patients for the sake of their mental health, and even then by other doctors, although confinement was regularly referred to.[25]

Yet, as the following analysis will show, this was by no means invariably the pattern. The Bethlem Apothecary, John Haslam, did not discount change of scene from the mad-doctor's armamentarium. Despite confessing that he was 'not enabled by sufficient experience to determine' 'in what particular cases, or stages of the disease, this may be recommended', he still recognised that 'many patients have received considerable benefit by change of situation'.[26] Other

30

physicians, with medical practices developed primarily outside the asylum walls, recommended travel for their mental patients with striking frequency and variety. For example, Alexander Morison, another one time Physician to Bethlem Hospital, recommended travel both at home and abroad for 'many patients, insane and otherwise'.[27]

It was only gradually and inconsistently that confinement became the common solution for the problems posed by insanity, relegating other alternatives to the background. Throughout the period confinement still had its critics. It was never the sole available option and was often invoked only for a limited time. There was no stark and absolute polarity between confinement and other options like travel for the mentally disordered. Nor was travel relegated to the dispensary ante-room as the apparatus of confinement advanced, even if it did tend to become more restricted to carefully selected cases. Travel continued to be embarked upon pre-, post- and instead of confinement in a wide variety of mental cases. Many institutions, including Bethlem, were quite active in utilising the therapeutic option of an excursion for their patients. Furthermore, doctors justified the confinement of the mad on grounds similar to those on which they justified travel: separating the afflicted from the objects and persons that had been formerly associated with their disease, and that might continue to interfere in its treatment. Confinement itself often presupposed a change of scene. William Battie, Physician to St Luke's Hospital, stressed that 'madness … requires the patient's being removed' to a 'place of confinement … at some distance from home'.[28] John Monro and John Haslam agreed in 'the necessity of confining' the mad away from their homes[29] (although frequently, of course, patients' friends preferred to keep them at home, an option that mad-doctors generally were disposed to discredit).

In the following century, this philosophy was fully intact in the advertising armoury of most asylums.[30] Removal from home, like travel, was additionally recommended, as Oppenheim has observed, as a means of imposing medical control, and freeing nervous and mentally disordered patients from the putatively indulgent and ignorant influences of families, whose subjective feelings would only impede patients' rational treatment, 'whose solicitude only intensified their self-absorption'.[31] The pathologising of solitude, sedentary habits and introspection in the eighteenth century, and moreover during the century that followed, so that, as Michael Clark has observed,[32] 'morbid introspection' became a bug-bear for Victorian alienists, had provided a dual justification for both removing sufferers to an asylum and for sending them away on trips. By the turn of the twentieth century, some practitioners were ranking the prevention of 'morbid introspection' (along with improving 'the physical constitution of the individual' and amending 'the association of ideas'), as one of the three most important rationales for recommending travel in mental cases.[33]

Outside of the asylum, however, it was for milder and convalescent cases that change of scene and travel were traditional and relatively standard remedies. For melancholia, hypochondriasis, spleen and other nervous afflictions, sufferers from which were deemed more manageable and responsive to pleasant new impressions, greater freedom of movement and kinder treatment, travel was very much a front-line cure. In his *Dissertation upon the Spleen* (1725), for example, the well-known physician and poet, Sir Richard Blackmore, recommended 'Change of Place' alongside a host of 'agreeable Diversions like riding, new Company … [and] variety of Objects'.[34] Towards the end of the century, William Cullen, prescribed travel for melancholics (and for a rather idiosyncratic category of insane persons with 'agreeable … emotions') in similar fashion:

> if … objects or persons … can call off their attention from the
> pursuit of their own disordered imagination, and can fix it a little
> upon some others … a journey, both by its having the effect of
> interrupting all train of thought, and by presenting objects engaging
> attention, may often be useful.[35]

Travel signalled a diversion from the pathological highways of mind. During the course of the following century, a train journey might put a stop, or entail an interruption, to a morbid train of thought.

While removal to an asylum invariably implied an imposition of medical control, and travel might be prescribed for similar reasons, more commonly the travel-cure was managed and resourced by the family, and was a means for the family to retain a certain degree of authority over a mentally deranged member. The way in which travel was employed in the case of the nonconformist Hannah Allen, as related in her own autobiographical account of 1683, presents a particularly vivid and revealing picture of its place in the treatment of melancholy amongst the well-to-do.[36] For Hannah, travel was utilised repeatedly on the advice of her friends rather than on that of medical men. While she was seen and prescribed for by medical practitioners, it was clearly Hannah's family who dominated her therapeutic regime and with remarkable forbearance and energy given that, as she herself admitted, 'I was but an uncomfortable Guest'.[37] The mainstays in her treatment were regular changes of scene and lay and religious counselling rather than medicine, ministers rather than mad-doctors. Initially, her family recommended sending her from her home in Snelstone, Derbyshire, up to London, both because it was there that might be found 'the best means both for Soul and Body', and because she had uncles and a brother living and working there.[38] Often such advice met with opposition from morbidly anxious patients, Hannah's family finding it 'hard work to perswade me to this Journey; for I said *I must go and dye by the way to please my friends*'.[39] The strain of such journeys was indeed not inconsiderable. Hannah's took place over a number of days, involving a horse-back ride to Tamworth, followed by nine miles by coach to Nuneaton, before reaching London. While her accompanying relatives complained of 'weariness', Hannah herself compounded the matter by arguing 'every Morning' with her mother about rising to proceed on the journey: '*had I not better dye in bed? Mother, do you think people will like to have a dead Corps in the Coach with them?*'[40] Indeed, Hannah's case is hardly an unmitigated endorsement of the benefits of travel. The sights along the road that medical theorists often envisaged as positive diversions to the senses might be torments for the deranged. A passing church was for Hannah (convinced, as she was, of her own sinfulness) 'a hell-house', while gathering 'black Clouds' and the rising wind were ominous portents of 'some dreadful thing' that would 'shew what an One I was'.[41] Unfamiliar places, sights and sounds could enhance rather than relieve disorientation: for Hannah, whilst lodging at her brother's, 'the lights that were in Neighbouring houses were apparitions of Devils', and neighbours' voices were devils berating her.[42] Hannah was later removed to a cousin's house in Newgate-Market,[43] before she returned home on 'an uncomfortable Journey – for by the way I would not eat sufficient to support Nature'.[44] The final journey Hannah undertook was 'to a good friend of mine, a minister, Mr John Shorthouse related to me by Marriage, who lived about Thirty Miles distance'.[45] Although initially she 'grew much worse' there, ultimately she regarded the combination of religious consolation and 'physick' Shorthouse was able to offer as crucial in her recovery.[46] Her case suggests how intimately the geography of travel for the mentally affected was linked to that of the extended family. It is also indicative of how, while patients themselves might strenuously resist journeys out of fear of dangers anticipated or unknown and out of anxiety at a further loss of control, *vice versa*, they might be impelled to travel by a desire for escape from their own demons and from the constraints they were under. Whilst in London, Hannah hired a coach with the intention of finding a place to do away with herself, although ironically her journey only made her more appreciative of the virtues of the companionship she was fleeing.

Despite their acute ambiguity, travel and change of scene clearly appealed to families, doctors and patients themselves as more pleasant and even safer alternatives to the asylum and to other common recourses, like shutting up patients in their rooms or houses. Of course, a journey might itself prove a diversionary ruse, or a prelude, to confinement. Transport to new lodgings in contemporary novels like Richardson's *Clarissa* had all the appeal of a kidnapping and imprisonment. Many documentary sources testify to the reality of patients being duped into confinement or a madhouse via a bogus journey, and some doctors even recommended such trickery. Nevertheless, the stigma attached to asylums and certification as a lunatic in this period rendered travel and change of scene desirable as alternative options, particularly for the better sort of families. They permitted respite and relief from a difficult family member, whilst also offering, to some degree, the possibility of preserving the family name from the taint of scandal. Many patients and families dreaded not only the stigma of the asylum and of insanity itself, but the very isolation, restraint and forms of treatment prevailing in the asylum. Indeed, it does seem that the lowly reputation of asylum care before the mid-nineteenth century provided plenty of encouragement for the mentally affected to travel, and for doctors to recommend it. W.A.F. Browne, the great proponent of the reformed asylum and of moral therapy, was certainly of this opinion. But he blamed it on what he understood asylums were, or used to be, rather than on asylums at their best, or as they ought to be. Writing in the 1830s, he declared:

> so indifferent is even now the repute of public asylums, that the physician in many instances recommends change of scene or of occupation, travelling, anything in fact rather than mere incarceration. And he gives this advice not from any preference of the step suggested, but from a conviction that mere isolation can do nothing.[47]

Evidence I present below may imply that Browne's cynicism regarding medical men's faith in salutary travel was little justified or shared by others in the profession. With the growing popularity of moral therapy amongst specialists during the early nineteenth century, and an often intensely critical attitude to the medical means of curing insanity, travel was being prescribed for more and more mental cases. Travel must have appeared all the more attractive to genteel families before 1850, when asylumdom and more interventionist forms of mad-doctoring offered such dubious attractions, tending to be conceived as more appropriate for the pauper than the gentleman. Nevertheless, because of its association with the moral rather than the medical treatment of insanity, and with an interpretation of insanity as more of a mental than a physical illness, many medical men saw the recuperative strategy of travel as carrying an implicit threat to the foundations of their nascent specialty. For, if it was too widely or exclusively touted that the mentally disordered could be restored through moral means like travel, the special claim of mad-doctors to an expertise in treatment through medicine, based on their understanding of diseases rooted in the body, would be undermined. Francis Willis, whose grandfather had famously treated George III's alleged madness, was strongly of this opinion. He complained in his *Treatise* of 1823 that:

> derangement has been considered by some to be merely and exclusively a mental disease, curable without the aid of medicine, by what are termed moral remedies; such as travelling and various kinds of amusements.[48]

And his comments reflect a concern that was broadly felt amongst contemporary mad-doctors.

As shall be shown, the rather blanket Burtonian endorsement of travel for mental cases (an endorsement that had sustained a currency in early modern times consummate with the numerous times Burton's *Anatomy* was reprinted), was to come under increasing fire as the nineteenth century wore on. Asylum doctors and other specialists in insanity strove to be more discriminating in their efforts to carve out new and widened realms of expertise over patients' disposal. Yet, as shall also be demonstrated, travel was to endure as a popular therapy for mental cases throughout the period and was far from invariably seen as a threat to orthodox psychiatry. While often undertaken as a real alternative to medicine and confinement for mental cases, travel was frequently prescribed as an adjunct to such treatment. It was advised in combination with medicinal remedies, as one of a range of first resorts prior to confinement, and as a means of engendering or aiding convalescence at the end of a period of residence in an asylum.

Travel as Airing Mental Problems:
Good Air, Bad Air, Changed Air and
Acclimatising as Cures for the Mind

Apart from its psychological benefits, a sojourn away from home might also be prescribed because it involved removing the afflicted to climes putatively more healthy for the general physical system, either out of the city into the country where the air was supposedly cleaner and fresher, or to some other foreign land where the climate was adjudged warmer, or more temperate. Theories about the benefits of air in mental disease had long been part of the medical corpus. The Burtonian heritage certainly emphasised 'change of aire' as one of the major virtues of travelling.[49] Indeed, change of air was accorded consummate importance with change of scene (they tended anyway to be interdependent), specialists having traditionally seen mental disorder as being caused or heightened by excessively warm, or cold air, or by the noxious and closed airs of urban spaces. For example, the 1746 *Treatise on Phrensy* by P. Frings recommended that:

> the Air ought to be contrary to this Distemper; that is temperate, pure, & inclining to be cold. Hot and dry Air is to be shunned, as it increases Phrensy, by over fatiguing the Animal Spirits ... Too cold Air is to be avoided; for, as it condenses the Pores, it insensibly puts a Stop to Perspiration.[50]

Similar views were particularly prominent in the early modern period, when certain types of mental affliction were actually conceptualised as bad airs. 'The vapours' became a major and fashionable diagnostic category for nervous patients (partially mitigating some of the stigma attached to the more serious diagnosis of madness), such patients being deemed to be suffering from the effects of internal gases and vapours rising into the brain.[51] Not even these views were consistent, however. Some regarded bad air as preferable to unchanged air, the Bethlem Physician, James Monro, telling Horace Walpole's father Sir Robert, 'that he scarce knew of anything that asses' milk and change of air would not cure, and that it was better to go into a bad air, than not to change it often'.[52]

During the nineteenth century, change of air became even more central in the motivations for invalids to travel, and a plethora of medical publications did much to propagate the gospel of fresh air.[53] While the pathological model of the vapours had been largely discredited by 1800, faith in zymotic theories of disease in general had actually widened with more research on diseases like malaria and tuberculosis. (The latter was itself identified with mental disorder by alienists like Thomas Clouston, the Edinburgh Royal Asylum Physician-Superintendent, who coined the term 'phthisical' or 'tubercular insanity').[54] As one constituent of a new emphasis on the effects of unhygienic and insanitary conditions on the physiological system as a whole, zymotic theories thus continued to provide support for the efficacy of removing patients (whether physically or mentally ill) to airier climes. Late Victorian alienists like Clouston spoke of change of air as a biblical commandment, or 'gospel of fresh air', for the depressed and melancholic.[55] Clouston regarded the 'fresh air' of the country as a natural pharmacopoeia: 'nature's great sleep producer, appetiser, and tonic'.[56] Although a virtual given throughout the period, this belief in the health-giving power of country air had clearly been encouraged by a general idealisation of 'the country life' and all it entailed that characterised nineteenth-century romanticism. Clouston distinguished 'a country life, with much fresh air' as 'no doubt the best [remedy], if it is possible' for melancholia.[57] For similar reasons alienists prized the bracing impact of 'mountain or sea breezes', with further encouragement from the 'magic mountain' cure so popular in the treatment of tuberculosis.[58] During the early 1900s, with zymotic theory sustaining its currency, the popularity of tent or open-air therapy for tubercular cases was transmitted to psychiatric circles, asylums too adopting such treatments with a view to airing mental illness.[59]

The Asylum and Travel: from Fresh Air to Airing Yards; from Seasonal Excursions to Convalescent Homes

The primacy given to fresh and changed air as a curative agent not only influenced the way in which travel was prescribed for mental disorders outside of the asylum. It also affected where asylums themselves were sited, the way in which they were designed and the way patients were managed within them. From at least the mid-seventeenth century until the 1900s, madhouses and asylums were designed with airing yards for patients to take air and exercise, and with wide galleries, corridors, wickets and vents helping to afford circulation of air. The provision of free flowing air, as Stevenson has shown,[60] was a particularly key principle behind Hooke's palatial remodelling in the 1670s of Bethlem Hospital. Partaking of an atmosphere of renewal and restoration after the Great Fire of London and the Civil War, New Bethlem became the symbolically revitalised architectural centre-piece of the airy expanses of a remodelled Moorfields. Many (although far from all) of the new 'reformed' asylums, including the York Retreat and Glasgow Asylum, were purposefully built in airy, expansive districts, at some remove from the atmospheric ills of the cities, set and depicted against a harmonious, bucolic background of sheep and cows. Throughout the period, conviction in the salutary qualities of air and spatial expanses repeatedly justified significant relaxations of the bounds of confinement. By the 1700s, hospitals like Bethlem were permitting patients leaves of absence in the country to take the air with a view to their recovery, and admissions might be delayed or avoided by recourse to the same strategy. Not only the moneyed classes, but metropolitan parishes and poorer families too occasionally sent mental cases into the country to procure the benefit of the air. Sending patients to the country might also be preferred because it offered a measure of quiet and exercise less available in the hustle and bustle and confined spaces of the metropolis.

A change of scene could seem a prudent and desirable option for families whose insane members showed little improvement in the asylum, especially if they were paying for such treatment. Asylum reports and case notes regularly record instances of friends who 'could no longer afford to maintain them'; who in cases 'of long duration ... thought that a change of place might be beneficial'; or who 'were prevailed upon, by the importunity of the Patients themselves, to consent to their removal'.[61] Asylum officers were often, however, critical of relatives for removing patients too soon and heeding patients' appeals for release against 'expert' medical advice. Even for these institutionalised patients, the initiative for therapeutic sojourns came less frequently, perhaps, from hospitals and doctors than from families, the former often merely sanctioning requests by relatives to try the country or travel alternative.

During the course of the nineteenth century, however, asylums and their medical officers began increasingly to initiate and resource regular outings for convalescent patients to the countryside or seaside, or even to foreign parts. The annual reports and case notes of Glasgow Royal Asylum show that such trips were generally restricted to the summer months and often to weekends; to 'small and select' groups of patients in convalescent or milder states; and, moreover, to patients from wealthy families who could afford them. Paupers had, at best, to make do with more modest excursions to sites in the city. Exceptionally, trips outside the asylum had an even more specific therapeutic object, as in 1816 when one patient under the delusion that Glasgow had been destroyed was taken to town by an attendant to convince her otherwise.[62] The ethos of moral therapy prevailing at most nineteenth-century asylums, which encouraged some staff to engage more sympathetically with the histories and delusions of their patients, clearly also provided extra impetus for the therapeutic use of excursions, in particular for their potential psychological impact. Magic lantern shows and public lectures before patients inside the asylum commonly involved outsiders and asylum officers giving presentations about the places they had travelled to, as when a Mr

Drysdale presented a photographic exhibition at Glasgow Royal in 1859 on Dr Livingstone's travels in Africa.[63] The object was evidently the standard one of diverting patients' minds from their current situations and troubles, while also affording them some sort of imaginative or vicarious escape. However, the insistence that these shows did not engage directly with mental illness itself, nor with morbid, potentially distressing or exciting subject matter, emphasises the limits of psychiatric empathy at this time.

Normally, the outings of asylum patients meant going to areas where the landscape and air was regarded as especially uplifting or health-giving. But occasionally they were special dispensations to individual patients whose families lived at great distances from the asylum. In 1858, for example, a Glasgow Royal party went on tour with their attendants to the West Highlands, while an Irish patient was permitted to visit his relations in Ireland.[64] The conduct of such trips emphasises how influential the family had remained in the provision of medical care, and how mediated and permeable the asylum could be.[65] In this more limited context of asylumdom, travel was clearly more purely an adjunct of moral therapy and diagnostic monitoring, of affording patients varying amounts of release from their situations of confinement, whilst rewarding them for 'good conduct' (and, *vice versa*, withdrawing the privilege if they behaved badly). For paupers there was evidently the added potential bonus of improving their productivity through such recreational incentives. These trips clearly also formed part of the asylum's advertising and public relations with its richer patrons, and administrators made efforts to normalise them and wrap them up in the standard language of society travel, recreational culture and general valetudinarian convalescence. Rather than employing loaded medical, legal or penal terminology like lunatics/inmates/patients or parole/probation, they referred to 'invalids', 'the season', 'residences' and 'tours'. Later reports spoke of 'ladies and gentlemen' taking 'summer quarters'.[66] The clinical aspects of such sojourns were still prominent, nonetheless, the former terms being used more regularly by medical officers. Asylums and their practitioners had been buoyed up in pursuing these policies by their forging of a more established and cohesive professional and institutional identity, granting them greater authority over the after-care of their patients. It was not until the last quarter of the century, however, that a formal After-Care Association was established in England for mental cases, with the first separate convalescent homes.[67]

Until the 1850s, occupational and recreational activity provided

39

for asylum patients had remained profoundly in-house, and outside excursions largely restricted to day-trips on walks and picnics in the country and by the sea, or visits to chapels, art galleries and other city sites. However, with increasing concerns in psychiatric circles about the institutionalising tendencies of confinement and growing recognition of a need to domesticate, hospitalise and open up the doors of asylums, more concerted efforts were made to provide patients with salutary trips outside the asylum walls. Temporary country and coastal residences were taken up at a number of the more adventurous British asylums, W.A.F. Browne of Crichton Royal, Dumfries, being one of the first to experiment with lodging convalescent patients at a neighbouring country house.[68] By the latter quarter of the century, convalescent homes in the country were becoming a relatively standard feature of asylum care. A real innovator in this respect, was Sir John Charles Bucknill.[69] As early as the 1850s, Bucknill was boarding-out quiet female patients in cottages just outside the Devon County Asylum he superintended and renting a seaside house near Exmouth for 40-45 of such. And this was despite considerable opposition from local residents worried about their own safety and about declining rentals and house prices, although the experiment was abandoned once available accommodation was found within the asylum.

Elsewhere, however, initiatives were more lasting, if taken rather later and equally hesitantly. Glasgow Royal, for example, hired a house for the use of convalescent ladies and gentlemen for two to three months every summer from around 1876, its Directors having emphasised three years earlier that 'many patients would benefit from a temporary residence at the coast in summer'.[70] Initially, such 'changes' remained highly restricted, Yellowlees wishing that excursions 'could be given more frequently, to larger numbers, and to a variety of places'.[71] Nevertheless, from this time until the 1920s, when a permanent convalescent home, Lyndhurst House in Skelmorlie, was purchased by the Hospital, Glasgow Royal provided temporary rented accommodation at quite a variety of resorts, including the Bridge of Allan, Helensburgh, Innellan, Moffat, Stirling, Arrochar, Ellie, Lunedin Links, Wemyss Bay and Skelmorlie. From c1892 a convalescent or 'country house' was being rented and used rather more extensively, it being 'occupied by detachments of patients for the greater part of the year'.[72] The benefits of such treatment continued to be conceived in psychological as well as physical terms. Sojourns were justified because they offered both release from the monotonous routine and familiar surroundings of

40

the asylum, and repose from the strains of asylum life and work and other noisy patients.[73] This option was also encouraged by the great influence in psychiatric circles of the so-called 'rest cure' being advocated from the 1870s by the prominent American neurologist, Silas Weir Mitchell, and disseminated in Britain most notably by the obstetrician, W.S. Playfair.[74]

Travel for Mental Cases to Spa Resorts and on Sea Voyages: Spa Resorts

During the period after 1700, trips to spa resorts as prescribed both for physically ill patients and for nervous patients were another custom combining travel with therapy which became particularly *à la mode*. This is a subject which has been well covered by historians and will therefore be only briefly referred to here.[75] The premier amongst such resorts in England were Bath and Tunbridge Wells. Here patients might either drink the health-giving mineral waters, or immerse themselves in the baths. Their ablutions were often combined with other medical prescriptions, including regimen, exercise, and tonic, purgative and other medicaments. Clearly, such options represented another soft cure for the wealthy and middling sort, a much preferred alternative to the starker forms of contemporary treatment for madness, such as bleeding, vomits, mechanical restraint and confinement in an asylum.

Writing in 1694, the London physician, Richard Morton, mentioned the case of a hypochondriacal and hysterical woman who 'recovered ... in the Spring with the timely use of Islington Waters, and the benefit of the Country Air'.[76] Prescribing for hysteria in 1693, Thomas Sydenham advised drinking 'chalybeate waters' and the 'sulphuric' waters of Bath, with intermittent bathing, for a period of between six weeks and two months.[77] The Scottish physician and author of *The English Malady* (1733), George Cheyne, advised the Bath waters as one amongst a host of largely physical remedies for 'the Spleen, Vapours, Lowness of Spirits, Hysterical and Hypochondriacal Disorders'.[78] In his famous treatise on vapours, John Purcell recommended that after a dietary of 'natural French wine with water, plus drams of volatile salts and spirit of lavender', some 'glysters' and a 'period of repose', the patient should 'be sent to the waters at Tunbridge or elsewhere' and 'afterwards to go to the Bath'.[79] The assumption, based on quasi-humoral pathological theory, was that the fluids and spirits of such patients had become sluggish and corrupted, and needed gentle purifying, fortifying and invigorating. Physicians like Purcell were convinced that patients' blood and bodily fluids lacked minerals, and argued that the 'iron in the waters will have the same effect as the chalybeat preparations' they often prescribed instead, while the 'salts' were 'good for the blood'.

Cold and warm bathing, douches, and other forms of hydro-therapy were standard remedies for the mentally (and physically) ill by the end of the seventeenth century, the writings of John Floyer and others having fanned enthusiasm for such therapies.[80] Towards the end of the eighteenth century, patients (mostly female) diagnosed with the fashionable disease chlorosis were also frequently sent to the spa waters. William Rowley, specialist in female nervous disorders, for example, observed in 1788 how 'the Bath waters have been known to cure the chlorosis when most other methods have failed'.[81] Quite apart from the health benefits, the enticement of fashion, the flavours of adventure, intrigue, mystery and quest surrounding trips to these and other health resorts clearly also attracted contemporaries. The extra financial and logistical problems involved in travelling some distance for the sake of health must have added to the air of exclusivity and promise, and may even have furnished a genuine placebo effect.

Trips to the baths or to take the waters continued to be advocated by doctors and undertaken by their nervous and depressed patients throughout the period 1700-1900, and a tide of publications on their health-giving virtues helped to spread the word.[82] As knowledge widened about salutary spa resorts on the continent, patients were encouraged to look even further afield for restoration. German mineral waters proved particularly popular with British invalids. An 1838 two volume book by the physician, Augustus Bozi Granville, entitled *The Spas of Germany*, claimed to be one of the first in English to give them publicity and a comprehensive medical coverage, previous accounts being confined to a selection of spas, or to geographical descriptions of all the mineral waters of the world.[83] In fact, German waters at Cleves and elsewhere had occasionally been recommended by British and continental doctors since at least the early eighteenth century.[84] Granville's book, like most early writings uniting travel and medicine, blended entertainment with science, tourism with medicine, including a variety of information on German institutions, buildings, cities, scenery and customs, being consciously aimed at a wide travelling/reading public. Indeed, Granville emphasised the failure of drier, more purely professional works, including an 1832 guide by the Edinburgh physician, Meredith Gairdner,[85] to be read. Ironically, it was the eclectic, unsystematic nature of such early works and the anecdotal, 'unscientific' way they often dispensed medical advice that was to be the subject of increasing criticism from the medical élite as the century progressed.

Nevertheless, Granville attempted to provide specific advice about travel to spas for specific diseases. Indeed, he criticised previous accounts for failing to do this. While adverting to considerable scepticism amongst contemporary medical men, whom he alleged tended to pooh-pooh every suggestion of sending an invalid to a foreign spa, he castigated them for their ignorance about foreign resorts, implying that their attitude had more to do with narrow-minded national prejudice:

> The leading medical men in London – those who are most likely to be consulted by such patients as can afford to, and would willingly, leave their home for a season to seek health on foreign shores – are avowedly little conversant with the subject.[86]

They were apt, claimed Granville, to favour native spas without appreciating the important differences between the mineral properties of different spas, and often sent the wrong sort of patients to spas both at home and abroad. Granville was also forthright in his criticisms of invalids and their families for rushing into such excursions without sufficient recourse to reliable medical advice, and his views echo and anticipate much in what was a growing medical critique of health advice for travellers in the nineteenth century. Even so, Granville offered a firm and comprehensive endorsement of the value of spas for a whole range of mental disorders. For example, while denying that Marienbad waters were much good for nervous, spasmodic cases,[87] he identified the waters of Cannstadt, Gastein, Toeplitz and Wiesbaden as good for 'hypochondriasis'.[88] Gastein waters he distinguished as beneficial for 'derangement of the nervous system ... depression of spirits ... anxiety of mind ... paralysis ... affections of the spine ... hysteric attacks ... sexual disturbances in females ... [and] erotic diseases, imperfectly cured'.[89] Carlsbad, however, was the real Mecca of spas for hypochondriacs, Granville describing how

> it is the despondent, dejected, misanthropic, fidgety, pusillanimous, irritable, outrageous, morose, sulky, weak-minded, whimsical, and often despairing hypochondriac ... that Carlsbad seems pre-eminently to favour.

here being a larger number of such patients there than anywhere else, except

the Constantinople Hypodrome.[90] Granville also sent those of his
splenetic patients who could afford it to Carlsbad. Whereas the
appeal of such resorts for mental as with physical cases was as much
about fashion as medicine, medical men like Granville plainly
contributed to this by, for example, taking quality clientele as good
evidence of the efficacy of the waters.[91] Granville's account was
followed by a growing crop of others on both continental and native
mineral waters, with a particular concentration from the 1850s to the
1870s.[92]

Partly informed by such literature and what was a vigorous fad
amongst nervous invalids, Victorian alienists routinely recommended
trips to such spas for their neurotic and melancholic patients, or else
espoused domestic versions of the same. Advising one gentleman
'about which continental spas to attend for his nervous debility',
Alexander Morison also investigated 'on his behalf ... a machine for
making artificial Carlsbad Waters'.[93] Thomas Clouston recommended
'the mineral waters of our own country', but more 'especially those of
Germany' as a great tonic for melancholia, distinguishing the springs
at 'Schwalbach, Wiesbaden, Carlsbad'.[94] Keen to stress the complexities
of their science, however, alienists like Clouston were careful to point
out the need to gauge particular types of waters to particular types of
diathesis, 'the purely chalybeate to the purely neurotic, the saline to the
gouty and rheumatic'.[95]

The virtues of going to the bath, as with other journeys for
health, had rarely been seen as purely physical. Granville emphasised
the psycho-social benefits of travel to continental spas as an
important auxiliary to the restoration of physical and mental health,
pointing to how:

> a difference in the previous mode of living ... a release from
> laborious occupation, and a leaving behind of every worry and
> anxiety of mind ... and lastly, the gaiety of the Spas, and the
> constant amusement to be found there amidst agreeable society, are
> viewed as additional causes of the recovery.[96]

At the beginning of the eighteenth century, Purcell and his
contemporaries had also emphasised the psychological, or rather
psychosomatic benefits of travel to the English baths:

> when the Patient goes thither, she, by the advice of her Physician,
> sets aside all Concerns and Cares, and gives herself wholly over to
> Mirth and Pastime, wherby the Blood is invigorated and rendered
> more lively.[97]

In fact, travel to such resorts and change of scene was advocated for the reasons of enlivening and diverting the mind that likewise persuaded physicians to advise recreation, change of company and change of occupation. [98]

The basic philosophy here was not just one of variety and diversion, but also one of confronting a pathological influence with one that ran directly opposite to it, a traditional medical approach to mental and physical illnesses that had been relied on since antiquity.[99] By the 1750s, specialists were becoming more critical of this approach in its more radical manifestations, warning of the dangers of excessively shocking the mind by the sudden alterations that substituting one passion for another could involve.[100] Nevertheless, over a century later, alienists and other practitioners were still speaking about the changes of scene they prescribed in terms that emphasise the continuities with these older models.[101]

Sea Voyages

Quite apart from the remedies of drinking the waters and hydro-therapy recommended for mental cases at spa resorts and elsewhere, various forms of transportation over water were also commonly recommended for such patients. Indeed, long sea voyages and shorter trips on yachts and other small boats became one of the most popular types of travel prescriptions for patients with mild mental disorders, and for mental cases in convalescence in this period. One of the earliest and most emphatic advocates of the remedial properties of sea voyages was the physician Ebeneezer Gilchrist, whose book on *The Use of Sea Voyages in Medicine* was reissued and enlarged in 1771.[102] Although mainly concerned with the use of sea voyages in cases of consumption, Gilchrist also espoused their efficacy in mental affections. He cited with approval the importance of such remedies in antiquity (the traditional way to lend authority to eighteenth-century medicine), when they were recommended in cases of 'passio stomachica' (i.e. 'the vapours'), as well as in 'lowness of spirits' and even in 'higher nervous disorders … such as epilepsy, palsy and maniacal affections'.[103] Gilchrist also presented a number of case histories from his own practice that he claimed showed the benefits of sea voyages in the vapours.[104] Conceptualising nervous disorders as profoundly located in the blood, internal vessels and stomach, and in need of evacuation, sea voyages and the sea-sickness they were so effective at provoking seemed an obvious good thing to such physicians. They appeared superior to medicinal emetics because of the putatively more natural and prolonged (but less extreme) way in which vomiting was induced.[105] Sea voyages and sailing were also supported because they could afford patients exercise.[106] They had the additional advantages of bringing patients into a better air,[107] and into warmer and more temperate climates, even if embarked on in 'less favourable seasons' and weathers. And Gilchrist stigmatised the air and climate of Britain as unfavourable because cold and changeable.[108]

Gilchrist concentrated mostly on the physiological rather than psychological affects of sea voyages. Nevertheless, he also mentioned that they helped to cheer the mind and discussed ways in which the sea was apt to act positively on the body through the mind.[109] Attempting to counter possible objections to this therapy, Gilchrist advised adjustments in its prescription for certain types of patients. He recommended trips closer to land, in smoother water, and in mild airs and seasons for 'those of greater delicacy, and liable to nervous spasmodic affections'.[110] Counselling modification of voyages as to length, vessel type, type of water and weather conditions, according to the nature of the affliction, he was careful again to point out that he was following the ancients.[111] On the other hand, Gilchrist was not entirely positive in his advocacy. Indeed, he anticipated some of the problems with sea voyages that later critics were to emphasise more forcefully, including the fear they provoked in passengers and the real danger of drowning, although generally concerned to reassure in this respect.[112] He also suggested how living by the sea might itself cause mental pathology, and provoke vapours and other nervous disorders.[113]

At the time Gilchrist was speaking about sea voyages the therapy was evidently 'suspected' and 'uncommon', and regarded as of doubtful efficacy, or else unsafe, even by most of his own patients.[114] During the course of the nineteenth century, however, sea voyages became one of the premier, if not, as George H. Savage pointed out in 1900, 'the ideal' form of travel cure for the mentally disordered.[115] Indeed, Victorian doctors helped turn the ocean into a veritable health resort, as William S. Wilson's 1880 book coining that title emphasised only too well.[116] As we shall see, however, by the end of the nineteenth century, medical professionals, and specialists in mental medicine in particular, were becoming steadily more critical of the way in which sea voyages of whatever duration were being advocated by families and by their own colleagues for all kinds of mentally disordered cases.

Travel Pathologised as Mental Disorder:
Climate and Sunstroke

Despite being seen as therapeutic, travel and mobility were often antithetically pathologised as mental disorder in this period. Indeed, travel was regarded as productive of mental pathology in a considerable variety of ways – whether as a consequence of the weariness and stress it might cause, the psychological threats it carried by potential confrontation with disturbing new experiences, or the physiological shocks it might bring upon the system through encounter with hostile climates, diet and diseases.

For some individuals, the nature of their travels was actually observed to have become part of the content of their delusions. The Bethlem Physician, John Monro, mentioned the case of a master of a Jamaican trading ship who believed:

> himself infected with the Venereal distemper, which he imagin'd he
> had contracted in his last voyage to Jamaica where, according to his
> own account, he had been familiar with some infected person ... had
> communicated [it] to his wife ... likewise infected his wife's mother
> aged about 90, and pretended to shew the marks of it in eruptions
> upon her face.[117]

Prevailing sensationalist interpretations of mental processes often meant that occasionally, rather than as purely symptomatic, the behaviour and ideas of such individuals might actually be conceived to be deranged, diseased or infected by their travelling. It was observed by John Haslam, for example, that the 'ideas' of John Archer, admitted to Bethlem Hospital in 1795, having:

> travelled with a gentleman over a great part of Europe ... ran
> particularly on what he had seen abroad; sometimes he conceived
> himself the king of Denmark, at other times the king of France ...
> he had some faint recollection of coming over to this country with
> William the Conqueror.[118]

Gulliver certainly returned from his travels in a state of derangement.[119] Swift (and variations on the theme by later writers) presented him as the archetypal Lockean madman, his mind overwhelmed by the strong impressions of his voyages, especially his final sojourn with the Houyhnhnms (so that he took to conversing with horses and found the sight, smell and company of his family and other humans repellent).

In addition to these more psychologically located threats to travellers were other somatically instigated perils to the intellectual faculties, the pathology of which resided in the actual process of travel and in the impact of foreign climates. Although mainly concerned with the physical illnesses incident to travellers, the anonymous *Practical Physician for Travellers, Whether by Sea or Land*[120] of 1729, by a member of the College of Physicians, also covered mental diseases such as 'phrenzies' and 'watching and ravings'. The latter and their consequent 'loss of senses', were attributed to 'want of Rest and Feeding', 'excessive Motion' and to the resulting 'Fatigue' and sleeplessness often involved in travelling.[121] The former were related to 'warmth of air, if join'd to an intemperate Way of Living'. The author also warned about the 'excessive Drinking of hot Liquors in hot Weather, on a Journey, so that a Lunacy succeeded a Phrenzy' and about mental disturbance arising from the sea air encouraging a 'saline state of blood'.[122] In general, this guide admonished readers as to how dangerous all sudden Changes are in our Way of Living', as well as all extremes of cold and heat.[123] It emphasised how 'on Journeys – the Sun-beams … falling perpendicularly on Travellers, never fail of putting the Blood into great Commotion and Elevations', advising for prophylaxis 'to avoid travelling in such Heats', to set out early, and to stop when the sun becomes powerful.[124]

Sunstroke, *coup de soleil* or 'insolation' had been recognised since antiquity as a cause of madness. Sunstroke was not surprisingly seen as particularly incident to sailors and travellers. The aetiology occasionally featured in eighteenth-century trials where witnesses testified in favour of an insanity plea.[125] Some medical practitioners offered detailed scientific explanations in their treatises. Most notably, Richard Mead explored the tremendous influence exerted by both the sun and the moon on human bodies in a 1708 treatise devoted to the subject.[126] Lay persons are also found proposing these same influences as causes for madness in eighteenth-century medical case books, and they were rarely contradicted by their doctors.[127] The frequent failure to explain or query such ascriptions is indicative of their broad, commonsensical, cultural acceptability. William Battie also emphasised how sunstroke could provoke mental disturbance. Because of the violent shock and derangement Battie felt sunstroke involved, he declared it 'generally of long duration and very often incurable'.[128] During the early modern period, madness was often understood generally as resulting from the blood, the spirits or the brain overheating, whether from influences without or within the body. Richard Blackmore observed that 'Madness and Distraction …

are frequently the Diseases of hot Countries', and P. Frings explained the cause of phrensy as 'the Overheating the Spirits, and an Effervency first in the heart and next in the Brain'.[129] Although classical medical theories about maniacs' animalistic nature had fostered a conviction in their partial immunity to extremes of temperature, these tended to focus on extremes of cold, rather than heat.[130] Mechanistic and sensationalist conceptualisations of madness emphasised how the condition could be caused by both temperature extremes and posited both heightened sensibility and insensibility as definitive of mental affections.[131] However, criticisms of this paradigm from medical men during the Enlightenment, including even Haslam, arising partly from a new appreciation of the sensibilities of the insane, undermined belief in it. This was despite the fact that types of medical care associated with the belief remained resilient at bastions of tradition like Bethlem and even amongst more modern thinkers like the Reverend William Pargeter.[132] Indeed, amongst both the laity and medical men, there is considerable evidence of the survival of folk beliefs in the animalistic immunities of the mad and the power of the sun (and other planets) over mental ailments well into the following century.

During the course of the nineteenth century, physicians and alienists grew more interested in the influence of climate on mental and physical diseases in general. Although the data they gathered often had conflicting results, most alienists continued to believe that temperature extremes and profound climactic changes caused mental illness. In France, Esquirol was certainly of this opinion, producing statistics to show an increase in admissions during the summer months. While some British alienists doubted that this was the case in the 'mild' climates of their own country, most expected climates in 'countries where the range of the thermometer is between extreme heat and extreme cold ... to have a marked effect upon the brain'.[133] Medical practitioners became distinguished as climatologists, often combining their analyses of climates with assessments of the comparative merits of various health resorts. Their publications further contributed to the medicalizing of the debate about climate, travel and mental health, although their work focused primarily on chronic physical ailments.[134] Widening experience and study of mental and physical illnesses in the British colonies, as well as growing concern at home and abroad with the importance of temperature in hygienic and sanitary measures,[135] also alerted medical men to the pathologies of changing climactic conditions. In asylums too, practitioners grew more appreciative of how 'sudden changes of temperature exert a most unfavourable influence on the sanatory condition of the inmates'.[136]

During the course of the nineteenth century, the failure of travellers and settlers to acclimatise was even more regularly cited as a cause of insanity, reports multiplying apace with the expansion of both the travel industry and the Victorian colonial empire, as well as of medical literature on the subject. More often than not change of climate was deemed to be merely contributory, or to have brought on a minor complaint. Patients' families and doctors repeatedly observed how they had 'gone to a trying climate ... and got a little run down'.[137] Occasionally, however, such encounters were seen as the major exciting cause of a mental disorder. Amongst various forms of such problems in acclimatising, sunstroke was perhaps the most universally accepted and ascribed in cases of madness. It was something that white tourists and settlers were deemed particularly prone to, the colonial presence of the English in India giving rise to the cliché 'mad dogs and Englishmen go out in the mid-day sun'. 'Warm climate' and 'sunstroke' appeared regularly in asylums' official tabulations of causes of disease. A few of such cases, of course, were thought to have succumbed to native temperature changes, in the manner, for example, of John Archer, who was admitted to Bethlem Hospital in 1795 after 'working in a garden, on a very hot day, without any covering on his head'.[138]

Earlier in the period, few disputed the prevailing view that Europeans going to the Tropics were peculiarly liable to nervous and mental disorders. Nevertheless, late Victorian psychiatry's rather more critical analysis of the causes traditionally assigned in mental cases inspired some alienists to be more dubious. Thomas Clouston, for example, thought it beyond doubt that 'sunstroke gets the credit of far more insanity than it produces', if only because 'few Britons become insane in hot climates in whom that cause is not assigned'.[139] This scepticism seems primarily to have been encouraged by the tendency for Victorian psychiatry to stress hereditary predisposition, underlying organic aetiology and degenerative diseases, rather than exciting, immediate and moral causes. New classifications of mental symptoms as resulting from neurologically-centred trauma and shock also tended to mitigate the concern with sunstroke *per se*. Following other Scottish alienists, including Francis Skae, Clouston certainly preferred to relegate 'the insanity of sunstroke' to an adjunct of the group of disorders he classified as 'traumatic insanity'. He played down the importance of both so much that he recorded only twelve instances (just 0.3% of admissions) during the nine years previous to 1887.[140]

At Glasgow Royal, sunstroke cases were also in decline towards the end of the period, after an early rise probably explained by improved information gathering as much as any growing awareness of the problem. As recorded in annual reports, sunstroke or hot climate was ascribed in 0.91% of all cases during 1862-72, but in just 0.67% of all cases during 1876-86. Throughout the period, climactic causes remained such a small proportion of the total that they rarely received any special attention from clinicians. What is particularly interesting, nonetheless, is that sunstroke was actually suggested as a significant aetiological factor more frequently and more straightforwardly by patients' relations than it was by the asylum's practitioners, the latter clearly recategorising some cases in line with their own pathological paradigms. For example, in annual reports during 1878-86 sunstroke was mentioned in just 11 cases, and in asylum registers in just 14 (in six of which other more standard late Victorian psychiatric causes were additionally assigned, from intemperance, heredity and previous attacks to overwork). In contrast, admission documents (where original ascriptions by friends and general practitioners were more faithfully recorded), mentioned sunstroke in 18 cases, and rarely referred to other underlying causes. Combining all sources one finds that sunstroke was somehow ascribed in 21 cases (1.3% of all admissions).

While partly explained by transcription errors and to some information being provided at later dates, these discrepancies are partly also due to differences between medical and lay views of insanity. Some testifiers expressed uncertainty in such ascriptions, and this seems to have discouraged asylum officers from accepting them. One patient's illness was explained as follows: 'uncertain perhaps sunheat or fright from being lost in a jungle where there were tigers'. While a few of these patients may have got sunstroke at home, most cases in which location was specified had succumbed in foreign climates, two in Australia, one in India, one in South America, one in Toronto and another in Havana. Not surprisingly, the vast majority (93%) of the Glasgow cases I have identified during 1814-86 where climate and change of scene was mentioned as a cause were men, the disparity being especially high in the sunstroke cases. More men than women, no doubt, were doing physical labour outdoors in inclement conditions, or had gone to work, settle or travel abroad in hot countries. Of the 1878-86 patients, for example, one had been an assistant tea planter in India; two had been in the army; three were employed in maritime service; while one had been a commercial agent. Not surprisingly, also, private cases predominated over paupers,

51

by 16:5 in the 1878-86 sample, the former being more likely to have the means and occupations to take them abroad, as well, perhaps, as a greater social imperative for understanding their illnesses as a result of an exogenous force more or less beyond their control.

The work of Waltraud Ernst has shown admirably that, amongst the British in India, climactic and environmental explanations for madness were also favoured owing to the exculpation they carried. If the susceptible were seen to have fallen victim to an alien climate and culture they were, to some extent, freed from blame for their conditions.[141] Ernst also delineates how the putative hostility of the Indian climate encouraged the early repatriation of European lunatics in India. Nevertheless, what Ernst failed to point out was that those who had travelled to India as a matter of free choice, heedless of their vulnerable constitutions, were sometimes held to be all the more culpable.

Another problem with travel, as well as the potential exposure to hostile climates and foreign diseases, was the very difficulty of obtaining medical advice in isolated situations abroad, or, at least, medical advice that travellers were prepared to trust. John Harriot, for example, related in 1815 how, when he caught a fever in the heat of Sumatra and 'apprehended approaching distraction', he effected his own cure. This was through combined treatment under a makeshift douche of his own devising and self-dosing with purgatives and tonics, and was 'in defiance' of native doctors who had predicted his death. Indeed, having noticed the ill-success of native remedies (and despite acknowledging his actions as rash), Harriot warned his readers sternly against following local medical advice.[142] In using this makeshift douche, Harriot was clearly implementing standard European medical prescriptions, which stressed hydrotherapy as a reliable treatment for sunstroke and mental and nervous disorders.[143] Literature published during the course of the century, both medical and lay, both military and civilian, on the hazards to health in tropical climates and the precautions that travellers should take, offered similar advice.[144] Such literature can also be seen as broadly located within the wider growth of 'domestic medicine' and self-help guides to medicine in this period. For example, an 1882 guide entitled *On Duty Under A Tropical Sun* by the Madras Army Major, S. Leigh Hunt and the London Surgeon and Anatomist, Alexander S. Kenny, sought to 'supply the traveller in hot countries with a little domestic medicine for his own use'.[145] Although generally keen to resist encouraging patients to treat themselves, medical authors tending to admonish travellers to 'avail themselves ...of the skill and experience of medical men', they were appreciative that this was often unavailable.[146] Such guides commonly contained separate sections on sunstroke, how to avoid it and how to treat its effects, the aforementioned book prescribing standard cures, including 'a cold water-douche ... applied to the head ... chest and spine', and evacuant remedies such as mustard plasters and enemas.[147] However, admissions that 'it is impossible to lay down any hard and fast rules calculated to meet each individual case'[148] pinpointed a basic irony with much of such literature, which licensed patients to pick and chose rather eclectically and randomly.

Travel Pathologised as Mental Disorder: Shock, Stress and Neurasthenia

As the quest for health in a natural setting, whether in the country or in spa resorts, had become a fashion during the early modern period, it had spawned its own sceptics amongst dissatisfied patients and rival practitioners. Some, demurring the impact of romanticism on this health culture, dismissed it as the illusory pastoral ideal of the rich urbanite and a medical con-trick. They alleged that such trips were more liable to make patients poorer and sicker, although carping practitioners often had their own commercial self-interest in mind.[149]

In another guise, the early nineteenth-century culture of Romanticism clearly encouraged the association of travel to foreign parts with mental (and physical) pathology, at least in so far as it involved artists travelling abroad. Nevertheless, for the artist, foreign travel constituted a confrontation with pathology that was an almost expected, if not desirable, eventuality, a kind of rite of passage encounter with dangerous and otherworldly sensations and experiences. Romanticism saw illness becoming a cultural and existential badge for the artist. As Wrigley and others have noted, the license it gave for bizarre behaviour, 'abnormal sensibility, and physical deterioration' reinforced 'the idea that artists were predisposed to a pathological state of mind when in Rome', or in other new environments.[150] This was especially so if such environments were perceived as radically different in the sense impressions, climatic conditions and pace of life that they imposed upon the newcomer.

Travel, and the yearned for otherness with which it was associated, also bred its own less welcome forms of mental illness. Most notable amongst these were the aforementioned traumatic illnesses and injuries, often associated with accidents and disasters during transport and travel. Some must have involved spinal and neurological damage, and others were probably precursors of that group of disorders now known as post-traumatic stress disorders. Marooning and survival from shipwreck, and the trauma, isolation and despair that often attended them, could also be harbingers of mental disturbance, something that was highlighted by literary inventions such as Ben Gunn of Stevenson's *Treasure Island*, and even by Defoe's *Robinson Crusoe* (before Man Friday arrived on the scene). However, such stories undoubtedly did more to communicate the allure and adventure of travel, than they did its threats – contemporaries, like Henry Matthews, actually being inspired by them to begin their travelling careers.[151] In medical writings, shipwreck became a metaphor for mental collapse and alienation that was commonly employed by specialists in psychological medicine. Yellowlees, for example, saw 'mental shipwreck' as a virtual concomitant of modern living, and the 'storms and turmoil of life'.[152]

Novel and widened forms of travel also engendered novel and widened forms of psychiatric illness. As Ralph Harrington explores admirably in this volume and elsewhere, the expansion of railway transport saw the emergence of a new type of neurological disorder known as 'railway spine'.[153] This diagnosis was one of a number of foci for Victorian cultural anxieties about the effects of new mechanized transportation systems and of the increasing stresses and strains of modernity. It also owed much to developments in neurological research, in particular the work of Marshall Hall, Thomas Laycock, David Ferrier and others on reflexology and localisation, and a growing medical literature on the wear and tear of modern civilization on the nervous system.[154] Greater reporting of such illnesses in Victorian times was also clearly encouraged by the expansion of the medical and accident insurance industry, which offered sufferers the benefit and enticement of financial compensation. However, these developments and the important recognition by alienists and neurologists that the psychological, emotional and physical consequences of trauma and shock might be delayed, or become progressively worse, posed difficult medico-legal problems. As alienists like Clouston and surgeons like James Syme warned, some patients were encouraged 'to exaggerate' their symptoms 'till the damages are paid by the company'.[155]

Much earlier than this, medical men had also stressed the dangers to mental (and physical) health inherent in standard forms of transportation such as stage-coaches and carriages. In 1816, for example, Thomas Bakewell attributed cases of 'madness' he had 'heard of which commenced while travelling in this manner' and others he had personally encountered who were 'seized while riding on the outside' to exposure to the extremes of the weather. He also blamed the psychological strains – 'watchfulness, and the excitement of terror' – involved in long and uncomfortable journeys.[156]

Whether travel was embarked upon for the purpose of socialising, recreation, vacation, work or health, contemporary medical literature was replete with warnings about the threats it carried to both mental and physical health, and the precautions that should be taken. The best laid travel plans could always be upset. Towards the end of the Victorian period in particular, medical men placed great emphasis on the manifold ways that travel might prove a strain on the nerves. It might be over-prolonged, prove exhausting and irritating; might place travellers in situations of considerable discomfort; or force them to share cramped spaces, with little air. Increasing concerns with the vulnerability of the nervous and delicate when travelling, ladies in particular, encouraged some practitioners to recommend that such people travel doped up with bromides, chlorals and other drugs. An 1881 article by the obstetrician, E. J. Tilt, for example, advised a 25-30 gram dose per day, claiming to 'have enabled such women to travel long distances, with comfort to themselves, and to the rest of the party'. He claimed that the drug's utility as a travel aid applied equally to men; and that it 'generally brings on the usual bromide sleep; or, at all events ... calms the system, and abates the irksome weariness of body and soul that follows long travelling in a cramped position'.[157] Others advised similar, although smaller doses for 'nervous and excitable' children.[158]

Such advice was clearly informed by the voguishness of stress, nervousness and neurasthenia that coloured medico-psychological discussions of travel for much of the second half of the nineteenth century. The diagnosis of neurasthenia, coined by Beard in America, is a striking example of how notions of mental illness were intimately bound up with a cultural and ideological construction of the ills of modern society in which travel played a role as both a therapy and a source of pathology. On the one hand, travel permitted a release from the pressures of life, and was a standard form of treatment for the neurasthenic. On the other hand, neurasthenia was articulated against a view of the progress of civilisation which posited the stresses of new forms of transport and travel as corollaries of the increasingly unhealthy, tiring and stressful pace of modern life. Thus the steam boat and the railway, in bringing with them increased mobility, stimulation, hustle and bustle, displacement, and new pressures of scheduling time and business, could themselves be regarded as vehicles of the nervous strain and exhaustion on which neurasthenia fed. The agitation and discomfort involved in such forms of transport were increasingly perceived by medical practitioners as damaging to the nerves of their patients. The medical climatologist, Symes Thompson, for example, claimed that 'no one in his senses would recommend a long railway journey for those whose nervous systems are in [an over-sensitive] ... condition'.[159]

Criticism of neurasthenia in Britain and elsewhere as a somewhat narrow definition of mental problems and somewhat culturally-specific to conditions across the Atlantic, encouraged many practitioners to talk more generally about stress when discussing the salubrity or pathology of travel. Symes Thompson, for example, viewed stress as at the root of a range of mental affections, and in so doing saw travel 'as of very great value' in offering sufferers 'changed surroundings' and climate.[160] Travel was prescribed as a particular antidote to the modern stresses of work. Thompson pointed in particular to 'professional occupation[s]', including 'the Stock Exchange', where (what many contemporary practitioners called) 'the nineteenth-century pressure is very great'. The world of such specialists was full of 'people whose nervous systems will go to pieces unless they can be taken away from the stress in which they are living'.[161]

Pathological models of mental affliction throughout the period 1700-1900 were commonly, to some degree, environmentally, culturally or racially mediated. Travel was often recommended in order to bring patients relief from the specific climactic, educational and social contexts with which their illnesses were held to be associated. The popularisation of neurasthenia, which encouraged many American mental patients to leave their homeland in search of a break from the pressures of modern life, also, however, encouraged some British alienists to interpret neurasthenia as itself a product of special native conditions across the Atlantic. Clouston, for example, believed that 'the air and climate, and the mode of life and education in some parts of America were so stimulating, that the brain there sometimes exhausted both its trophic and energising power, and paid the penalty by prolonged periods of "Neurasthenia"'. He regarded 'the natural cure' for this as 'change to a more sleepy climate'.[162] It was on similar grounds of specificity that Clouston resisted the applicability of certain American plans of treatment like massage. More pertinently, this suggests how medical notions of travel might be premised on prevailing national and racial prejudices.

Sometimes, of course, nervous or neurasthenic states were themselves (or were conceived to be) fostered by the shock and stresses of encounter with a disparate culture and society. This aetiological interpretation must have been encouraged just as much by contemporary biases towards the manners, conditions and customs of supposedly 'primitive' societies, and by common associations of mental disorder with an atavistic, savage, or pre-civilised state, as by the genuinely disturbing effect of problems in assimilating. Gender disparities are also pertinent in this connection, women often being conceived as more vulnerable than men to problems of adjustment to the harsh conditions and social indignities of a new world, a view that clearly referred back to traditional models of women as frail in sensibilities and tender in minds. Commenting, whilst in White's Town, along the Mohawk River, on an apparent prevalence of insanity amongst English women 'in the back settlements' of America, John Harriot, for example, declared:

> I am firmly persuaded it arises from a depression of spirits, occasioned by so great a change from civilized to an almost savage state of society ... A man will struggle through much easier, yet not without many heart-aches, though his pride may not permit him to confess it. But it falls with tenfold weight on the mistress of a family, who, having experienced the benefits of servants in the mother country, is under an unavoidable necessity of being the greatest, drudge, and a slave to the very indifferent help she can, with difficulty, procure in America[163]

In fact, Harriot had little to go on, having only encountered two such cases.

Lay Versus Medical Travel Guidance

One thing that is noticeable in most medical practitioners' writings about salutary travel for the mentally disordered is their regular insistence that trips should be made strictly in accordance with medical advice, as Purcell instructed in 1702.[164] Other medical authorities, emphasised how 'it is the Business of a Traveller to be well appriz'd of his Condition, to apply to proper and learned Assistance, and not to trust himself, unless he can't be supplied with any better'.[165] Thus, medical advice about travel can be seen as another example of the profession's attempts to establish its status and expertise. Patients' own views of the matter were often dismissed as irrational. Nevertheless, this was far from invariably the case, and some patients, particularly those from higher social circles, were able to exert more influence over where they went and were treated. Moreover, if they were to sustain a lucrative and successful private practice, medical practitioners were thoroughly dependent on gaining the good will and co-operation of wealthy families. Often against their better discretion, they were obliged to abide by the will of the family when advising on the travel, form of treatment and appropriate residence of a mentally disordered member. Yet neither medical practitioners nor families could be relied upon necessarily to agree on such matters. And many had passionate and divergent opinions about the conditions and treatment appropriate for a mental case. As is only too clear from fictional cases like Clarissa and real cases like Mrs Clerke[166] or George III, the contentiousness of madness as a diagnosis and the power of family, political and other interests turned medical consultations on mental cases into an arena of conflict more regular and profound than any other area of contemporary medicine. This was especially the case before say 1850, when the status of mad-doctors and their specialty was so insecure.

In cases like that of Hannah Allen discussed earlier, it was clearly the family that called the tune in deciding on changes in residence and general treatment. Yet changes of scene for Hannah were also carefully negotiated with the patient herself. Hannah required regular coaxing to get her to travel. And such patients often had their own reasons for preferring a country (or city) residence. While, for example, Hannah related how 'my Aunt resolved to take me down again into the Countrey', it was far from irrelevant that Hannah herself 'was very glad of [this]; for there I thought I should live more privately, and be less disturbed'. On her arrival home, Hannah felt herself 'where I would be; for there I could do what I pleased, with little opposition; there I shunned all Company tho' they were my near Relations'.[167]

It would not do, however, to exaggerate patients' powers of determining their care, or the frailties of medical authority, or indeed the conflicting nature of lay-medical relations in this period. Some families displayed great determination to stick to medical advice (conscious that they had gone to some trouble to procure it and were paying for it through the nose), particularly if such advice coincided with their own views and interests. As much as between medical men and families, conflicts were intra-familial or intra-lay. In this context, the aforementioned case of George Walpole (1730-91), third Earl of Orford, nephew of Horace Walpole (1717-97), fourth Earl, is especially illustrative. This case also highlights the dangers with which removing the sick were, or were deemed to be, attended, and how lodging a deranged individual with his friends in the country might encourage the concealment of his illness. Walpole seems to have made some effort to secure 'the best advice' for his nephew, including that of John Monro, William Battie, and the London private practitioner, John Jebb (1736-86). When advised by Drs Monro and Jebb that his 'very mad' nephew should 'be brought immediately to town' from the parsonage in Eriswell where he was staying, however, Walpole encountered staunch opposition from 'his mistress, his steward and a neighbouring parson', who 'cried out I should kill him if I conveyed him [to London] from that paradise'. Orford's accountant, Carlos Cony, also objected. Walpole's imperious response was that they had 'concealed the illness to the last moment they could'; that he 'had never heard of a madman being consulted on the place of his habitation', and that the doctors were 'not to be doubted'. Walpole clearly believed Eriswell (which was 'on the edge of the fens'), to be an unhealthy and inappropriate habitation for a sick man, referring to it as:

> that wretched hovel … one of the most improper places upon earth … being so out of the way of all help [it seems to have been 40 miles from the nearest doctor] … built of lath and plaster [so that] … he might escape with the greatest ease … [with] not a decent lodging room, and … ponds close.

However, Walpole also appears to have had other motives. Evidently stung by certain society gossip about his conduct towards Orford, he wanted to make a public display of his concern for his nephew, declaring that he 'would place him in the face of the whole town, where everybody might see or learn the care that was taken of him'. Ultimately, however, Orford's friends had their way, with the assistance of extra medical advice. A Norwich physician declared that 'my Lord Orford has so considerable a degree of fever and flux … [that] he cannot be removed at present' and Orford soon made an almost complete (if temporary) recovery.[168]

Specialists in mental cases not only stressed the need for deranged individuals to obey their doctors when changing their residences and travelling, but this conviction also prompted and informed their advice on the companions travellers should keep. Clouston recommended 'a cheery, sensible companion' for melancholics, evidently someone who would help ensure the trip was well managed and enlivening to the spirits. However, he distinguished 'travel … with a … companion' as 'twice as valuable if he is a doctor'.[169] Yet such advice represented more of a medical ideal than a common practice. Although, like Purcell before him, Savage also felt that travel should always be undertaken with relatively thorough attention to medical advice, he actually recommended 'travelling with a companion *or* [my emphasis] doctor'.[170] Lay companions were the common preferences of sick travellers themselves, and the ease of obtaining the services of a travelling doctor was limited by the pragmatics and economics of travel and of medical practice. Thus nervous patients travelled rather more seldom with medical professionals than with lay companions, or with a nurse.

Nevertheless, for private practitioners, in an age when the wealthy expected to be able to purchase a highly personalised form of medical care, being employed as a travelling doctor was not an unusual occurrence. Whether undertaken (as was more often than not the case) at the beginnings of their careers, when private custom was harder to come by, or when more established as society doctors needing less to forge than to sustain their social connections and patronage, service as a travelling physician to gentry or aristocracy might present an attractive and lucrative option. Soon after qualifying in medicine, for example, W.A.F. Browne was 'entrusted with the care of a well-to-do lunatic who was to be treated through travel and change of scene' for two years, journeying through Belgium, France and Italy.[171] Browne regarded this experience and the knowledge of continental asylums he gathered whilst abroad as of sufficient value to mention it in his subsequent successful application for the Superintendent's job at Montrose Royal Lunatic Asylum in 1834. In similar fashion, while trying to establish his own medical career in the 1820s, Alexander Morison called upon well-connected friends to attempt to procure him a post as a travelling physician to nobility. Subsequently, he was to spend over two years accompanying Lady Bute, Lady Guildford and an entourage of children and their tutor around Europe, on a typical 'medical version of the Grand Tour made by invalids'.[172] While Lady Bute seems to have been suffering from a physical rather than a mental complaint, Morison's grumbling as to her 'dithering about travel arrangements' emphasises the frustrations such posts carried for physicians and the extent to which their advice was subject to the whims of their wealthy clients.[173]

Travel Medicalised?
Late Victorian Travel Guidance for Mental Cases

As travel became increasingly *à la mode* after 1700, it was accompanied by a growing glut of travel literature. While much of this was in the nature of descriptive tour guides and adventuring, many of these travel guides also gave specific advice to invalids on how to procure and safeguard their health. And medical practitioners, keen to establish new areas of expertise and worried about the dissemination of bad advice, sought increasingly to control, if not monopolise, this literature. The trouble was that there was often no general consensus on where and when people should go, or what types of people should go, in search of health. It was not just that people travelled in ignorance, or followed allegedly fallacious, or observably discrepant advice, but that what knowledge they had was often so empirically and subjectively based. There were genuine vicissitudes over time in the climactic and social conditions of the countries people travelled to. Differences in travellers' mental baggage – their experiences, predilections and cultural background – meant considerable variations in the dissemination of health knowledge about travel. For example, Henry Matthews found it 'difficult to conceive how Montpellier ever obtained a name for the salubrity of its climate', but offered the explanation that:

> the climates of Europe are but little understood in England, nor indeed is it an easy thing to ascertain the truth, with respect to climate. Travellers generally speak from the impression of a single season, and we all know how much the seasons vary.[174]

The growth of an increasing literature on climatology in the nineteenth century was, in part, an attempt to put such apparent misapprehensions right. Even when people were offered supposedly good advice, however, they were not always in a position to take it. Travel often entailed considerable limitations of choice over timing, destination and logistics, and was subject to a large degree of chance in what might be encountered once away.

By Victorian times the travel industry had expanded well beyond its early modern levels. Yet while more and more mentally and physically sick people were (metaphorically) getting the travel bug, travel itself seemed to be becoming increasingly pathological. Alienists were particularly concerned that, as a result of the growing and rather indiscriminate recommendation and use of travel as a treatment for mental disease, people were actually damaging their mental health. People who they regarded for health reasons as wholly unfit for travel were doing so for the sake of their health, while the wrong types of people were going to the wrong types of climate. Medical practitioners had long striven to ensure that travel advice was geared to individual constitutional and mental types. By the 1880s and 90s, as part of a general move in psychiatric circles to make knowledge about the preservation of mental health more available to the public at large, and as part of a wider explosion in healthy travel guides, a spate of psychiatric publications began to deal more comprehensively with the proper use and abuse of travel.

Part of the problem then, as Oppenheim also observed,[175] was that alienists themselves tended to be inconsistent and ambivalent, if not downright contradictory, about advice on travel for mental cases. As well as in the process of travel itself, there were deep uncertainties inherent in medical knowledge about travel, climate and pathology. In his *Clinical Lectures on Mental Disease* (1887), however, Clouston declared that 'there is scarcely a point on which I have so much difficulty in the early treatment of melancholia as whether to send patients away to travel or not, and, if they go from home, where to send them to'.[176] Whilst observing how 'usual' was 'the plan of travel and change of scene' for melancholics, he alleged that (apparently because of its too indiscriminate adoption) they were 'often the worse for it'.[177] Yet for milder, incipient cases, 'who merely have the temperament and the tendency', he regarded such recourses as 'most effective in warding off attacks'.[178] Though forced to confess 'that no definite rules can be laid down on this subject', he did attempt to offer some basic guidelines. Convinced that a certain amount of peace and calm was requisite, he condemned 'quick travelling – going to many places in a short time – big noisy hotels and an exciting life' as 'nearly always bad for a patient'.[179] Anything overly 'fatiguing', or that might make the mind overly excited or restless was anathema for such alienists. Travel needed to be 'slow', unhurried, organised, restful and pleasurable, not hectic, exhausting and stressing.[180] The Grand Tour was definitely out. Influenced by American-style rest-cure strategies, Clouston and other late Victorian alienists normally prescribed travel as a form of restful diversion, often combining it with recommendations for 'mental, affective, motor, and sexual rest' in general and avoidance of 'any expenditure of nerve energy'. Thus, Clouston recommended a combination of 'regular changes of scene, "breaks" in occupation, and long holidays'. Of course, by definition, travel required a temporary or more prolonged suspension of work.

Clouston also counselled against travelling for other types of patient. 'If the bodily condition is very weak and exhausted', he claimed, it would do 'more harm than good'. Similarly if the patient was suffering from paranoia (or strong 'delusions of suspicion'), 'the quieter he is kept the better'.[181] Clouston tried to establish a distinction between the type of travel that was best for incipient, or 'less serious' mental disease, as opposed to that which would suit more advanced cases. This distinction was based fundamentally on a judgement as to fragile, but divergent, levels of attention span, as well as of bodily vigour. For incipient cases he recommended 'travel abroad', whilst stressing that it should be 'done in a systematic, methodical, leisurely way'. For more chronic patients, whose 'power of attention is much impaired', he advised 'a quiet country place, where there are few visitors'.[182] Trips to the country (and seaside) were often combined with other changes to patients' diet, social interaction and intellectual and spiritual input, designed to counter previous regimen and associations, and to afford them a calming, more naturalistic, naturopathic setting. In such settings, the artificial disharmony and agitation of patients' former lives was to be countered by return or retreat to a putatively harmonious realm of basic physiological functioning. Whereas some depressed patients were offered diverting activities, other nervous, distraught patients were made to lead an uneventful, if not monotonous existence. Plant-like, they were to be nourished by wholesome foods and minerals: literally, both mentally and organically, they were to 'vegetate'.[183] One melancholic adolescent girl, prone to religious agonising, was required whilst in the country 'to take aloes, iron, and quinine, to read little, [and] not to go to church for a short time'.[184]

Despite his attempts to be a little more schematic than some of his colleagues, however, Clouston fundamentally favoured an *ad hoc*, empirical approach – convinced that the prescription had to be made case by case, and that 'in many cases we must try experimentally to see whether travel is to do good or harm'.[185] Occasionally, he advised trips both to the country and abroad, the latter being favoured if the patient showed signs of convalescence and a return of energy, or what Clouston referred to as a 'tendency to romp'.[186] For example, Clouston sent the aforementioned melancholic girl 'at once to the country, to ride, walk, live in the open air'. However, when after 'a month or two' she 'got girlish, romping and quite well', a tour to Switzerland was prescribed, from which 'she returned fat, cheerful, and vigorous, with no undue religious emotionalism'.[187]

Clouston prescribed travelling in a considerable variety of ways for a wide range of mental cases who often had very little in common with each other. While generally he favoured peace and 'quiet in most cases', 'rest from exhausting or irritating work', and 'above all, escape from worry', 'in a few of the less serious cases', he counselled 'active travel and bustle'.[188] Beside melancholics and hypochondriacs, Clouston also advised travel as a form of treatment for cases of 'delusional insanity' such as monomania, at least 'at the beginning' of the affliction, when the delusions were 'not ... quite fixed'.[189] His advice to his patients on their travelling was often painstakingly detailed and regularly adjusted. Apart from prescriptions concerning his diet and medicine, one patient who consulted Clouston was advised 'absolute rest, a sea voyage, almost no company – to live out in the fresh air', and not to expend any 'nerve energy whatever, either in seeing company, travelling too fast, walking or talking'. His friends were warned not to exhaust him by adherence to that old (and, as Clouston believed, misconceived) chestnut that melancholics needed 'cheering up'. Clouston also integrated travel into his prophylaxis, telling this patient for example 'to weigh himself every month, and whenever he found he had lost 3 lbs to stop work and take a change or sea voyage'.[190] The over-protective tone adopted by such doctors reflects those new levels of anxiety about nervous illness in late Victorian psychiatry charted so incisively by Oppenheim.[191] Their prescriptions represent an idealised health regime that would hardly have been available to a working-class patient; their strategies were primarily reserved to wealthier patients whose employment and financial options were sufficiently flexible. Therapeutic travel thus continued to be profoundly socially demarcated: a visa or badge of membership for a rather exclusive valetudinarian club. This suggests the continuing relevance of Jewson's argument about (eighteenth-century) medical theory and practice being highly conditioned by the interests, demands and capabilities of a superior sort of clientele.[192] Indeed, the culture and fashion of travel, for the invalid as much as for the adventurer, had long been quintessentially the domain of the genteel classes. Henry Matthews referred to 'travelling' as 'the best receipt I know for curing a fine gentleman'.[193] Nevertheless, more modest trips were clearly freely embarked upon by a wide variety of persons from the middling sort, amongst whom ambitions for social climbing and the shadowing of fashion were part and parcel of their demands as consumers in a growing market for health.

Including a couple of pages of advice about travelling in mental cases in his textbook *Insanity and Allied Neuroses* (1896), the former Superintendent of Bethlem Hospital, George Henry Savage, 'protest[ed]' even more 'emphatically' than had Clouston against the way in which it was being used. In particular he objected to its indiscriminate prescription for 'all kinds of nervous disorder', which he regarded as more the result of 'fashion' than knowledge.[194] He suggested that patients tended to be 'sent away from their homes' with more hope than forethought, 'on the [mere] chance of some of them deriving benefit'. By contrast, Savage recommended travelling only for carefully selected cases, emphasising that the destination and type of such travel should be geared to the particular nervous system in each case. Yet his advice was in a number of important respects rather different in bias from that offered by Clouston. Most of all he believed 'travelling is useful in many young cases suffering from weakness, bodily or mental, especially in those suffering from morbid self-consciousness, and [like Clouston] for those with hypochondriacal tendencies'. His justifications for such views highlight the survival of earlier sensationalist interpretations of mental disorder, overlaid by an enhanced and rather gendered onus on relieving the stresses of work and education (the latter being an especial concern in female cases). To 'the self-conscious girl' who had 'spent years in hard monotonous book-learning', he emphasised the benefits of 'a course of fresh sense impressions, which travel and change supply'. Likewise, painting a picture typical in contemporary medico-psychological texts of 'the over-worked student' who 'continues to work', ignoring 'the warnings' of 'indigestion and sleeplessness' and 'neglecting exercise', and 'breaks down under some trifling physical or moral shock', Savage counselled removal 'from old surroundings and occupations' as a necessity against the risk of insanity. Here the enemies to the psychiatrist were monotony and overwork (as well as its opposite 'dissipation'); the friends were variety, exercise and 'comfort'.

Such alienist's stress on travel as a form of exercise contrasts considerably with their general identification of travel with the rest cure, and once again spotlights the contradictions and ambiguities inherent in the medicalisation of travel. While exercise had long been an important cure for madness, it had rather less often been used as a justification for the benefits of travel for mental cases. Burton's *Anatomy* had associated variation of air and scene with variation of work, relaxation and exercise, but had not identified travel itself as a form of exercise.[195] Mead certainly saw travel as a form of exercise, recommending it for madness under this head in his *Medical Precepts* (1751), where he referred to 'travelling by land and sea' as a means 'to strengthen the constitution'.[196] Less emphatically, an anonymous 1769 guide to medical practice prescribed 'long journeys' for the treatment of hysteria, alongside 'agreeable company, daily exercise ... and amusements'.[197] Of course, certain forms of travel had long been seen as forms of exercise, in particular travel by horse and by carriage, and had regularly been recommended by practitioners for mental cases. In an 1833 book on the treatment of mental disturbances, Ralph Fletcher, Consulting Surgeon to the Gloucester Lunatic Asylum, prescribed rapid riding on a horse or stage coach, as well as long walks. His belief was conventional: that the motion and passage 'through the air, invigorates the body', and that 'the constantly varying objects amuse [or employ] the mind' and 'snap the chain of gloomy associations'.¹⁹⁸ Such therapies proved popular both inside and outside Victorian asylums, carriage exercise for higher class patients being provided daily within many asylum precincts.¹⁹⁹ On the domestic front, mechanical horses for indoor use were one of a number of innovations in medical technology that were infiltrating a growing home market for exercise, slimming, and the prophylactic treatment of hysteria and other nervous and physical diseases. Models such as Vigor's Horse-Action Saddle manifest how intimately contemporary medicalisation and commercialisation of transport and exercise were entering into people's lives.²⁰⁰ Early nineteenth-century specialists often conceived of such techniques as a form of shock therapy, designed to shake the physiological system out of its torpor. Thomas Bakewell, for example, who espoused a new American-style design for carriage travel, advocated the use of 'violent motion', such as 'making a patient fast in a cart, and driving smartly over a rough road', in the same breath as 'sudden shocks' like Joseph Mason Cox's swing.²⁰¹ By the later nineteenth century, however, clinicians had in general grown more critical of shock tactics as applied to mental diseases.

Exercise was not only highlighted by late Victorian alienists in prescribing travel, but travel was often medically defined as itself a form of salutary exercise for mental cases. Savage spoke of 'the active exercise of travel' and recommended it especially for young male adolescents who were 'developing unhealthy religious ideas'. 'Six months' knapsack work' was thus seen as a kind of worldly initiation rite into healthy masculinity, ideal for bringing down to earth morbid 'fear of the unpardonable sin'. A means of reducing excessive sensibility and emotionalism via controlled manly exertion, such prescriptions speak volumes about Victorians' identification of health and manliness with the great outdoors and the traditional rustic, Arcadian, recreational world of the country gentry. Savage was himself an incarnation of this philosophy. He was a keen cyclist, golfer, fisherman, gardener and fencer (establishing the 'Savage Shield'), as well as a regular walker (being one of the 'Sunday Tramps'). His enthusiasm for mountaineering made him a member of the Alpine Club and brought him a record ascent of the Matterhorn.²⁰² This implies a strong personal and gendered bias to his medical prescriptions of exercise and travel. Yet it was a bias that was substantially shared by many of his professional colleagues,²⁰³ while concurrently a means of cementing associations and seeking social parity with their gentrified clientele. Despite Clouston's view of travel as essentially a form of rest cure for melancholia, he too was not averse to pointing out the benefits 'in most cases' of combining such with 'occupation', and in 'certain cases' with a degree of recreational exertion. The important thing for Clouston was that the occupation should be 'a pleasure', not a chore, and that recreations such as 'fishing ... mountaineering, shooting, boating, [and] out-door games' should be 'easy' on the system.[204] Furthermore, Clouston's identification of healthy femininity with vigour, 'romping' and fatness, and with sober religiosity, obtained or restored through travel and the modulation of diet, air, exercise and occupation in an outdoor or pastoral setting, reminds us that prescriptions were issued for both sexes in ways that were not necessarily so far apart as might be supposed.

Like Clouston, Savage strove to be more precise in the advice he gave, recommending specific types of travel for specific cases. He additionally stressed the need to gear destinations to the right seasons, recommending 'the sunshine of the south of Europe ... during winter and early spring', and the mountains 'in summer and autumn'. The putative salubrity of the warm south was well known to contemporaries and has been much discussed by historians, including some contributors to this volume. Mountain regions seem to have been favoured because of their 'bracing' physiological qualities, and the psychological impact of their 'scenery'. In his *Diary of an Invalid*, Henry Matthews had waxed lyrical on the health-giving properties of the air and scenery of the Swiss and Italian Alps, which he thought mostly mental and 'moral, rather than physical'.[205] Apart from the mountains, Savage also recommended Australia 'for a long voyage', although he regarded the Cape as 'more handy'. Harriet Deacon's chapter in this volume, however, emphasises the more negative or ambivalent contemporary evaluations of the environs of the Cape.

Despite his genuine reservations about the universal benefits of travel and efforts to render medical advice about such more specific and therefore 'scientific', Savage still made great and often rather vague claims for the virtues of travel. Of course, in such a short piece he could hardly be especially explicit about where and which patients should travel. Savage followed up and expanded on these comments in a 1900 paper delivered before the Medico-Psychological Association (MPA), which appeared in the *Journal of Mental Science* for 1901.[206] In this paper Savage was even more caustic in his criticisms of the use of travel in the treatment of mental disorders, confessing to having been feeling 'for years past ... more and more strongly that travel as a treatment was being carried too far' and regarding it as 'essential' in a 'very small' number of cases.[207] He censured the motives of both families and even his professional colleagues in endorsing its irresponsible use.[208] With limited self-reflexivity, he observed how prone his fellow practitioners were to being influenced by their own peculiar 'habits, fads, or fancies' in deciding whether and what kind of travel to advocate.[209] That such trips were being embarked upon not only by those 'able to afford the luxury', but also by people who had only a 'slender capital' to 'draw on', was a clear sign, suggested Savage, that things had got out of hand.[210]

The paper was specifically focused on travel abroad (rather than domestic sojourns) and moreover on the contemporary penchant for sea voyages, about which Savage was especially dubious. Conceding that sea voyages might provide 'rest and removal from the daily worries of the business or family, and from the old surroundings', he declared a profound difference in this between cases of 'nerve exhaustion' and others of 'mental perversion'. And he dismissed Weir Mitchell's rest cure as of 'little or no good, but often harm' in cases of confirmed mental disease.[211] Often, furthermore, according to Savage, travel involved, and was advocated for reasons of, stimulation rather than rest. And most melancholics required the latter 'much more' than the former, Savage dismissing antique lore as to stimulation as often 'painful' bullying of the melancholic.[212]

However, as is indicated by Savage's (and other doctors') treatment of Virginia Woolf's nervous illness early on in the twentieth century, British doctors' versions of the rest-cure had their own harsher side. The treatment might itself appear to be a form of bullying to those it did not suit. It would be inappropriate to go into Woolf's case in great detail here. A number of points are worth making nevertheless. Woolf's 'banishment' from London to a house and a nursing home in the country, her isolation from family and friends, and the restrictions imposed on her reading, writing, diet and patterns of rest (modulated by sleeping draughts) were strategies that she detested. She perceived them as impositions on, if not insults to, her autonomy and her physical, emotional and intellectual identity as an artist and a woman. And such treatment, carried on over many months, alongside Savage's dismissive attitude to her objections, made Woolf characterise him as brusque, over-confident, 'tyrannical and shortsighted'.[213] On the other hand, modern accounts of Woolf and her treatment,[214] have varied between two extremes of seeing her as simply mad, or *vice versa* as a victim of male medicine. And such analyses seem themselves rather anachronistic and monochromatic, tending to over-identify with the artist's perspective to the exclusion of other views, and/or to fail sufficiently to contextualise her doctors' views. It does appear that Savage pursued a therapeutics which strongly observed the gods of social, moral and gender conformity.[215] Yet his prescriptions, which also included country and coastal breaks, were relatively conventional fare for less severe forms of mental (and physical) illness amongst the moneyed classes in late Victorian times. They were also relatively mild by comparison with other contemporary strategies towards nervous breakdown. As Oppenheim has argued,[216] it is significant that Woolf was treated as nervous rather than as mad. The relationship between her diagnosis and her class ensured that she was not consigned to a lunatic asylum, as, more than likely, a similarly affected lower-class patient would have been. Furthermore, Savage's earlier treatment of Vanessa, Virginia's sister, shows that the stricter, isolationist aspects of the rest-cure might be mitigated for 'milder' cases of exhaustion.[217] Finally, Virginia's own reaction to her treatment regime was itself prejudiced by a personal social and cultural disdain for Savage and his circle, whom she regarded as 'dreary' and tasteless.[218]

In general, as his aforementioned MPA paper makes clear, Savage preferred to keep nervous patients at or near their homes. 'Many patients', he contended, 'are sent travelling who had better be at home', and would be better off 'left alone or kept in bed' than provided with 'excitement and … so-called stirring up'.[219] Even in cases of convalescence and remission, Savage much preferred to keep patients nearer home, or to send them 'to vegetate in some out-of-the-way spot than [to] run the risk of explosions in distant parts'.[220] He particularly stressed the great risks of sending melancholics travelling, emphasising the impossibility of guaranteeing favourable conditions on sea voyages and the liability of patients to accidents, whether because they could not be adequately controlled, or because local medical attendance was inadequate or unavailable. On sea voyages melancholics might be starved because artificial feeding was inoperable, or else were apt to throw themselves overboard. Savage was especially concerned about the latter risk: 'every melancholic should be treated as a possible suicide'.[221] Sleeplessness was just as often, claimed Savage, the concomitant of travel as sleep, ships tending to be noisy and uncomfortable places. He was even more damning of 'railway travelling' and the Grand Tour for melancholia. Suggesting and possibly exaggerating the considerable amount of compulsion in such treatment, Savage shuddered at 'the misery of patients I have known dragged from one so-called pleasure to another', whether 'driven early about garden parks', or 'later being made to sit out plays or operas'.[222] He condemned also the sending of general paralytics, hysterics and 'delusional cases' on trips. The excitement of hysterics, he felt, would only be increased by travel; given that delusional cases were apt to 'appropriate every fresh impression ... the fewer new and strange impressions such people have the better', while general paralytics tended to 'suffer most of all' and 'ought never to be sent abroad'.[223]

The comments of other participants in the MPA debate, including contemporary experts on climatology like Sir Hermann Weber and Dr Symes Thompson, largely endorsed Savage's views. They signal something of a medical backlash against the fashion of therapeutic travel in late Victorian times. Despite their reservations, however, most were still keen to champion travel, if far from in all cases, then for 'preventive ... and convalescent purposes', for which it was declared 'of immense value'.[224] Furthermore, regularly prescribing travel for his own mental patients, Savage was himself far from being a heretic in this respect. For certain patients, Savage felt voyages and other forms of travel of 'great utility'.[225] If Savage went further in his doubts about travel than many of his contemporaries, the generally guarded tone of his own and Clouston's writings was echoed by many other contemporary discussions, distinguished as much for being critical as for being advocational in their advice about the salutary benefits of travel. Editorials and articles in the *Lancet* and *BMJ* during the 1880s and 90s had been especially censorious of the way travel was being pursued, whether for health or pleasure.[226] This may appear paradoxical in an era when, as recent historiography has evinced,[227] many alienists were becoming increasingly negative about asylum solutions to mental illness. That men like Savage, who had built up successful private consultancy careers outside of the asylum, could be so ambivalent towards non-institutional treatments like travel further highlights the lack of any simple or absolute distinction between the private and public spheres of mental medicine in this period.

Conclusion

A number of general conclusions arise from the preceding analysis of travel. Firstly, this account has reiterated something Roy Porter underlined some time ago[228] – the considerable trouble and expense contemporaries were prepared to incur to shop around for health care. It has indicated how the period 1700-1900 is marked by the development of a considerable marketplace linking travel to the procurement of health. And, far from confined to the physically ill, this market offered a wide range of treatments for a variety of nervous, hysterical, hypochondriacal, melancholic patients and mental convalescents, whether at home or abroad, on land or at sea, in the country or at the seaside, in spas or health resorts, in asylums, sanatoria or convalescent homes.

Nevertheless, being associated with, or perceived as a corollary of, moral therapy and the non-institutional, non-medical treatment of mental disorders, travel was frequently, also, regarded as a threat to medical practitioners' claims to special expertise in the treatment of insanity. The popularity of alternative therapeutic strategies like travel could be seen as both undermining of the status of medical and asylum solutions, as well as symptomatic of the low repute in which they were held in many quarters. This was particularly the case before 1850, when the establishment of psychiatry as a specialty and the programme of asylum reformers was still very much in doubt. Even after this date, like a host of other alternative treatments including massage, hypnotism and 'Weir Mitchelling', often adopted as first resort strategies by moneyed families, travel might be viewed as questioning the wider programme of mental science. It could be interpreted as a symptom of the profession's continuing self-doubt and of the public's continuing lack of faith in asylumdom and mental medicine.[229] Indubitably, the popularity of travel as a remedy points to the continuing vigour of forms of mental medicine that were operating significantly outside of the asylum in this period. If not actively dubious about the benefits of travel, many asylum practitioners admitted to having little experience of trying it as a therapy. Despite his wide experience of the travel cure as a private consultant, George Savage conceded that 'when at Bethlem, I had no chance of sending patients on such trials'.[230]

Yet, this article has also shown that there was no total division between the prescription of travel and more mainstream medical and institutional strategies, and that travel was not necessarily the kind of 'departure from orthodoxy' in treating the mentally disordered that some have portrayed it as.[231] Travel and change of scene were commonly recommended for mental cases both within and without the asylum, and were, perhaps, as commonly combined with other traditional medical agents as they were seen as a substitute for them. An increasing emphasis on travel as a resort in incipient, mild and convalescent cases, both prior to and at the end of an asylum stay, tended to articulate travel as an adjunct, as well as an alternative, to asylumdom. Travel was rarely seen as a viable option for more serious, full-blown cases of mental illness, so that it would always imply a

71

significant place for medical and institutional treatment – although, in the opinion of many alienists, it was apt to be one of a number of first resorts which seemed to limit their province too much to treating chronic and incurable cases. Travel was often predicated on the same bases of providing patients with a set of conditions – whether removal from unhealthy domestic situations, psychological distraction, or rest/exercise – that were generally themselves deployed to sanction confinement in an asylum. Some specialists and some general practitioners, like Weatherly, certainly seem to have felt that asylum care and therapeutic travel were on opposite sides of the medical spectrum. Moreover, they felt that properly constituted asylums could provide most of the benefits offered by travel and actually mitigate the excessive resort to it. Weatherly claimed that:

> if our asylum physicians will get places erected where they can keep their patients out almost all day, and if they will only allow them free access of fresh air to their bedrooms and living rooms, they will ... not necessitate the rush for travel which, in so many cases, leads to great disaster.[232]

It is tempting, in this light, to see the increasing deployment within Victorian asylums themselves of travel to the country and the sea, and of convalescent homes, as a means for alienists to absorb and nullify non-asylum alternatives. While this would certainly be a plausible view, however, it would tend to treat the motives of asylum practitioners too suspiciously, to deny their genuine sympathies for the benefits of travel in mental disorders and to fail to appreciate the space for evolution, dialogue and negotiation between asylum and non-asylum-based medicine. If Victorian critics of travel as mental medicine came more from the asylum sector, their doubts were often shared by specialists in the private sector. This point seems well illustrated by hybrid figures like George H. Savage, who pursued a career in both asylum medicine and in private practice, and who was both an advocate of travel for mental cases and one of its staunchest critics. And the real divisions and disagreements over the way in which travel was being prescribed for the mentally disordered may have been more between those on the one hand who were specialists in insanity and/or members of the medical élite, and those on the other hand who were in the rank and file, or on the fringes of orthodox medicine, and those members of the laity who dared to offer advice on travellers' health.

The growth of a vigorous, significantly lay-authored and oriented travel literature in the eighteenth and early nineteenth centuries, offering often contradictory, questionable and anecdotal self-help and domestic medicine to travellers on how best to preserve their mental and bodily health indubitably posed a challenge to medical authority. However, this literature was increasingly matched, and was itself influenced and suffused by, a wide and expanding range of medical writings on travel, climate and health. Traditional Burtonian advice for melancholics to seek the comforts and distractions of travel, and the subsequent romanticisation of travel during the late eighteenth and early nineteenth centuries, were replaced, or rather tempered, by a much more discriminating and ambivalent medical endorsement of travel for mental cases in the Victorian age. While Burton argued that travel 'availeth howsoever' it was conducted,[233] nineteenth-century specialists imposed a whole host of qualifications on such an endorsement. Nevertheless, the emphasis in Victorian psychiatric literature on the appropriateness of travel for only a select group of cases may be seen as an attempt to contain the resort to alternatives outside of the mainstream of asylum and medical care for mental cases. The highly critical attitude taken by mad-doctors and other medical experts during Victorian times to the type of advice being routinely dispensed to mental invalids for being indiscriminate and ignorant, and the deep concern in psychiatric literature with the need for patients to travel either with a doctor, or in strict accordance with medical advice, was clearly a conscious attempt by the profession to shore up its own authority in such matters. The problem was, of course, as the profession itself conceded, that it was difficult, if not impossible, to lay down general rules for healthy travel. Each individual might require a different prescription; the circumstances of travel were liable to extreme vicissitudes; and medical knowledge about climate, pathology and physiology was still so open to debate. In isolated regions abroad, it was often impossible to obtain the kind of medical advice one wanted or needed.

The importance of travel as a prophylactic and remedial prescription for mental cases in this period indicates how profoundly the early roots of mental medicine were formed within the context of private, consultative practice upon the moneyed classes. Medical men emphasised how 'expensive' were 'the agents' at the mad-doctors' disposal, and how dependent the prescription of travel was on patients' social circumstances (as well as their conditions).[234] Throughout the period, travel was a strategy for the nervous and hypochondriacal amongst the upper and middle classes most able and eager to procure it, to afford it, and to secure the kind of individualised medical attention on which it largely depended. Travel was much less available as a health-seeking option for the poorer sort.

Quite apart from how travel advice was dispensed by medical practitioners and applied by patients and families, this article has sought to explore the flip side of how travel and mobility were pathologised in this period. Analysis has tended to stress the national, gender and racial biases in such medical ideologies. All of these biases were plainly involved, for example, in the attribution of the mental afflictions of Europeans to sunstroke, which served to explain away and excuse susceptibilities and to preserve the national and racial integrity and superiority of white male travellers, settlers and colonisers. I have also shown how broad changes in ideas about the pathology of mental illness affected the ways and the extent to which various mental afflictions were seen as both treatable and ascribable to various forms of travel. For instance, sunstroke was redefined at the end of the period as a subordinate form of shock, or a secondary/exciting cause (often with other organic and hereditary causes underlying), as much as it was the cause of insanity in its own right. Examples such as mental trauma, railway spine and neurasthenia have also been cited to indicate how new forms of travel and transportation, alongside the cultural and social consequences and anxieties they brought with them, spawned new or newly articulated mental diseases.

Notes

1 William Shakespeare, *The Tragedy of Hamlet, Prince of Denmark*, v, i, 150-58.

2 *Ibid.*, iii, i, 173-7.

3 *Ibid.*, iii, ii, 1-4.

4 Plato, *Laws*, Book IX, cited in Daniel N. Robinson, *Wild Beasts and Idle Humours: The Insanity Defense from Antiquity to the Present* (Cambridge, Massachusetts and London: Harvard University Press, 1996), 21.

5 Thomas G. Benedek, 'The image of medicine in 1500: theological reactions to The Ship of Fools', *Bulletin of the History of Medicine*, 38 (1964), 329-342; Michel Foucault, *Madness and Civilisation. A History of Insanity in the Age of Reason* (London: Tavistock, 1967), chap. 1, 3-37, trans. and abridged by Richard Howard from *Histoire de la folie à l'âge classique* (Paris: Librairie Plon, 1961).

6 Andrew Scull, Charlotte Mackenzie and Nicholas Hervey, *Masters of Bedlam. The Transformation of the Mad-Doctoring Trade* (Princeton, New Jersey: Princeton University Press, 1996), 137.

7 John Monro, *Remarks on Dr Battie's Treatise on Madness* (London: Clarke, 1758), Richard Hunter and Ida Macalpine (eds) (London: Dawsons, 1962), 37.

8 George H. Savage, 'The use and abuse of travel in the treatment of mental disorders', *Journal of Mental Science* (henceforth, *J. Ment. Sci.*), 47 (April, 1901), 236-42, 236-7.

9 *Ibid.*, 237.

10 Scull *et al.*, *Masters of Bedlam*, 137.

11 *Horace Walpole's Correspondence*, ed. W.S. Lewis (48 vols, New Haven: Yale University Press, 1954), xxxvi, 295, letter dated 28 April 1777.

12 *Ibid.*, xxiv, 372, letter dated 9 April 1778.

13 E.g. Basil Clarke, *Mental Disorder in Earlier Britain* (Cardiff: University of Wales Press, 1975), 43-5.

14 Robert Burton, *The Anatomy of Melancholy* (reprinted from 16th edn of 1836, itself reprinted from folio edn of 1651) (Oxford: Thornton, 1997), 338.

15 Ian Hacking, 'Les aliénés voyageurs: how fugue became a medical entity', *History of Psychiatry* (henceforth, *Hist. Psy.*), 7, 27 (Sept., 1996), 425-50.

16 Burton, *Anatomy*, 338.

17 *Ibid.*, 338-9.

18 *Ibid.*, 591.

19   John Locke, *An Essay Concerning Human Understanding* (London: printed by Elizabeth Holt for Thomas Basset, 1690), ed. John W. Yolton (London; New York: Dent; E. P. Dutton and Co., 1961), Book II, chap. 11, paras 12 and 13, 127-8; William Battie, *A Treatise on Madness* (London: printed for John Whiston and B. White, 1758), Richard Hunter and Ida Macalpine (eds) (London: Dawsons, 1962), 6, 68.

20   German E. Berrios, *The History of Mental Syndromes* (Cambridge: Cambridge University Press, 1996), chaps 5 and 6.

21   Monro, *Remarks*, 3-5; William Cullen, *First Lines of the Practice of Physic* (Edinburgh: printed for W. Creech; J. Murray; London: J. Williams, 1777-84), in *The Works* (2 vols, Edinburgh: William Blackwood, 1827), i, 521-23.

22   Cullen, *Practice of Physic*, 521-3.

23   Richard Mead, *Medical Precepts and Cautions* (London: printed for J. Brindley, 1751), 75, 89; *idem*, *Medica Sacra* in *The Medical Works of Richard Mead* (London: printed for C. Hitch and L Hawes, 1762), 626 and 628.

24   See e.g. William Battie, *Treatise*, 68; John Haslam, *Observations on Insanity* ...(London: printed for F. and C. Rivington, 1798), 133.

25   MS Casebook of John Monro (1766), in private possession of the family of Dr F. J. G. Jeferiss, 85-6, 112-3 and 121-2. See forthcoming modern edition, Jonathan Andrews and Andrew Scull (eds), *Customers of the Mad-Trade. The 1766 Casebook of Dr John Monro, Physician to Bethlem Hospital* (London: Athlone).

26   Haslam, *Observations*, 135.

27   Scull *et al.*, *Masters of Bedlam*, 135.

28   Battie, *Treatise*, 69.

29   Monro, *Remarks*, 37; Haslam, *Observations*, 133.

30   *Twenty-third Annual Report* (henceforth AR) *of the Directors of the Glasgow Royal Asylum* (henceforth GRA) (Glasgow: James Hedderwick and Son, 1837), 5.

31   Janet Oppenheim, *"Shattered Nerves". Doctors, Patients and Depression in Victorian England* (Oxford: Oxford University Press, 1991), 125.

32   Michael J. Clark, '"Morbid introspection", unsoundness of mind, and British psychological medicine, c1830-c1900', in W.F. Bynum, Roy Porter and Michael Shepherd (eds), *The Anatomy of Madness* (3 vols, London and New York: Tavistock, 1985-88), iii (1988), 71-101.

33   Weatherly in *J. Ment. Sci.*, 47 (April, 1901), 245.

34   Sir Richard Blackmore, *A Critical Dissertation Upon the Spleen, so far as Concerns the Following Question; Whether the Spleen is Necessary or*

Useful to the Animal Possess'd of it (London: J. Pemberton, 1725), 174.

35 William Cullen, *First Lines of the Practice of Physic*, 531.

36 Hannah Allen, *A Narrative of God's Gracious Dealings with that Choice Christian Mrs Hannah Allen* (London: printed by John Wallis, 1683), in Allan Ingram (ed.), *Voices of Madness* (Thrupp, Gloucestershire: Sutton, 1997), 1-22.

37 *Ibid.*, 11.

38 *Ibid.*, 10.

39 *Ibid.*

40 *Ibid.*

41 *Ibid.*

42 *Ibid.*, 11-12.

43 *Ibid.*, 11.

44 *Ibid.*, 16-17.

45 *Ibid.*, 7.

46 *Ibid.*, 7, 18-19.

47 W.A.F. Browne, *What Asylums Were, Are and Ought To Be* (Edinburgh: A. and C. Black *et al.*, 1837), Andrew Scull (ed.) as *The Asylum as Utopia. W.A.F. Browne and the Mid-Nineteenth-Century Consolidation of Psychiatry* (London and New York: Tavistock/Routledge, 1991).

48 Francis Willis, *A Treatise on Mental Derangement* (London: Longman, 1823), 2, quoted in Scull *et al.*, *Masters of Bedlam*, 96.

49 Burton, *Anatomy of Melancholy*, 339.

50 P. Frings, *A Treatise on Phrensy Wherein the Causes of that Disorder, as Assigned by the Galenists, is Refuted* (London: T. Gardner, 1746), 41.

51 John Purcell, *A Treatise of Vapours, or Hysteric Fits* (London: 1702; 2nd edn, London: E. Place, 1707); Roy Porter, *Mind-Forg'd Manacles. A History of Madness in England From the Restoration to the Regency* (London: Athlone, 1987), 50-51, 86, 105-6; Jonathan Andrews, '"In her Vapours [or] ... in her Madness"? Mrs Clerke's case: an early eighteenth-century psychiatric controversy', *Hist. Psy.*, 1, 1 (1990), 125-43.

52 *Horace Walpole's Correspondence*, xxxiii, 254, letter dated 17 Dec. 1780.

53 E.g. James Johnson, *Change of Air, or, The Pursuit of Health* (London: Highley, 1831).

54 Thomas Clouston, *Clinical Lectures on Mental Disease* (London: J. and A. Churchill, 1887), 465-81; *idem*, 'Illustrations of phthisical insanity', *J. Ment. Sci.*, 10 (1864), 220-29.

55 Clouston, *Clinical Lectures*, 82.

56 *Ibid.*, 39.

57 *Ibid.*, 137.

58 *Ibid.*, 131; Linda Bryder, *Below the Magic Mountain* (Oxford: Clarendon, 1988).

59 E.g. Jonathan Andrews and Iain Smith (eds), *"Let There Be Light Again". A History of Gartnavel Royal Hospital* (Glasgow: Gartnavel Royal Hospital, 1993), 59, 71.

60 Christine Stevenson, 'Robert Hooke's Bethlem', *Journal of the Society of Architectural Historians*, iv (1996), 252-73; and Jonathan Andrews *et al.*, *The History of Bethlem* (London: Routledge, 1997), chapters 14 and 15.

61 34th AR of GRA (1838), 7.

62 Greater Glasgow Health Board Archives, 13/5/1, 19, 28 May 1816, case of Janet Craig.

63 45th AR of GRA (1859), 11-12. See, also, e.g. 44th AR of GRA (1858), 12.

64 44th AR of GRA (1858), 11-12.

65 The 'usual' *modus operandi* is described in the 1864 Annual Report; 50th AR of GRA (1864), 11-12.

66 69th AR of GRA (1883), 12.

67 For reports on this association, see e.g., 'The After-Care Association', *J. Ment Sci.* (Jan., 1887), 535-9; (July, 1896), 556-7. See, also, Rev. H. Hawkins, 'After Care', *ibid.* (Oct., 1879), 358-67; *idem*, 'Dr. Hack Tuke and the "After-care" Association', *ibid.* (July, 1895), 556-7; *idem*, 'Reminiscences of "After-care" Association, 1879-1898', *ibid.* (April, 1898), 299-304; Robert Jones, 'The After-care Association for befriending persons discharged from asylums for the insane', *ibid.* (July, 1906), 623-5; and Jonathan Andrews, 'Notions of mental health and prophylaxis in nineteenth-century Britain', forthcoming in Jonathan Andrews, Helen Bartlett and John Stewart (eds), *Historical and Contemporary Perspectives on Health Care in Britain since the Seventeenth Century* (Oxford: Oxford Brookes University, 1998), 13-34.

68 *18th Annual Report of Crichton Royal Asylum* (1857), 5; cited in Scull *et al.*, *Masters of Bedlam*, 116.

69 Scull *et al.*, *Masters of Bedlam*, 209.

70 60th AR of GRA (1874), 41. See, also, 63rd AR (1877), 16-17; 68th AR (1882), 12; 69th AR (1883), 12; 70th AR (1884), 12.; 74th AR (1888), 12.

71 64th AR of GRA (1878), 16-17; 67th AR (1881), 12.

72 79th AR of GRA (1893), 14; 80th AR (1894), 12; Andrews and Smith (eds), *Let There Be Light*, 36.

73 Yellowlees spoke of this 'change' as 'a most welcome and healthful

break in the monotony of their lives'; 63rd AR of GRA (1877), 16-17.

74   Silas Weir Mitchell, *Wear and Tear, Or Hints for the Overworked* (Philadelphia: J. B. Lippincott, 1871); *idem, Fat and Blood,* 6th rev. edn (Philadelphia: J. B. Lippincott, 1893; orig., 1877); W.S. Playfair, *The Systematic Treatment of Nerve Prostration and Hysteria* (London: Smith, Elder, 1883).

75   For historical surveys, see e.g. Roy Porter (ed.), *The Medical History of Waters and Spas* (London: Wellcome Institute for the History of Medicine, 1990), *Medical History,* supplement no.10; Roger Rolls, *The Hospital of the Nation: The Story of Spa Medicine and the Mineral Water Hospital at Bath* (Bath, Avon: Bird Publications, 1988); Michael Raymond Neve, *Natural Philosophy, Medicine and the Culture of Science in Provincial England: The Cases of Bristol, 1790-1850, and Bath, 1750-1820* (University of London PhD, 1984); R.S. Neale, *Bath 1680-1850: A Social History, or, A Valley of Pleasure, Yet a Sink of Iniquity* (London; Boston: Routledge and Kegan Paul, 1981); Charles Mullett, 'Public baths and health in England 16th-18th century', *Bulletin of the History of Medicine,* supplement no. 5 (Baltimore: 1946); George D. Kersley, *Bath Water: The Effect of the Waters on the History of Bath and of Medicine* (Bath: Victor Morgan Books Ltd, 1979). For contemporary accounts, see e.g. Robert Hutchinson Powell, *A Medical Topography of Tunbridge Wells* (Tunbridge Wells: J. Colbran, 1846); William Seaman, *On Vapour Bathing Conducted at the Royal Baths, Tunbridge Wells* (Tunbridge Wells: J. Clifford, 1832?); Charles Scudamore and Thomas Thomson, *An Analysis of the Mineral Water of Tunbridge Wells, With Some Account of its Medicinal Properties* ... (London: Longman, Hurst, Rees, Orme, and Brown, 1816); Anon., *Experimental Observations on the Water of the Mineral Spring near Islington; Commonly Called New Tunbridge Wells* (London: J. Robinson, 1751); Joseph Browne, *An Account of the Wonderful Cures Perform'd by the Cold Baths. With Advice to the Water Drinkers at Tunbridge, Hampstead and all the Other Chalibeate Spaws* (London: printed for J. How and R. Borough, and J. Baker, 1707).

76   Richard Morton, *Phthisiologia: Or, a Treatise of Consumptions* (London: printed for S. Smith and B. Walford, 1694), 223.

77   Thomas Sydenham, *Processus Integri* (London: S. Smith, B. Walford and J. Knapton, 1693), in *The Works of Thomas Sydenham, M.D.,* trans. R. G. Latham (London: The Sydenham Society, 1850), 234.

78   George Cheyne, *The English Malady...* (London: printed for G. Strahan and J. Leake, 1733), 207.

79   Purcell, *A Treatise of Vapours,* 144.

80 John Floyer, e.g. *An Enquiry into the Right Use and Abuses of the Hot, Cold and Temperate Baths in England* (London: R. Clavel, 1697).

81 William Rowley, *A Treatise on Female, Nervous, Hysterical, Hypochondriacal, Bilious, Convulsive Diseases; Apoplexy and Palsy; with Thoughts on Madness and Suicide* ... (London: printed for C. Nourse, E. Newbery and T. Hookham, 1788), 14. For modern studies of chlorosis, see e.g. M. Rosenthal, '150 Years of a Disease Called Chlorosis' (University of London, B.Sc. diss., 1989); Robert P. Hudson, 'The biography of disease: lessons from chlorosis', *Bulletin of the History of Medicine*, 51 (1977), 448-463; Karl Figlio, 'Chlorosis and chronic disease in nineteenth-century Britain: the social constitution of somatic illness in a capitalist society', *Social History*, 3 (1978), 167-197; Irvine Loudon, 'The diseases called chlorosis', *Psychological Medicine*, 14 (1984), 27-36.

82 E.g. Augustus Bozzi Granville, *The Spas of England, and Principal Sea-bathing Places* (3 vols, London: Henry Colburn, 1841).

83 A. B. Granville, *The Spas of Germany* (2 vols, Brussels: Belgian Printing and Publishing Society; Hauman and Co., 1838), i, vii-viii.

84 Diederick Wessel Linden, *A Treatise on the Origin, Nature and Virtues of Chalybeat Waters, and Natural Hot Baths. With a Physico-chemical Analysis, and Medicinal Description of the Mineral Waters at Tunbridge, Islington, and Shadwell with Others in England and at Cleves in Germany* ... (London: T. Osborne, 1748); Lewis Rouse (Rowzee), *Tunbridge Wells: Or, a Directory for the Drinking of Those Waters* ... *With a Particular Account of the Virtues of the German Waters*, trans. from the Latin original (London: J. Roberts, 1725).

85 Granville, *Spas of Germany*, I, x; Meredith Gairdner, *Essay on the Natural History, Origin, Composition, and Medicinal Effects of Mineral and Thermal Springs* (Edinburgh: W. Blackwood, 1832).

86 Granville, *Spas of Germany*, i, xx-xxii.

87 *Ibid.*, ii, 120.

88 *Ibid.*, i, 145; ii, 336.

89 *Ibid.*, i, 307-8.

90 *Ibid.*, ii, 51-2.

91 *Ibid.*, ii, 45.

92 E.g. John Aldridge, *A First Trip to the German Spas and to Vichy* (Dublin: McGlashan and Gill, 1856); Sigismund Sutro, *Lectures on the German Mineral Waters and on their Employment: With an Appendix Embracing a Short Account of the Principal European Spas and Climatic Health-resorts* (2nd edn, rev. and enl.; London: Longmans, Green, 1865); Dayrell Joseph Thackwell Francis, *Change of Climate Considered as a Remedy in Dyspeptic, Pulmonary, and Other*

Chronic Affections (London: John Churchill, 1853); Sir Erasmus Wilson, *A Three Weeks' Scamper Through the Spas of Germany and Belgium* (London: J. Churchill, 1858); Alfred Donne, *Change of Air and Scene: A Physician's Hints, with Notes of Excursions for Health Amongst Watering-places* (London: H.S. King, 1872); Julius Rohden Braun, M.D., *On the Curative Effects of Baths and Waters: Being a Handbook to the Spas of Europe* ... (abridged translation, with notes), ed. Hermann Weber (London: Smith, Elder, 1875); Fortescue Fox, *Strathpeffer Spa, its Climate and Waters* (London: Lewis, 1889).

93 Scull *et al.*, *Masters of Bedlam*, 147.

94 Clouston, *Clinical Lectures,*.130.

95 *Ibid.*

96 Granville, *Spas of Germany*, i, xxxv.

97 Purcell, *A Treatise of Vapours*, 145.

98 *Ibid.*

99 Richard Mead and most other eighteenth-century mad doctors shared the same conviction that in treating the mentally affected 'it ought to be a standing rule, to inculcate notions directly contrary to those with which they were long possessed'; Mead, *Medical Precepts*, 98; *idem, Medica Sacra*, 623.

100 E.g. Monro repudiated Battie's hesitant espousal of substituting fear for joy, and sorrow for anger, condemning 'the doctrine of substituting one passion for another' as one of 'the errors of antiquity'. See Monro *Remarks*, 45; Battie, *Treatise*, 84.

101 Clouston, *Clinical Lectures*, 131-2.

102 Ebeneezer Gilchrist M.D., *The Use of Sea Voyages in Medicine; And Particularly in a Consumption: with Observations on that Disease* (New enl., rev. and corr. edn, London: printed for T. Cadell, 1771).

103 *Ibid.*, 85-6.

104 *Ibid.*, e.g. 47-9, 262.

105 *Ibid.*, 87-8.

106 *Ibid.*, 12-20.

107 *Ibid.*, 1-11.

108 *Ibid.*, 79, 153 and 155-6.

109 *Ibid.*, 67, 150, 182, 289.

110 *Ibid.*, 156.

111 *Ibid.*, 150.

112 *Ibid.*, 151-3.

113 *Ibid.*, 38, 79-80, 156, 261.

114 *Ibid.*, viii.

115 Savage, 'Travel in mental disorders' (1901), 238.

116 William S. Wilson, *The Ocean as a Health-resort: A Handbook of*

Information as to Sea-voyages for the Use of Tourists and Invalids
(London: J. and A. Churchill, 1880).

117 John Monro, Casebook (1766), 48-9.

118 Haslam, *Observations*, 64-5.

119 Jonathan Swift, *Gulliver's Travels*, ed. Paul Turner (Oxford and New
York: Oxford University Press, 1986), 1735 corrected edn; orig.
1726.

120 *The Practical Physician for Travellers, Whether by Sea or Land ...By a
Member of the College of Physicians...* (London: printed for Fran.
Fayram, 1729).

121 *Ibid.,* 190-1.

122 *Ibid.,* 125-30.

123 *Ibid.,* 1-2, 4.

124 *Ibid.,* 72-3.

125 Joel Peter Eigen, *Witnessing Insanity: Madness and Mad-doctors in the
English Court* (New Haven and London: Yale University Press,
1995), 104.

126 Richard Mead, *A Treatise Concerning the Influence of the Sun and
Moon upon Human Bodies and the Diseases Thereby Produced*
(London: printed for J. Brindley, 1748), trans. of the second edition
by Thomas Stack; originally, *De Imperio Solis Ac Lunae in Corpora
Humanis* (London: s.n., 1708).

127 Casebook of John Monro (1766), 16, 42 and 120.

128 Battie, *Treatise on Madness*, 47. Uniquely exposed to severe climactic
changes, sailors were deemed to be particularly vulnerable to such
problems. William Battie recounted the story of 'a Sailor, who
became raving mad in a moment while the Sun beams darted
perpendicularly upon his head'; *ibid.*

129 Blackmore, *A Critical Dissertation*, 258; Frings, *A Treatise on Phrensy*,
20-1.

130 E.g. Thomas Tryon, *A Discourse of the Causes, Natures and Cure of
Phrensie, Madness or Distraction* from *A Treatise of Dreams and Visions*
(London: Andrew Sowle, 1689), ed. Michael V. Deporte (California:
University of California, L.A.: William Andrews Clark Memorial
Library/The Augustan Reprint Society, No. 160, 1973), 279-81;
Richard Mead, *Medica Sacra*, 619; *idem, A Mechanical Account of
Poisons* (London: J. M. for R. Smith, 1708; orig., 1702), in *Medical
Works*, 135.

131 E.g. Battie, Treatise, 36, 45, 47, 63, 79-80, 99; Monro, *Remarks*, 6,
43, 56.

132 Rev. William Pargeter, *Observations on Maniacal Disorders* (Reading
and London: J. Murray; Oxford: J. Fletcher, 1792), ed. Stanley W.

Jackson (London and New York: Routledge, 1988), 8; Haslam, *Observations*, 35-6.

133   Jean Etienne Dominique Esquirol, *Mental Maladies: A Treatise on Insanity*, trans. with additions by E. K. Hunt (Philadelphia: 1845); 50th AR of GRA (1864), 30.

134   E.g. Alex Taylor, *A Comparative Enquiry as to the Preventive and Curative Influence of the Climate of Pau and of Montpellier, Hyeres, Nice, Rome, Pisa, Florence, Naples, Biarritz etc., ... with a Description of the Watering Places of the Pyrenees ...* (New edn considerably altered and enl.; London: John W. Parker, 1856); Thomas More Madden, *On Change of Climate: A Guide for Travellers in Pursuit of Health ...*(London: T. C. Newby, 1864); Isaac Burney Yeo, *Climate and Health Resorts* (New edn; London: Chapman and Hall, 1885).

135   See e.g., Sir James Clark, *The Sanative Influence of Climate: With an Account of the Best Places of Resort for Invalids in England, the South of Europe, and c.* (3rd edn; London: J. Murray, 1841; 4th edn, 1846); *idem, The Influence of Climate in the Prevention and Cure of Chronic Diseases ... Comprising an Account of the Principal Places Resorted to by Invalids ... and General Directions for Invalids While Traveling and Residing Abroad ...* (London: T. and G. Underwood, 1829).

136   55th AR of GRA (1859), 27.

137   Clouston, *Clinical Lectures*, 81.

138   John Haslam, *Observations*, 64.

139   Clouston, *Clinical Lectures*, 421.

140   *Ibid.,* 425; F. Skae, 'On insanity caused by injuries to the head and by sunstroke', *Edinburgh Medical Journal* (Jan., 1866), 679-94. Other medical authorities also tended to stress the nature of sunstroke as 'shock', and the traumatic impact of the sun 'on the brain and spinal cord' ; e.g. Major S. Leigh Hunt and Alexander S. Kenny, *On Duty Under a Tropical Sun* (London: W.H. Allen and Co., 1882), 14; Andrew Duncan, *Remarks on Some Recent Theories on the Action of Heat in the Tropics* (London: John Bale, Sons and Danielsson, 1908). See, also, William Pirrie, *On Insolatio, Sun-stroke, or Coupe-de-soleil* [sic] (Aberdeen: A. King, 1861); E. T. Renbourn, *Life and Death of the Solar Topi: Protection of the Head from the Sun: A Chapter in the History of Sunstroke* (Farnborough, England: s.n., 1961); Graham A. Edwards, 'Sunstroke and insanity in nineteenth-century Australia', in Harold Attwood and Geoffrey Kenny (eds), *Reflections on Medical History and Health in Australia* (Parkville, Victoria: Medical History Unit, University of Melbourne and the Medical History Society, AMA (Victorian Branch), 1987), 35-42.

141 Waltraud Ernst, *Mad Tales From the Raj. The European Insane in British India*, 1800-1858 (London and New York: Routledge, 1991), esp. 41, 162, 169-70.

142 John Harriot, *Struggles Through Life, Exemplified in the Various Travels and Adventures in Europe, Asia, Africa, and America of John Harriot ...* (3rd edn, 3 vols, London: For the Author, 1815), i, 327-32.

143 E.g. John W. Williams, *An Essay on the Utility of Sea Bathing, in Preserving Health, and as a Remedy in Disease: Especially in Nervous, Scrophulous, Bilious, Liver, and Cutaneous Complaints: with Directions for Employing the Warm, Cold, Vapour, Shower, and Medicated Baths. Also, Observations on Mineral Waters, Natural and Artificial* (Portsmouth: S. Mills, 1820); John Murray, *Descriptive Account of a Shower Bath ...* (Glasgow: W.R. M'Phun, 1826); Andre Pamphile Hippolyte Rech, *De la douche et des affusion* [sic] *d'eau froide sur la tête, dans le traitement des aliénations mentales* (Montpellier: J. Martel, Snr., 1846); Horatio Mahomed, *The Bath: A Concise History of Bathing, as Practised by Nations of the Ancient and Modern World ...* (London: Smith, Elder and Co., 1843).

144 E.g. James Africanus Beale Horton, *Physical and Medical Climate and Meteorology of the West of Africa: With Valuable Hints to Europeans for the Preservation of Health in the Tropics* (London: J. Churchill, 1867).

145 Hunt and Kenny, *On Duty Under a Tropical Sun*, 9.

146 *Ibid.*

147 *Ibid.*, 10-21.

148 *Ibid.*, 11.

149 Wilson, *The Philosophy of Physic ...* (Dublin: 1804), cited and discussed in Ginnie Smith, 'Prescribing the rules of health: self-help and advice in the late eighteenth century', in Roy Porter (ed), *Patients and Practitioners. Lay Perceptions of Medicine in Pre-Industrial Society* (Cambridge: CUP, 1985), 249-82, p.265.

150 Richard Wrigley, 'Infectious enthusiasms: influence, contagion, and the experience of Rome', in Chloe Chard and Helen Langdon (eds), *Transports: Travel, Pleasure and Imaginative Geography* (New Haven; London: Yale University Press, 1996), 75-116, p.85.

151 Matthews averred 'I took my first bias for traveling, or going to sea, from reading Robinson Crusoe', and was himself to be shipwrecked later, Henry Matthews, *The Diary of an Invalid. Being the Journal of a Tour in Pursuit of Health in Portugal, Italy, Switzerland and France in the Years 1817, 1818 and 1819* (2 vols, London: John Murray, 1822), ii, 15 and 96-116.

152 E.g. *63rd Annual Report of Glasgow Royal Asylum for Lunatics, Gartnavel* (Glasgow: James Hedderwick, 1877), 15, 'the danger of

mental shipwreck in the storms and turmoil of life'.

153   See Ralph Harrington, 'The railway journey and the neuroses of
      modernity' in this volume; *idem*, 'The neuroses of the railway', *History
      Today*, xliv, 7 (Jul. 1994), 15-21; *idem*, 'The "railway spine" diagnosis
      and Victorian responses to PTSD', *Journal of Psychosomatic Research*, xl,
      1 (Jan. 1996), 11-14; *idem*, article in Mark Micale and Paul Lerner
      (eds), *Traumatic Pasts* (forthcoming, Yale University Press). See, also,
      Wolfgang Schivelbusch, *The Railway Journey: Trains and Travel in the
      Nineteenth Century* (Oxford: Blackwell, 1980); *idem, The Railway
      Journey: The Industrialization of Time and Space in the Nineteenth
      Century* (Leamington Spa: Berg, 1986); George F. Drinka, *The Birth of
      Neurosis: Myth, Malady and the Victorians* (New York: Simon &
      Schuster, 1984), ch. 5; Thomas Wharton Jones, *Failure of Sight from
      Railway and Other Injuries of the Spine and Head ...* (London: James
      Walton/ Bradbury, Evans and co., 1869); John Eric Erichsen, *On
      Railway and Other Injuries of the Nervous System* (London : Walton and
      Maberly, 1866); Edwin Morris, *A Practical Treatise on Shock After
      Surgical Operations and Injuries: With Especial Reference to Shock Caused
      by Railway Accidents* (London: R. Hardwicke, 1867); John Charles
      Hall, *Medical Evidence in Railway Accidents* (London: Longmans,
      1868); 'Railway injuries', *Medico-Chirurgical Review*, lvii (1876), 1-20;
      Herbert William Page, *Railway Injuries; with Special Reference to Those
      of the Back and Nervous System: In their Medico-legal and Clinical Aspects*
      (London: Griffin, 1891); Allan McLane Hamilton, *Railway and Other
      Accidents with Relation to Injury and Disease of the Nervous System: A
      Book for Court Use* (New York: W. Wood and Company, 1904).

154   E.g. W.F. Bynum, 'The nervous patient in eighteenth- and nineteenth-
      century Britain: the psychiatric origins of British neurology', in Bynum,
      Porter and Shepherd (eds), *Anatomy of Madness*, i (1985), 89-102, esp.
      94 and 96; Oppenheim, *Shattered Nerves*; Edward M. Brown, 'Post-
      traumatic stress disorder and shell shock', 'Social Section', in German
      Berrios and Roy Porter (eds), *A History of Clinical Psychiatry. The Origin
      and History of Psychiatric Disorders* (London: Athlone, 1995), 501-8; Sir
      Geoffrey Jefferson, 'Marshall Hall, the grasp reflex and the diastaltic
      spinal cord', in E. Ashworth Underwood (ed.), *Science, Medicine, and
      History: Essays on the Evolution of Scientific Thought and Medical Practice
      Written in Honour of Charles Singer* (London; New York; Toronto:
      Geoffrey Cumberlege, Oxford University Press, 1953), 2, 303-20; Weir
      Mitchell, *Wear and Tear*; Robson Roose, *Wear and Tear of London Life*
      (London: Chapman and Hall/J. S. Virtue, 1886).

155   Clouston, *Clinical Lectures*, 423-5; James Syme, 'Compensation for
      railway injuries', *Lancet*, i (5 Jan., 1867), 2-3.

156 Bakewell, Letter, *Monthly Magazine*, xlii (1816), 2.
157 E. J. Tilt, 'Bromides in relation to travelling', *British Medical Journal* (henceforth *Brit. Med. J.*) (2 July 1881), 11; Edward Drummond, 'The bromides in relation to travelling', *ibid.* (15 Oct. 1881), 627.
158 Arthur W. Edis, 'Hints for travelling in the case of children', in *ibid.* (30 July 1881), 149-50.
159 *J. Ment. Sci.*, 47 (April, 1901), 243.
160 *Ibid.*, 243-4.
161 *Ibid.*, 244.
162 Clouston, *Clinical Lectures*, 46.
163 Harriot, *Struggles Through Life*, ii, 256-7. For more of Harriot's views on the progress from savage to civilised life, see 294-9.
164 Purcell, *A Treatise of Vapours*, 144.
165 *The Practical Physician for Travellers*, 3 and 67.
166 Andrews, 'Mrs Clerke's case'.
167 Allen, *Narrative*, 16-17.
168 For this account, see *Horace Walpole's Correspondence*, xxxvi, 118-21 and 293, letters dated 21, 22 and 29 April 1777 and note 4, 118.
169 Clouston, *Clinical Lectures*, 132.
170 Savage, *Insanity and Allied Neuroses*, 478.
171 W.A.F. Browne, 'Application and Testimonials for the Superintendency of the Montrose Royal Lunatic Asylum' (1834), iv, in Crichton Royal Museum and Archives, Montrose; Scull *et al.*, *Masters of Bedlam*, 88.
172 *Ibid.*, 134.
173 *Ibid.*, 134-5.
174 Matthews, *Diary of an Invalid*, ii, 155.
175 Oppenheim, *Shattered Nerves*, 126-7.
176 Clouston, *Clinical Lectures*, 56.
177 *Ibid.*
178 *Ibid.*, 137.
179 *Ibid.*, 56.
180 *Ibid.*, 56, 132 and 137.
181 *Ibid.*, 56.
182 *Ibid.*
183 *Ibid.*, 186
184 *Ibid.*, 44.
185 *Ibid.*, 56.
186 *Ibid.*, 44.
187 *Ibid.*
188 *Ibid.*, 131.
189 *Ibid.*, 265.

190   *Ibid.*, 39-40.
191   Oppenheim, *Shattered Nerves.*
192   N. Jewson, 'Medical knowledge and the patronage system in eighteenth-century England', *Sociology*, xii (1974), 369-85.
193   Matthews, *Diary of an Invalid*, ii, 176-7.
194   For this reference and ensuing discussion, see Savage, *Insanity and Allied Neuroses, Practical and Clinical* (London: Cassell and Co., 1896), 478-80.
195   Burton, *Anatomy of Melancholy*, 338.
196   *Op. cit.*, 100-101.
197   Anon., *The London Practice of Physic. For the Use of Physicians and Younger Practitioners* (London: ? 1769), 230.
198   Ralph Fletcher, *Sketches from the Case Book, to Illustrate the Influence of the Mind on the Body* ... (London: printed by J. Barfield and sold by Longman and Co., Simpkin and Marshall, and Gumm, Gloucester 1833), 129, 145-6.
199   42nd AR of GRA (1856), 8-9; Andrews and Smith (eds), *Let There Be Light.* See, also, C. Crommelinck, *Rapport sur les hospices d'Angleterre, de la France et de l'Allemagne* (Courtrai: ?, 1842), 113-4; Lincolnshire Asylum Archives, *LAWN 1/1/4*, 14 Oct. 1839. I am grateful to Len Smith's generosity in providing me with these last two references.
200   E.g. 'Horse Exercise at Home', advertisement for Vigor and Co. (of London) Horse-Action Saddles (Innerleithen: R. Smail and Sons, 19th century, undated).
201   Thomas Bakewell, *The Domestic Guide in Cases of Insanity* (Stafford: 1805), 74-5; *idem*, letter in *Monthly Magazine*, xlii (Aug., 1816), 2. I am once again grateful to Len Smith for these references.
202   Savage, Obituaries and biographical sketches, *Lancet*, ii (1921), 155; *Brit. Med. J.*, ii (9, 16 and 30 July, 1921), 63, 98-9 and 174; R. Percy Smith, 'Sir George Henry Savage, M.D., F.R.C.P.', in *J. Ment. Sci.*, lxvii (Oct., 1921), 393-404; G. H. Brown, *Lives of the Fellows of the Royal College of Physicians* (London: 1955), 307.
203   See e.g. Elaine Showalter, *The Female Malady. Women, Madness and English Culture, 1830-1980* (London: Virago, 1988), 117.
204   Clouston, *Clinical Lectures*, 131.
205   Matthews, *Diary of an Invalid*, ii, 116-7.
206   George H. Savage, 'The use and abuse of travel in the treatment of mental disorders', *J. Ment. Sci.*, 47 (April, 1901), 236-42 and discussion 242-5; *idem*, 'Travel; its use and abuse in the treatment of mental diseases', *BMJ*, ii (1900), 1526.
207   Savage, 'Travel in mental disorders' (1901), 236 and 238.

208 *Ibid.*, 236-7.
209 *Ibid.*, 238.
210 *Ibid.*, 236.
211 *Ibid.*, 238-9.
212 *Ibid.*, 239 and 242.
213 Nigel Nicholson and Joanne Trautmann (eds), *The Letters of Virginia Woolf* (6 vols, London: The Hogarth Press, 1975-80), i, 147. See, also, *ibid.*, 153, 175, 179, 198, 239-40, 430-2; ii, 34; iv, 325-6; vi, 77 and n.1; Anne Olivier Bell (ed.), *The Diary of Virginia Woolf* (5 vols, London: The Hogarth Press, 1977-82), esp. i, 31 and n.90; iii, 333 and n.10; v, 273 and n.11.
214 Quentin Bell, *Virginia Woolf: A Biography* (2 vols; St Albans, Herts: Triad/Paladin, 1976); Stephen Trombley, *All That Summer She Was Mad. Virginia Woolf: Female Victim of Male Medicine* (New York: The Continuum Publishing Company, 1982). See, also, Showalter, *Female Malady*, esp. 4, 126, 134, 143-4, 164, 181, 193.
215 E.g. Trombley, *All that Summer*, 81; Showalter, *Female Malady*.
216 Oppenheim, *Shattered Nerves.*
217 Woolf, *Letters*, i, 240; Trombley, *All that Summer*, 84-5.
218 Woolf, *Letters*, i, 179; Trombley, *All that Summer*, 82.
219 Savage, 'Travel in mental disorders' (1901), 242.
220 *Ibid.*
221 *Ibid.*, 240.
222 *Ibid.*
223 *Ibid.*, 241.
224 *Ibid.*, 244.
225 *Ibid.*, 237, 239, 240-1.
226 See e.g. *Lancet*, 15 Nov. 1890, 1039-40; 16 March and 25 May 1895, 714-5 and 1344-6; 18 and 25 July, and 8 Aug. 1896, 196-7, 252-3 and 410-11; 18 Dec. 1897, 1634; *Brit. Med. J.*, 29 Nov. 1879, 870-1; 10 July 1880, 55 and 69.
227 E.g. Scull *et al.*, *Masters of Bedlam.*
228 Roy Porter, *Health for Sale. Quackery in England 1660-1850* (Manchester: Manchester University Press, 1989); Scull *et al.*, *Masters of Bedlam*, 147.
229 *J. Ment. Sci.*, 51 (1905), 144, cited in Scull, *Masters of Bedlam*, 272.
230 Savage, 'Travel in mental disorders' (1901), 240.
231 Scull, *Masters of Bedlam*, 209.
232 *J. Ment. Sci.*, 47 (April, 1901), 245.
233 Burton, *Anatomy of Melancholy*, 338.
234 Fletcher, *Sketches*, 145-6.

2

The Continental Journeys of Andrew Duncan Junior: A physician's education and the international culture of eighteenth-century medicine

Malcolm Nicolson

Eighteenth-century medical men travelled in a multitude of guises – as military and ship's surgeons, as the tutors and bearleaders of Grand Tourists, as the attendants of ambassadors and explorers, as tourists or explorers in their own right, and indeed as patients.[1] In the eighteenth century's Republic of Learning, established physicians could cross frontiers to consult with wealthy clients, to take up teaching appointments, and set up practices.[2] At the lower end of the professional scale, young and would-be physicians and surgeons journeyed the length and breadth of Europe in search of education and experience. Of all the types of medical travellers those who travelled abroad to study were probably the most numerous and the most footloose.[3] What motivated so many aspiring physicians and surgeons to subject themselves to the expense, discomforts, dangers and distempers of journeying to distant universities in unfamiliar cities? What did they seek to gain from their travels? What impact on their future careers and practices, on their perceptions of illness and therapy, did their foreign experiences have? The present essay attempts to illuminate some of these issues by a scrutiny of the youthful journeys of Andrew Duncan junior.

Born in 1773, Andrew Duncan was the eldest son of a famous father. Andrew Duncan senior occupied the chair of the Institutes of Medicine in Edinburgh University from 1790 until 1821.[4] The author of several volumes including *The Elements of Therapeutics*, Duncan senior also edited the periodical publication, *Medical Commentaries*.[5] Physician to the King and the Prince of Wales in Scotland, founder of the Edinburgh Royal Public Dispensary and the Royal Edinburgh Asylum, Duncan was, at various times, President of the Royal Medical Society and the Royal College of Physicians of Edinburgh. He remained a major figure within the Edinburgh medical establishment until his death in 1828.

Andrew Duncan junior began his medical education in 1787 with a surgical apprenticeship.[6] He later attended Edinburgh University, graduating first with an M.A., in 1793, and then, in the following year, with an M.D. From 1791 he assisted his father with the editing of the *Medical Commentaries*, writing analyses of recently published books.[7] After graduation, Duncan junior continued his education by travelling, at his father's expense and direction.[8] He went first to London and then to many of the major medical centres of Continental Europe, including Göttingen, Vienna, Pavia, and Padua, returning to Scotland in 1796. In the next year he set out on another European journey, this time in the capacity of medical attendant to a Scottish nobleman. As a grateful and dutiful son, Andrew regularly wrote long letters home to his father. The bulk of this correspondence has survived.[9]

In the eighteenth century, there were very few essential educational prerequisites to medical practice. Medical students could devise and select their own curriculum, according to what their financial resources would allow and what form of medical career they wished subsequently to pursue.[10] The aspiring eighteenth-century practitioner, thus, enjoyed the opportunities and responsibilities of *Lernfreiheit*. As the travels of Andrew Duncan exemplify, the existence of this degree of educational freedom of choice enabled and impelled the ambitious young physician to travel abroad for some part of his medical education. But, as we shall also see, Duncan did not go to the Continent merely to increase his technical knowledge of medicine. He sought also to improve his general education, to learn European languages, and to make the acquaintance of eminent men. Duncan hoped, moreover, that his Continental experience would aid his career chances by enhancing his gentlemanly poise and social *savoir faire*. Thus his journeys served Duncan both as postgraduate education and as finishing school.[11]

The market for medical services in the eighteenth century being an open and pluralistic one, the successful practitioner was by necessity an entrepreneur.[12] The Duncan letters vividly highlight the social settings which gave meaning and structure to particular entrepreneurial strategies. A vital component of medical success was the effective exploitation of the support systems provided by family connections, patronage, scholarly and collegial acquaintance, and other sources of social obligation and mutuality. Secondly, individual entrepreneurship took place within an economy that was firmly centred upon household and family units.[13] In an instructive essay, Roy Porter has shown how William Hunter was the quasi-patriarchal head of what was, in effect, a family business of anatomy teaching.[14] Similarly it is useful to regard the Duncans, father and son, as being involved in a single economic enterprise, with the elder Duncan concerned, not just to provide for his son, but also to train and equip him to take his place in the Duncan family business of physicking, university teaching, journal editing, and medical power-broking.[15] Furthermore Duncan did not travel merely as an individual and as a member of an eminent medical family; while abroad he also acted as a representative of Edinburgh's medical school and its associated institutions.

One must, of course, recognise the limitations of the Duncan correspondence as a historical source. It would, indeed, be a remarkable young traveller who provided his father with a full and candid account of his activities on the Continent. Robert Burns, who was only fourteen years older than Duncan and who died when Duncan was abroad on his first journey, satirised the escapades of the affluent young Scotsman, who

> ... maybe, in a frolic daft,
> To Hague or Calais takes a waft,
> To make a tour an' take a whirl,
> To learn bon ton an' see the worl'.
> There, at Vienna or Versailles
> He rives his father's auld entails.[16]

The Continental tour, the poet noted, exposed the young traveller to many temptations and dangers, physical, financial and moral. Some suffered 'the consequential sorrows, Love gifts of Carnival signioras'.[17] Of these and other personal experiences of the pathologies of travel, Duncan junior is, for whatever reason, silent. The letters often read, moreover, like the first draft of the account of his travels that Duncan intended to prepare for publication but never actually did. They are, in other words, structured throughout by both filial and literary conventions. Nevertheless, Duncan's letters provide us with interesting insights into why the eighteenth-century medical student travelled, what he did while he was abroad, and what personal and professional benefits Continental experience might bring.

In London

Andrew Duncan's first journey began in the autumn of 1794. He was accompanied from Edinburgh to London by his father. The Duncans stayed at the house of Mr Barclay, the well-known Scottish anatomist, and went visiting together.[18] Duncan senior was thus able personally to effect the introduction of his son to many of the leading learned men of the capital. As a result the younger Duncan quickly gained access to London's medical, scientific and literary circles. He went to meetings of the Royal Society and the Medical Society, and made the acquaintance of such luminaries as Joseph Banks, Matthew Baillie, John Coakely Lettsom and Gilbert Blaine.

Duncan junior enrolled for classes at the Great Windmill Street School, where he enjoyed Dr Baillie's 'very excellent demonstrations'.[19] In his first letters to his father, now returned to Scotland, we can see what was to be a constant feature of their correspondence – the making of comparisons between the medical institutions Duncan saw on his travels and those he knew in Edinburgh. He routinely considered how experience of the former might complement the education to be had in the latter:

> I have now begun business in earnest at Windmill Street, so that from 8 a.m. to 4 p.m. I have not a moment unemployed. But I find so much of benefit from it already that if another of your sons were to choose the same profession I should advise that he should spend his first winter in London. He would then be able to understand and derive infinitely greater advantage from the incomparable physiological lectures of Dr Monro.[20]

Even when the Windmill School was closed, Duncan occupied his days with dissection and learning to make preserved specimens. He felt he was gaining skills that would be valuable to him in later life – 'I hope to acquire as much of the art as will enable me hereafter to make a tolerable collection of comparative anatomy'.[21] Human material was difficult to obtain but he appreciated that London was a good place to which to come to learn practical anatomy.

Other aspects of medical education in the capital he found less attractive. He was disappointed in what he saw as a lack of opportunities for the study of clinical practice – '[e]xcept seeing operations nothing is to be learnt at the hospitals here'.[22] He attended and addressed the student society, the Lyceum Medicum, but found it 'wonderfully inferior to our medical societies'.[23] Little was done to provide educational facilities for medical students and their general level of culture and learning did not impress:

> There is nothing in the way of literature which I miss so much as the library of the Med. Soc. Students here have no access to books of value and are therefore, in general, extremely illiterate. The whole knowledge of the most learned of them consists in the origin and insertion of a few

of the muscles or the course of the blood-vessels and nerves.[24]

Duncan was careful to reassure his father that his own educational endeavours were not being adversely affected by the prevalence of such philistinism. He was reading what medical books he could lay his hands on (without, of course, running the unnecessary expense of buying them for himself) and also improving his general accomplishments. He recorded that, one evening at Joseph Bank's house, he had heard a discussion 'amongst critics of polite literature' concerning 'the authenticity of some manuscripts of Shakespere [sic]', found among some old papers belonging to a Mr Ireland. Duncan expressed the urbane hope that Mr Ireland 'has not yet examined all his old papers, and that, like Chatterton, he may find as many as he chooses'.[25]

While in London Duncan assiduously cultivated the acquaintance of the learned and the eminent men of the capital, not only in order to increase the social and educational value of his visit but also in preparation for travel further afield. Many of the men to whom he paid his compliments gave him letters of introduction to their academic colleagues on the Continent. As we shall see, this network of personal contact was to be crucial in enabling Duncan to fulfil his father's intentions as to how he was to spend his time abroad. He knew that the elder physician considered:

> my principal objects are to acquire the languages, get a knowledge of the medicine and literature and form acquaintances among the learned of each country ... [26]

In December 1794, however, Duncan received an offer which caused him to reconsider his plans. Dr Pearson, a friend of his father, suggested to Duncan that he had interest to get him a position on the medical staff of a London hospital or, alternatively, as a hospital mate in the Army. Duncan promptly wrote to ask his father's opinion. Of the two possibilities, he evidently favoured the latter, which would entail a foreign posting and would not deny him the opportunity of learning German:

> The pay of a hospital mate is 7sch and 6d a day ... This, I think, would be sufficient to pay my expenses and at my period of life and in my profession to spend a few years without expense is certainly an object ... It is also the best field for acquiring experience that can possibly exist.[27]

His father, however, did not consider that, whatever its practical or

financial advantages, a background in military surgery was quite
what he had in mind for his eldest son and protégé.[28] The Army
scheme was quickly dismissed.

By 4 January 1795 Duncan considered 'my objects in coming to
London are pretty well attained, while the frost continues dissection
is at an end and there is nothing else I can study here'.[29] He had
begun actively to look for a passage across to the Continent – an
uncertain and difficult business since the Channel and the southern
North Sea were still a theatre of war. In the meantime he had to
discuss with his father the financial arrangements for his travels:

> I am afraid that my expenses on the continent will be more than you
> are aware of. I can find nobody here that spent less than £250 a year.
> But I shall endeavour as much as possible to avoid the society of
> Englishmen and to adopt the manners of the natives.[30]

One of the means by which Duncan hoped to repay the investment
being made in his education was by writing about his Continental
experiences:

> a work in German which I am impatient to be able to read is 'Travels
> thro' Italy chiefly with a view to the state of medicine in that
> country'. A similar work in English with respect of Germany as well
> as Italy would be of use. As far as I can I shall collect materials for
> such a one …[31]

There was, at the end of the eighteenth century and the beginning of
the nineteenth century, a great demand for travel books and guides
of all sorts. Charles Este, for example, recorded that he had sold the
rights of his *A Journey in the year 1793* before he had left England or
opened a notebook.[32] Duncan was, moreover, aware that appearing in
the public prints was an important means by which a young
physician could make his name more widely known and thereby
improve his career prospects. While on his travels Duncan, as we
shall see, gave much thought to publication as a means by which his
foreign experience could advantageously exploited.

In Germany

On the 16th of March 1795, after several false starts and many
delays, Duncan sailed from Yarmouth to Hamburg. Shortly
afterwards he travelled on to Brunswick. In both cities Duncan paid
social calls on all the learned men to whom he had an introduction.
He was so pleased with the warmth of his reception in Brunswick
that he dared to depart from the itinerary laid out for him by his

father, who had intended that he should travel directly to Göttingen:

> On Saturday I called upon Prof. Eschenburgh [sic] and came at last
> to a determination which I hope will not displease you, that of
> remaining here a month. I can live here at no great expense and I
> have the best opportunity of learning German. I have got a very
> good room and bed closet at 4 dollars a month. I dine with Prof.
> Eschenburgh, who is the only one of his family that can speak
> English and I get a lesson from him every day.[33]

Eager to cultivate the role of the scholarly connoisseur, Duncan was
particularly concerned to view the cabinets of famous collectors. On
a visit to Haldstedt, he:

> delivered a letter of introduction to Prof. Beireis [who] ... possesses
> collections in no less than eleven different branches. He began by
> showing me the very minute anatomical preparations of Lieberkuhn,
> reckoned the finest in the world ... I saw injections of the bone and
> enamel of the teeth, of the vessels of the liver and kidney, almost
> detecting nature in its process of secretion ...[34]

Duncan did not, moreover, confine his connoisseurship solely to the
medical sphere. He cultivated a wider interest in natural history and
philosophy:

> we called upon Hoffrath Ebel to see his collection, and got an
> admirable lecture of two hours upon petrifactions. I was never more
> pleased with a cabinet. He did not expose his specimens like a
> showman, but explained them like a philosopher ... the pride of his
> collection is a table of slate containing pentacrinites.[35]

He was also concerned to exhibit a gentleman traveller's taste in
landscape, gardens and curiosities:

> At Cassel we ... made a party to go to the Landgraff's palace at
> Weisser Stein. Its situation is naturally beautiful but much improved
> by art. The house ... lies a little way up the side of a beautiful hill,
> whose surface is entirely converted into pleasure grounds. Artificial
> ruins and other buildings are thrown in with great taste, wherever
> they can please the eye most ... After we descended a little way we
> entered a grotto in the side of the building in which statues of Fawns,
> Nereids, etc. We were immediately surprised by most beautiful
> music and a hundred streams of water sprung up amongst our feet.[36]

However, evidently anxious not to give his father the impression that
he had altogether abandoned his Scottish proprieties and given

himself entirely over to luxury and sensuality, Duncan concluded:

> Altho at first the whole struck me as the most stupendous work of
> man I ever saw, yet I could not help regretting that so much labour
> and money should have been wasted in a manner which benefits no
> living soul.[37]

In late June or early July, Duncan moved on to Göttingen. He arrived
with letters of introduction to, among others, Arneman, Wrisberg,
Feder, Richter, Blumenbach, Lichtenberg, Gmelin, Persoon, Meyer
and Stromeyer.[38] All these men knew his father by reputation; many
had met Duncan senior in London or in Edinburgh. It is not
surprising therefore that, despite the language barrier, Duncan very
quickly accomplished an entry into Göttingen's learned community.
He proudly wrote to tell his father of dinners with Blumembach and
Wrisberg, of teas and suppers with Arneman, Gmelin and Osiander.

By early August, Duncan was enjoying himself so much in
Göttingen that he again became reluctant to follow his father's
itinerary:

> If I were to pass this winter in Italy, I must set out very soon and I
> have not yet by any means acquired so much of the language that I
> could trust my accuracy of translation, so much as to allow the
> public to judge of it and I flatter myself with the hopes that a good
> knowledge of German and a great deal of industry will enable me to
> repay my whole journey.[39]

He hoped to be allowed to spend the winter of 1795-96 attending
classes at the University. He suggested to his father that, apart from
the direct educational benefit of such a period of study, his improved
knowledge of German would enable him to prepare a revised and
annotated translation of Johann Peter Frank's *System einer
vollständigen medicinischen Polizey* (Complete System of Medical
Police).[40] Duncan's hope that his father would look favourably upon
this plan would seem to have been a very reasonable one. Quite apart
from any financial benefits, such a scheme would have
complemented and developed the elder physician's own interest in
medical police. It was in this same year, 1795, that Duncan senior
began to devote a portion of his teaching effort in Edinburgh to
lectures on medical jurisprudence.[41]

Andrew Duncan's outline of his plans for his studies in Göttingen
provide an instructive exemplification of the travelling medical
student's *Lernfreiheit.*

I read German at 8 a.m. with Mr Beneke four times a week and mean to attend Arneman's materia medica at 11, to go to Richter's hospital on Mondays and Thursdays, and to Stromeyer's clinicals Tuesdays and Fridays at one, to hear Lichtenberg's natural philosophy at two, Richter's diseases of the eye at three, and Wrisberg's medicina forensis four times a week at six p.m. I chose the hospital and clinicals to see the German practice, in preference to the practical lectures, where I would hear a good deal I already know ... Since I have been here I have attended the hospital regularly ... it is really very practical, for Richter exercises the students in questioning the patients and prescribing, while he points out their failures and amends them.[42]

But, as we have already seen, Duncan's foreign 'postgraduate' education did not consist solely of attending classes and clinics. His twenty-second birthday, in late August, provided him with occasion to reflect about his progress toward becoming both a learned physician and an accomplished gentleman. He took, as he put it, 'a retrospective view of my education, of my life':

My knowledge of anatomy is much increased and in the German language, I have entered upon an inexhaustible field of improvement ... My time, I believe, can be better employed than in attempting to regain a knowledge of Greek or ... Latin. But I must not let any time be lost in learning to speak French ... and in increasing my practical knowledge of medicine, particularly in the forms of prescriptions and doses of medicines. The less necessary accomplishments, which I wish I possessed, are to draw well, to play tolerably various games at cards, and to ride well. For this last alone I cannot blame myself ... But if you will permit me to offer you any advice, do not let your other sons be defective in that art, for the sake of a few half crowns. Many a one it might have saved me.[43]

He then returned to the question of where he should spend the winter. Friends had informed him that the University of Pavia was 'in disorder'. The Italians had opposed Johann Peter Frank's innovations and the distinguished professor had decided to remove himself to Vienna. Due to the political situation, travel in southern Europe was difficult and exorbitantly expensive. Besides 'there is no book published in Italy, which is not translated into German in six months':[44]

This has almost determined me to pass the winter in Germany, which I had already begun to regret the thoughts of quitting, just as

97

I was beginning to understand the language and before I had learnt
it sufficiently to prevent me from forgetting it in a year or two.[45]

But 'in this as in all other cases' the final decision remained with his
father.[46] Duncan senior must have insisted on his original itinerary
being adhered to. Duncan junior remained in Göttingen for only
three months and, in September, he left to begin his journey to Italy.[47]

The first few letters in the Edinburgh collection of Duncan
correspondence exemplify how an eighteenth-century student
physician could construct his own education. But they also show us
that Duncan was not wholly a free agent. The overall plan of his
itinerary was not his to decide. Nor did he act only on his own
behalf. Some of his time had to be devoted to the requirements of
what I have called the 'Duncan family business'. He worked to
consolidate his father's relationships with the Continent's learned
men by conveying to them the elder Duncan's good wishes and by
presenting them with complimentary copies of the *Medical
Commentaries* or some other Edinburgh publication.[48] In turn
Duncan forwarded to his father compliments and sometimes letters,
books or journals from the scholars he met. Duncan senior wished to
keep up with European medical politics and was always eager for
medical intelligence from the Continent. His son supplied him with
up-to-date information about new publications and appointments so
that notices of the latest events could be included in his journal.
Duncan junior seems also to have spent a considerable time going
through the catalogues of libraries and booksellers, sending back to
his father detailed listings of the Continental medical literature.
Another of Duncan's tasks was to buy books for his father and for
some of his colleagues in Edinburgh. He was also engaged in this
capacity by Edinburgh's Royal Medical Society. He also sought to
appoint commercial agents in several of the major cities he visited –
who, on behalf of Edinburgh University Library and/or the Medical
Society, would buy and despatch the new Continental medical books
as they appeared.

In Italy

On his way to Pavia Duncan visited Ratisbon, Vienna and Milan.
Again he sought out all the learned men to whom he had letters of
introduction and endeavoured to view whatever was of medical,
philosophical or cultural interest. In Ratisbon he saw:

> what alone would have repaid me for my journey here, I mean the
> Museum of wax preparations belonging to the military surgical

school ... It baffles all description and would be well worth young
Monro's coming here to see.[49]

In Milan he called upon Dr Locatelli and accompanied him on his
visit to the 'great hospital', taking particular note of the clinical
arrangements:

> [Locatelli] gave a short account of each patient to the students in
> Latin and the reports were kept in a kind of tabular form by two
> clerks. The last ward he visited was the clinical. Here the case of each
> patient was entrusted to some advanced student who took their cases
> in Latin, but he prescribes himself. After his visit he shewed me the
> hospital. The wards were in general remarkably clean, and
> completely free from smell: but what seemed to me most remarkable
> were the two large wards, each containing 360 patients.[50]

By November Duncan had reached Pavia. Here again he had a ready
introduction to the eminent men of the University. Having presented
several letters to Professor Brugnatelli, he was offered lodging in the
professor's house. Duncan senior had also prepared the ground by
writing to tell Antonio Scarpa to expect a visit from his son. The
famous anatomist offered to help the young Duncan if he wished to
dissect. But, notwithstanding the cordiality of his immediate
reception, Duncan found that his earlier misgivings about Pavia were
quickly confirmed:

> At present I feel myself more awkwardly situated than I was at any
> time in Germany, for though Scarpa has been in England and
> Brugnatelli translates English, yet neither of them converse in it, and
> I dislike extremely speaking bad French. I have also been obliged to
> employ a Frenchman as my language master, for there is none here
> who understands English ... It is now too late to change, but I am
> afraid we have been wrong in choosing Pavia for the situation of my
> longest stay in Italy, because the language, even of the better class of
> people, is very bad ... so that I shall be almost deprived of the
> advantage of living in the country where the language is spoken.[51]

The University of Pavia was indeed, as Duncan had feared, in
turmoil. The prospect of invasion by the French armies loomed. The
students were disaffected. The vacancy created by the departure of
Johann Peter Frank had been filled temporarily by his son, Joseph,
'but I perceive that he is thought too young and unequal to the
charge'.[52] Of the remaining professors only Scarpa was held in much
esteem. Duncan came to the conclusion that Italian medical

scholarship was moribund:

> With regard to the medicine of the Italians, I shall be able to learn
> their hospital treatment. But of medical literature they have very
> little. I have asked many of the students to inform me of the late
> works of reputation published, and they give the names of
> translations ... I have not heard of a single author of reputation in
> the lines of theoretical or practical medicine. Pavia is, however, the
> best university in Italy, and the opportunities for dissection are
> superb.[53]

Apart from Brugatelli and Scarpa, the faculty were inhospitable. He
was not invited to the other professors' houses. He explained to his
father:

> You need not be astonished at the want of attention in the Pavians.
> Hospitality is not a part of the Italian character and £100 a year are
> not the means. Besides the Professors are independent of the
> students and do not seek after popularity.[54]

Duncan occupied himself exploiting the anatomical facilities,
preparing his 'annotated translation of Frank', and attending clinical
classes. Here again his perspective was a comparative one:

> The management of the clinical wards is very different from that at
> Edinburgh. When a new patient comes in any student takes care of
> him. When Frank comes to that patient, that student examines him
> and is assisted by Frank who then asks what he thinks the disease to
> be, what his opinion of the prognosis, and what he would prescribe.
> Having approved or rejected the student's opinion, he gives a clinical
> lecture upon the disease. Next visit the student reads a Latin history of
> the case, the future reports he writes at his leisure, and after the disease
> is finished, gives the complete history to Frank. At each visit he also
> writes his prescription on a tabular paper which hangs at each bed.[55]

By January 1796, Duncan was on the move again. He set out on
what was virtually a Grand Tour of Italy, visiting first Bologna,
Sienna, Rome and Naples, before returning north to Leghorn, where
he arrived in early April.[56] The letters he wrote during this part of his
Continental excursion make it abundantly clear that his intention in
visiting Italy was not solely to increase his technical knowledge of
medicine. Indeed once he gets south of Bologna, discussion of
medical matters virtually disappears from his correspondence. As he
wrote to his father:

> You will think it strange that I have attended so little to medicine
> since I have been in Italy. I think it strange myself and cannot well
> account for it. All that I observed of the Roman hospitals was
> looking into one of the men's wards at S. Spirito, as I passed one day.
> At the door was hung a printed list of the lectures, one of which was
> to be given every Sunday night by a different person. I intended to
> have heard one but forgot to go.[57]

He reserved his energies for such activities as touring the architectural
and artistic sights of Rome and spectating, in a sceptical Protestant
manner, at the celebrations of Holy Week.

At Leghorn Duncan had a friend in residence, Mr Grant, who
could introduce to local society. Duncan set out wholeheartedly to
enjoy himself – so much so that he had to apologise to his father for
the length of time he remained there:

> You will perhaps think that I have made my stay here too long, as it
> is not a literary place. But I can only say that I have seen more of the
> Italians here than in all the rest of Italy. I have been at
> conversaziones, concerts and plays in the Italian fashion and at
> dinners, tea and cricket in the English manner. Every night … I have
> drunk tea at Mr Grant's, who … is never without visitors. After tea,
> we either go to the play, conversation, or concert. In the play house
> there are no operas at present, but comedies and tragedies … They
> are in general sad stuff, but as each box is a separate little company,
> it is not of much consequence. When we enter the theatre we go to
> the pit to see what ladies are in the boxes and then go up and spend
> the evening with them.[58]

The natives were, he had discovered, 'more sociable than in other
parts of Italy'.[59]

Eventually Duncan dragged himself away from Leghorn. He
travelled on, through Pisa, Padua and Florence to Venice, arriving
there on the first of May – just in time to see the Doge celebrate the
marriage between the city and the sea. Again he had something to
apologise to his father for – he had not fulfilled the parental
instruction to make the acquaintance of the learned men of Padua.
He was handicapped, he explained, by having no letters of
introduction:

> To tell the truth, the reception I have meet with from Italian
> philosophers, to whom I carried the best recommendations, was
> such that I could not prevail upon myself to wait upon any of them
> entirely without introduction …[60]

Moreover his plan to return to Pavia had had to be abandoned because the French had invaded and the university was closed. Duncan was forced to 'idl[e] my time away here in Venice'.[61]

The first of June found Duncan in Vienna and, once back across the Alps, he took up the study of medicine seriously again:

> as I wished to attend particularly to the hospital, I fixed my residence in the suburbs, although in most respects very inconvenient on account of its great distance from the town. In the mornings at eight Frank goes round the clinical ward and at nine gives his practical lecture ... He speaks a great deal at the bedside of the patient, generally in Latin, but sometimes in German, and as was to be expected from him much to the purpose ... I have seen the lying-in part of the hospital, which is clean, and everything very naturally conducted.[62]

Later in the same month Duncan visited the hospitals in Prague.

Duncan now felt able to offer to his father the following comparative generalisation:

> The medical practice of Italy and Germany is, in general, not so simple as ours, which on the whole Continent is dignified with the name of empiric, because you do not give medicines as resolvents, inspissants, attenuants, &c., and do not talk of a bilious-phlegmatic-pituitous pain in the big toe. I must, however, except from this remark the Franks, whose practice is extremely plain and simple. These, however, tried no new remedies, and in their choice they were principally directed by cheapness and efficacy[63]

He had evidently fulfilled part of his father's plan. He had learned something of Continental medical practice.

A Second Trip to Italy

Duncan's letter from Prague, dated June 22, 1796, is the last one from his first journey which is extant in the Edinburgh collection. The next letter dates from 19 July, 1797. It was written in London and relates to Duncan's second Continental trip. There are several indications in the correspondence of the first journey that it had long been a part of Duncan senior's plans for his son that he should travel abroad again – this time as a medical attendant. Duncan junior had initially been rather sceptical as to the feasibility of this venture:

> We may still keep the travelling scheme in view, but I hardly think it will take place. My youth will be an almost insuperable objection

and I should be afraid to trust myself with the care of an invalid.[64]

Nevertheless his father's plan had come magnificently to fruition. He had succeeded in getting Duncan junior engaged by the Earl of Selkirk to travel to Florence to take care of his son, Lord Daer, and accompany him back to Britain.[65] This must have been a considerable coup for the Duncan family business since the Earl of Selkirk was one of Scotland's leading noblemen.

Duncan originally intended to use his outward trip to fill an important gap in his education, both medical and gentlemanly – to visit Paris.[66] Lord Selkirk was however unable to obtain a passport for him to travel through France and he was thus forced to go via Germany and Switzerland. Duncan had reached northern Italy before he discovered that Lord Daer would have no need of his services. He had died before Duncan had left Britain. The principal purpose of his journey being thus tragically removed, Duncan was again free to devote his time in Italy to the pursuit of his own ends. He had, by this time, begun to practice physic on his own account and he was evidently proud to tell his father that he was occasionally consulted by expatriates or Grand Tourists. But, as on his first visit, the improvement of his practical or theoretical knowledge of medicine was not Duncan's only, nor indeed his major, preoccupation while in Italy. He had, as he put it, 'no precise object in view except general improvement'.[67]

His father had again cause to chide him for not making the acquaintance of Italy's learned men. But a second experience of the country had not improved Duncan's opinion of Italian scholarship:

> You will naturally imagine that I am now busy studying medicine. I would do it, [word indecipherable] I found Italian authors that retained my attention. But it is inconceivable how trivial they are in general, how hypothetical and how ignorant of the laws of nature and the science of reasoning. In the branches of juridical and political medicine I have not met with a single book.[68]

Nor, although he still posed as a man of taste, was he as interested as he had been in scholarly connoisseurship:

> I have lost all taste for the study of pictures, statues, etc. I think it absurd to be in raptures with a copy when we can have the original before our eyes.[69]

Duncan's lack of enthusiasm for Italian medicine and art should not however be written off as merely a manifestation of a young man's pleasurable idling. Duncan knew that humanistic learning, knowledge of medical theory, and clinical experience were not the only personal accomplishments to which the would-be physician should aspire to gain on his travels:

> I believe if you were on the spot to judge you would rather have me keep company with genteel people here, both natives and strangers, than with the literati. I am convinced that it will in the end be more to my advantage by improving my manners and knowledge of the world, articles essential to success in my profession.[70]

In other words Duncan consciously determined to use his time in Italy more to improve his social grace and acumen rather than to increase his professional or decorative knowledge. He sought, by making the acquaintance not of the learned but of the polite, to acquire skills which would enable him to mingle easily with the class of person from which he would later be seeking professional patronage.

In September, he repaired again to his friend Mr. Grant in Leghorn, where he could not 'keep company with the literati, for there are none',[71] but where there were excellent opportunities for pursuing a broader, more social form of education:

> The second night I supped with Mr Filippi, the third with Mr Armario, and the last with Mr Fluddart, in their different boxes at the theatre. These entertainments were overall as elegant as possible and hilarity prevailed universally. Champaign [sic] is indeed a magic draught. Its influence is irresistible. It strips the most reserved prude of her mask and affectation cannot stand its fumes.[72]

After several weeks pleasantly and, no doubt, instructively socialising in Leghorn, Duncan moved to Florence, and on to Pisa, for some more of the same. In January he returned to Leghorn.

In November 1797, he was still hoping, in vain as it turned out, 'that in Spring I may take in Paris on my way home'.[73] But he was aware that his travelling and his education were approaching their end. He must now think seriously about how he was to earn his living:

> When once returned I hardly expect that any offer will be made sufficient to tempt me abroad again. On the contrary, it is time to determine, in some measure upon my future plans. Whether it will be better for me to fix at Edinb, or elsewhere. My profession is of that kind that for years yet, I must rely upon your support, for although by writing I might earn something yet it is but uncertain

and interferes much with laying the basis for a more certain income. I feel myself without many things necessary for enduring success in the struggle for riches and advancement.[74]

Duncan's doubts were however soon resolved. His father commanded him to make great haste in the latter part of his journey and he arrived back in Britain in June 1798. The surviving correspondence does not specify any reason for this urgency other than it related to 'so important a business'.[75] From the context the letters provide, it is, however, reasonable to assume that the younger man's professional advancement was involved. At this time Duncan senior was engaged in an attempt to persuade the Town Council to create a new chair of medical jurisprudence at Edinburgh University. Shortly after his return to Edinburgh, Duncan junior was made a Fellow of the College of Physicians of Edinburgh and a physician to the Royal Public Dispensary, an institution which, as noted above, his father had founded. Duncan junior began to assist his father in editing their new periodical venture, the *Annals of Medicine*. However, the initiative to found the new chair did not succeed, on this occasion.

Back in Edinburgh, perhaps waiting until something more substantial came his way, Duncan junior began to write. He began to publish the results of a series of investigations into the chemistry of pharmacologically active substances.[76] He was also developing research interests in anatomy, following the approved Continental clinico-pathological model.[77] In 1803, Duncan published a new edition of the *Edinburgh New Dispensatory*, in which he displayed his knowledge of European scientific innovation. The edition incorporated, for example, an 'introductory Epitome of Modern Chemistry'.[78] A review in *Nicholson's Journal* acknowledged the range of his expertise, concluding that: 'Dr Duncan appears to have availed himself of every thing in the field of modern discovery, or in the best foreign Pharmacopoeias, that was consistent with the plan of his work'.[79]

Duncan junior's work on the *Dispensatory* should be seen as another aspect of the family business – Duncan senior had been responsible for three earlier editions of the work. Two years after its publication, the mantle of journal editorship was formally passed from father to son, Andrew Duncan junior becoming founder editor-in-chief of the successor to the *Annals*, the *Edinburgh Medical and Surgical Journal*. With his wide acquaintance among the leading medical men of Britain and Europe, his working knowledge of more than one European language, and his experience of anatomical, clinical and chemical research, Andrew Duncan junior was very well qualified to be the editor of a medical journal. Under his guidance *Edinburgh Medical and Surgical Journal* became the leading British medical periodical, publishing a wide variety of research papers and providing authoritative reviews of the latest scientific and clinical developments taking place in Britain and Europe.

In 1807, the Duncans manufactured and seized another important opportunity for career advancement, fulfilling an ambition born in the previous decade. Duncan senior managed to persuade his friends in the new Whig administration to act upon his scheme for instituting a chair of 'Medical Jurisprudence and Medical Police' in Edinburgh.[80] Duncan junior became the first holder of the new professorship. He never published his long-promised translation of Frank's *System* but his study of its contents provided him with the basis of his course of lectures. In addition to his professorial duties, Duncan was appointed, in 1809, to the salaried position of Librarian to the University, a post for which his knowledge of Continental libraries and the international book trade equipped him well.[81]

Andrew Duncan's chair in Medical Jurisprudence was held in the Faculty of Law. But, in 1819, he transferred to the Medical Faculty to occupy the chair of the Institutes of Medicine jointly with his father – another success for the family business. In 1821, Duncan junior was elevated to sole possession of the chair of Materia Medica. By this time the Duncans could be said to have unequivocally succeeded in their joint enterprise – the son, like the father, had become a leading member of the Edinburgh medical establishment.

A Typical Traveller?

This essay has, so far, concerned itself with only one itinerant and aspiring physician. A question is thus begged – how typical or representative an eighteenth-century medical traveller was Andrew Duncan junior?

In his letters to his father, Duncan regularly mentioned encounters with other British medical students, many of whom were engaged in itineraries very similar to his own. In London he met young men who had already been on trips to the Continent and others who were still to go. An example of the latter was Dr Tayleur, an Edinburgh graduate, with whom Duncan dissected at the Great Windmill Street School. Duncan and Tayleur travelled together to Göttingen. There they made the acquaintance of another three Britons – Carpenter, Kinglake and Palmer. Duncan left Göttingen in the company of Carpenter and Palmer, parting from them in Vienna. In Pavia, Duncan met another Briton, Charles Este, and they shared a dissecting room. Later Duncan was joined in Pavia by Palmer, who accompanied him on his tour of southern Italy.

It is evident therefore that the sort of itinerary undertaken by Duncan was by no means unique. Moreover, not only did Duncan's acquaintances travel to the same universities and for broadly similar reasons, their education was also under similar direction and control – namely that of their fathers. For example, Duncan wrote that his friend Charles Este was tired of Pavia and was 'going to endeavour to prevail upon his father to let him pass the next winter in Halle'.[82]

An extended comparison can be made between the travels of Duncan and those of Charles Este because Este's father was Parson Charles Este, erstwhile editor of the *Courier*, who accompanied his son to Italy and who published an account of their Continental journey 'in search of science'.[83] In his *A Journey in the year 1793*, the elder Este explained in some detail how he had decided where his son should pursue his medical education. They were forced to look abroad because Oxford and Cambridge were too expensive and he did not consider either Edinburgh or London to be wholly suitable. Edinburgh:

> for what we wanted offered only partial aid. Of science, philosophical, contemplative, there might be enough. But art was wanting. There is no mechanical supply – The superstitious prejudices of the place forbid it.[84]

The younger Este did, however, intend to go to Edinburgh to graduate, after he had completed his period of study on the Continent.

The Duncans did not, of course, hold the merits of an Edinburgh education quite so lightly but, to some extent, they agreed with Este's perception as to where its shortcomings lay. It will be remembered that the elder Duncan deemed it necessary for his son to compliment his formal University education both with a practical apprenticeship in surgery and with further study of anatomy and clinical practice.

London was likewise dismissed by Pastor Este – again for reasons very similar to those cited by Duncan:

> from the nature of the market, with talents in such demand, and at such prices for them, there must be ever many accomplished men in it; but where is ... there any systematic establishment for popular instruction? Where are there public libraries generously open to all? Where are there any Medical Schools? – as far as it offers to be a school, it seems challengeable on the various objections of being loose

and disjointed; therefore probably impracticable, certainly very dear.[85]

Este would have preferred his son to have gone to Paris but 'France alas! ... seemed daily less and less likely to retain for foreigners that free reception and repose hitherto so amiably imparted to all'.[86] His 'clever and experienced' friends recommended the Italian Universities. Padua was in decline, Bologna was good only for the 'imitative arts', Florence was 'pre-eminent as a museum' – therefore he decided upon Pavia.[87]

On their way to Italy, the Estes visited the universities and museums of the Low Countries, Germany and Switzerland – much as Duncan was to do on his journey, two years later. Parson Este published detailed impressions of these places. Here is his assessment of Cologne:

> As a school for elegant learning, belles lettres and for medicine, it does not seem auspicious. The chymistry is the best part, the anatomy is the worst. Anatomical preparation fails, and the subjects to supply them, are I believe, fewer still. A hospital, on a good plan, is in contemplation. But till it be executed, that part of the medical study must continue wanting in the extreme. There [are] ... two small wards to receive strangers ... but ill-ordered, as to cleanliness and air ... As a student of any class, rank and in any line, the expenses at Cologne are very moderate; the greater number of young men do not spend more than forty or fifty pound a year ... What they can get for their money, may not be so much, nor so well made as at better places ... But what they may get is by no means insufficient, for the more obvious purposes of ... practice ...[88]

A Journey contains similar descriptions of the institutions of learning at Ghent, Liège, Leiden, Mannheim and Louvain. It will be noticed that there is a strong resemblance between Este's published accounts of the Continental medical schools and those which Andrew Duncan provided for his father. This similarity is not accidental. Este included this material in his text, partly at least, so as to assist his readers in the making of informed choices about the education of their own sons. It was assessments such as these which sustained the elective, 'pick-and-mix', character of eighteenth-century medical education.

But, while the journeys of the younger Este and the younger Duncan together represent and exemplify a general pattern of eighteenth-century medical travelling, it must also be noted that they differ from one another in several respects. Many of the details of each man's European experience are explicable only in terms of individual circumstances. Both Este and Duncan were able to exploit the possibilities of *Lernfreiheit* but their initial opportunities were not equal, nor were their career strategies identical.

Many of the differences between Este and Duncan may be understood in terms of the contrasting social situations of the two men's fathers. Parson Este was not a member, far less a prominent member, of the medical profession. Accordingly he was not very ambitious or knowledgeable in respect of his son's medical education. He sought simply to give him a qualification, suitable to a young man of his class and adequate for practice, at as reasonable a cost as possible.

Edinburgh medical professors were, by contemporary standards, comfortably well-off.[89] Duncan senior was sufficiently well-positioned to be ambitious for his eldest son. He had the money and the know-how to set about equipping Andrew Duncan junior to be recruited into the ranks of élite Edinburgh physic. The younger Duncan was able to have a longer and deeper medical education and to travel more extensively than the younger Este. Furthermore, having a famous medical professor as a father was a major advantage in achieving an entry into academic society. Unlike Este, Andrew Duncan junior travelled, for the most part, well-equipped with introductions to the eminent men of his profession and made their social acquaintance relatively readily.

As we have seen, both the Estes and Duncan took note of the arrangements for clinical teaching in the various cities they visited. However, Duncan's interest was more intense and better informed. His especial concern with that aspect of medical education may be understood in the light of his father being himself a leading clinical teacher. Moreover, in Edinburgh, the facilities for clinical teaching were both an object of pride and a subject of controversy. There was, around the turn of the century, considerable discussion as to how good clinical teaching in the Infirmary actually was and how and whether it could be improved.[90] Duncan's interest in comparing Continental arrangements for clinical teaching with those available in Edinburgh must thus be seen as a product of the concerns prevailing at his home base. Likewise Duncan's concern to study Continental developments in forensic medicine follows on from his father's active involvement in that subject. As Stephen Jacyna has observed, accounts of medical travel not only tell us something about what the travellers saw, they are also instructive about who the travellers were and about the character of the medical centres whence they had come.[91]

Duncan's correspondence makes clear, for example, the extent to which the élite, late eighteenth-century, Scottish physician still valued and cultivated social graces and ornamental learning, as well as technical knowledge and skill. Physic remained, in other words, integrated within a wider humanistic culture. The views of the Duncans on this point are very similar to those of another Scottish medical traveller, John Moore.[92] Moore, a Glasgow surgeon and later a physician, travelled several times to the Continent – as an Army surgeon, to study anatomy in Paris, and, in 1772, as medical attendant to the young Duke of Hamilton. Over a period of five years, the ducal party journeyed through France, Switzerland, Germany, Austria and Italy. In 1779, Moore published *A View of Society and Manners in France, Switzerland and Germany*, which was followed in 1781 by *A View of Society and Manners in Italy*. In the latter text, Moore articulated very clearly the perceived need for a physician to display social as well as technical skills. The relevant passage is worth quoting at length:

> Your account of our Friend's state of health gives me much concern ... You say the doctor, under whose care he is at present, has employed his mind so entirely in medical researches, that he scarcely displays a grain of common sense when the conversation turns to any other subject, and that although he seems opinionative, vain and ostentatious in his profession, and full of false and absurd ideas in the common affairs of life, yet he is a very able physician and has performed many wonderful cures. Be assured ... that this is impossible; for medical skill is not like the rod of an inchanter ... which transfers its miraculous powers indiscriminately to a blockhead or a man of sense ... The profession of medicine is that ... in which the generality of mankind have the fewest lights by which they can discern the abilities of its professors; because the studies which lead to it are more out of the road of usual education, and the practice more enveloped in technical terms and hieroglyphical signs. But I imagine the safest criterion by which men, who have not been bred to that profession, can form a judgement of those who have, is the degree of sagacity and penetration they discover on subjects equally open to mankind in general, and which ought to be understood by all who live in society.[93]

Moore explicitly recommended the undertaking of a Grand Tour as a means whereby young physicians might develop the requisite general abilities of discourse and deportment.[94]

It is perhaps also worth noting that the Duncan correspondence supplies insights not only into medical travel by British students but into the internationalism of eighteenth-century medical culture more generally. It was, for instance, not only the British that were itinerant. In Pavia, Duncan studied with Poles, Greeks and Swiss as well as Englishmen and Italians. Moreover his letters indicate that not only did many Britons travel to the Continent but large numbers of Continental physicians travelled to Britain. Many of the medical men Duncan met either had visited London and/or Edinburgh or were planning to do so in the near future. Thus, for example, he remarked to his father that he had met Dr Locatelli, 'whom you have known in Edinburgh'.[95] Duncan describes a total of thirteen of the Continental physicians he met as having, at one time or another, visited Edinburgh. Letters received by Duncan following his return to Scotland confirm the existence of a steady stream of foreign visitors to Edinburgh.[96]

We noted earlier that, while on the Continent, Duncan functioned as his father's agent supplying him with medical intelligence from abroad. Like the movement of personnel, this transfer of information was not, by any means, one-way traffic. The Continental professors Duncan met quizzed him about what was happening in British medical and academic circles. This questioning was, it is my impression, most assiduously pursued by those who were, like his father, editors of, or regular contributors to, periodical publications. Thus, while at Göttingen, Duncan was closely questioned by Dr Steiglitz, one of the reviewers of medical books for the *Allgemeine Literatur-zeitung*. Dr Steiglitz was, Duncan recorded, 'very eager in his inquiries about Dr Beddoes' plans'.[97] Professor Crell, also at Göttingen, engaged Duncan 'to give occasionally a letter of the chemical [words obliterated] Edinburgh for his journal'[98]. Duncan also received several commissions to supply private or institutional libraries with books or theses published in Edinburgh. And he contributed, in a small way, to the trade in medical artefacts. On one occasion, for example, he wrote to ask his father to send elastic gum catheters to an acquaintance in Italy – for the ones available 'here are by no means good or durable'.[99]

Conclusion

Duncan's letters home to his father provide us with insights into why the aspiring physician of the eighteenth century travelled, what he did while he was abroad, and what personal and professional benefits exposure to Continental learning, culture and society might bring. The letters also effectively demonstrate the internationalist character of eighteenth-century medicine – which both encouraged the free movement of personnel and was sustained by it. They give us an indication of how travel, in the eighteenth century, was centrally constitutive of the discourse of medicine, of health and illness. Throughout the modern era, throughout Western civilisation, the discourses of disease, and of lay and professional responses to it, were characteristically the products of an essentially mobile society – as the latter essays in this collections explore more specifically.

Notes

1   For entries into the literature on medical travel, see I.A. Bowman, 'Books by Physician Travellers', *Bookman*, xi (1984), 3-9; G.S.T. Cavanagh, 'Medical Travel Books', *Bulletin of the Medical Library Association*, xlvii (1959), 315-8; R.M. Goldwyn, 'The Physician-Traveller', *Harvard Library Bulletin*, xvii (1969) 410-24; M.C. Meehan, 'Physician Travellers', *Journal of the American Medical Association*, ccxx (1972), 97-102. For interesting examples, J. Bell, (J.L. Stevenson (ed.)) *A Journey from St Petersburg to Peking, 1719-22* (Edinburgh: Edinburgh University Press, 1965); M. Lister, *Journey to Paris in the Year 1698* (Urbana: University of Illinois Press, 1967); H. Avery, 'John Bell's Last Tour', *Medical History*, viii (1964), 69-77; J.D. Spillane, *Medical Travellers: Narratives from the Seventeenth, Eighteenth, and Nineteenth Centuries* (Oxford: Oxford University Press, 1984); J.Z. Bowers, 'Engelbert Kaempfer: Physician, Explorer, Scholar and Author', *Journal of the History of Medicine*, xxi (1966), 237-259; B. Chance, 'Richard Bright – Traveller and Artist', *Bulletin for the History of Medicine*, viii (1940), 909-33.

2   Archibald Pitcairne, for example, an Edinburgh physician, was called to the chair of medicine at Leyden in 1692; see D. Guthrie, 'The Influence of the Leyden School on Scottish Medicine', *Medical History*, iii (1959), 108-22.

3   It is estimated, for example, that as many as a third of the students taught by Boerhaave in Leiden were English speakers; see R.W. Innes-Smith, *English-Speaking Students of Medicine at the University of Leyden* (London: Oliver and Boyd, 1932). See also A. M. Luyendijk-Elshout, 'The Edinburgh Connection, William Cullen's Students and the Leiden Medical School', in H. de Ridder-Symoens and J.M. Fletcher (eds), *Academic Relations between the Low Countries and the British Isles* (Ghent: Studia Historica, 1989), 47-63. Unlike previous Edinburgh travelling scholars, however, Duncan was unable to visit Leiden, due to it being occupied by the French in 1795.

4   For biographical information on Andrew Duncan senior, see L.
    Rosner, 'Andrew Duncan, M.D. F.R.S.E. 1744-1828', *Scottish Men
    of Science Series* (Edinburgh: History of Medicine and Science Unit,
    1981); R. Chambers, *A Biographical Dictionary of Eminent Scotsmen*
    (Glasgow: Blackie, 1855); J. Comrie, *History of Scottish Medicine* (2
    vols; London: Bailliere, Tindall and Cox, 1932), ii, 481.

5   For remarks about the nature of the *Medical Commentaries*, and
    about the eighteenth-century medical periodical press as a whole, see
    Roy Porter, 'The Rise of Medical Journalism in Britain to 1800', in
    W.F. Bynum, S. Lock, and R. Porter (eds), *Medical Journals and
    Medical Knowledge. Historical Essays* (London and New York:
    Routledge, 1992), 16-28.

6   The best source for biographical information on Andrew Duncan,
    junior, is A. Grant, *The Story of the University of Edinburgh* (London:
    Longmans, Green, 1884), 445-7.

7   W.S. Craig, *History of the Royal College of Physicians of Edinburgh*
    (Oxford: Blackwell, 1976), 29.

8   For another example of an ambitious Edinburgh father directing his
    son's travels to London and the Continent, see H.D. Erlam,
    'Alexander Monro, Primus, Autobiography', *University of Edinburgh
    Journal*, xvii (1955-56), 80-3.

9   A. Duncan, 'Letters, 1794-1798', Mss. Dc 1.90, Edinburgh
    University Library. A selection from these papers has been published
    by W.A. MacNaughton, 'Extracts from the Correspondence of
    Andrew Duncan, jr., M.D., F.R.C.P.E., Professor of Materia Medica
    in the University of Edinburgh from 1821 until 1832', *Caledonian
    Medical Journal*, ix (1914), 203-8, 262-265,307-315,370-377, 426-
    429, 456-470; x (1915) 23-27, 84-90, 104-114, 129-146, 165-178,
    194-200. MacNaughton was more interested in Duncan as a tourist
    than as a trainee physician and thus quotes at length from his
    descriptions of landscape and scenery – most of which I have
    omitted from my own account.

10 See L. Rosner, *Medical Education in the Age of Improvement:
    Edinburgh Students and Apprentices, 1790-1826* (Edinburgh:
    Edinburgh University Press, 1991).

11 Christopher Lawrence has classified Edinburgh medical men, earlier
    in the eighteenth century, in the two divisions of 'ornate physicians'
    and 'learned artisans'; see C. J. Lawrence, 'Ornate physicians and
    learned artisans: Edinburgh medical men, 1726-1776', in W.F.
    Bynum and R. Porter (eds), *William Hunter and the Eighteenth-
    Century Medical World* (Cambridge: Cambridge University Press,
    1985), 153-76. He argues that, as the century progressed, these two

categories coalesced. Certainly Duncan junior sought, or was directed by his father, to seek, both ornamental and practical learning. See also S. Lawrence, 'Anatomy and Address: Creating Medical Gentlemen in Eighteenth-century London', in V. Nutton and R. Porter (eds), *The History of Medical Education in Britain* (Amsterdam: Rodopi, 1995), 199-228.

12 D. Porter and R. Porter, *Patient's Progress: Doctors and Doctoring in Eighteenth-century England* (Cambridge: Polity Press, 1989); N.D. Jewson, 'Medical Knowledge and the Patronage System in Eighteenth-Century England', *Sociology*, viii (1978), 369-85; M. Nicolson, 'The Metastatic Theory of Pathogenesis and the Professional Interests of the Eighteenth-Century Physician', *Medical History*, xxxii (1988), 277-300.

13 P. Laslett, *The World We Have Lost* (London: Methuen, 1971); P. Laslett, *The World We Have Lost: Further Explored* (London: Methuen, 1983).

14 R. Porter, 'William Hunter: a Surgeon and a Gentleman', in W.F. Bynum and R. Porter (eds), *William Hunter and the Eighteenth-Century Medical World* (Cambridge: Cambridge University Press, 1985), 7-34.

15 The Duncans might be compared with the Thomson clan, in early nineteenth-century Edinburgh, who have been the subject of a sensitive study by L.S. Jacyna, *Philosophic Whigs: Medicine, Science and Citizenship, 1789-1848* (London: Routledge, 1994).

16 Robert Burns, 'The Twa Dogs: A Tale', in J. Kinsley (ed.), *Burns: Poems and Songs* (Oxford: Oxford University Press, 1971), 110-16. To 'rive' is to tear up.

17 *Ibid.*

18 For a recent discussion of Barclay, see C. Lawrence, 'The Edinburgh Medical School and the End of the "Old Thing"', *History of the Universities*, vii (1988), 259-86.

19 Letter, A. Duncan, junior to A. Duncan, senior, London, 13 October 1794, see note 9 above. In the following notes I have referred to the individual letters only by place and date.

20 Letter, London, 20 October 1794. 'Dr Monro' was presumably Alexander Monro secundus, Professor of Anatomy and Surgery at the University of Edinburgh from 1758 to 1808. For the Monro dynasty, see Comrie, *op. cit.* (note 4).

21 Letter, London, 22 January 1795. A collection of comparative anatomical specimens might prove a useful aid to university or extra-mural teaching, see Jacyna, *op. cit.* (note 15).

22 Letter, London, 13 January 1795.

23   Letter, London, 24 October 1794.

24   Letter, London, 1 December 1794. For the Royal Medical Society,
see J. Gray, *History of the Royal Medical Society, 1737-1937*
(Edinburgh: Edinburgh University Press, 1952); J.R.R. Christie,
'Edinburgh Medicine in the Eighteenth Century, the View from the
Students', *Society for the History of Medicine, Bulletin*, xix (1976), 13-
15; and Rosner, *op. cit* (note 10). Attempts were shortly made in
London to remedy the deficiency Duncan identified, see S.
Lawrence, '"Desirous of Improvements in Medicine"', Pupils and
Practitioners in the Medical Societies at Guy's and St Bartholomew's
Hospitals, 1795-1815', *Bulletin of the History of Medicine*, lix (1985),
89-104.

25   Letter, London, 9 February 1795.

26   Letter, London, 4 March 1795.

27   Letter, London, 8 December 1794.

28   Duncan senior had himself spent some time in the relatively lowly
position of a ship's surgeon. This may have contributed to his being
initially perceived as an outsider when he first attempted to establish
himself within the élite circles of Edinburgh physic, Rosner, *op.cit.*
(note 4). Duncan senior evidently wanted his son to labour under
no such stigma.

29   Letter, London, 4 January 1795.

30   Letter, London, 4 March 1795.

31   *Ibid.*

32   C. Este, *A Journey in the Year 1793 through Flanders, Brabant and
Germany to Switzerland* (London: 1795).

33   Letter, Brunswick, May 1795, no day given. For Eschenburg, who
was a philologist and a distinguished translator of Shakespeare, see
G.A. Lindeboom, 'Historisches zum begriff "Enzyklopädie" – Die
Wissenschaftskunde von Johann Joachim Eschenburg (1743-1820)',
in R. Toellner and M.J. van Lieburg (eds), *Deutsch-Niederländische
Beziehungen in der Medizin des 18. Jahrhunderts* (Amsterdam:
Rodopi, 1985).

34   Letter, Brunswick, May 1795, no day given.

35   Letter, Göttingen, 6 July 1795.

36   Letter, Göttingen, 1 September 1795.

37   *Ibid.*

38   The University of Göttingen was at this time the foremost centre for
scientific learning in Germany, see Timothy Lenoir, *The Strategy of
Life: Teleology and Mechanics in Nineteenth-century German Biology*
(Dordrecht and Boston: Reidel, 1982).

39   Letter, Göttingen, 18 August 1795.

40   For Frank's system of medical police, see L. Baumgartner and E.M.
     Ramsey, 'Johann Peter Frank and his "System einer vollständigen
     Medicinischen Polizey"', *Annals of Medical History*, v (1933), 525-32.

41   For the early history of forensic medicine in Scotland, see M.A.
     Crowther and B. White, *On Soul and Conscience: The Medical Expert
     and Crime: 150 Years of Forensic Medicine in Glasgow* (Aberdeen:
     Aberdeen University Press, 1988); and B. White, 'Training Medical
     Policemen: Forensic Medicine and Public Health in Nineteenth-
     century Scotland', in M. Clark and C. Crawford (eds), *Legal
     Medicine in History* (Cambridge and New York: Cambridge
     University Press, 1994).

42   Letter, Göttingen, 1 September 1795.

43   Letter, Göttingen, 7 August 1795.

44   *Ibid.*

45   *Ibid.*

46   *Ibid.*

47   MacNaughton states that Duncan spent a winter studying in
     Göttingen. This would seem to be an error.

48   'You mentioned having sent to me ... some pickled herrings and two
     copies of the Commentaries.' Letter, London, 9 February 1795.

49   Letter, Ratisbon, 3 October 1795. 'Young Monro' is presumably
     Alexander Monro tertius (1773-1859) who was to inherit his father's
     chair in anatomy and surgery in 1817, see Comrie, *op.cit.* (note 4). I
     have retained the names Duncan used for Ratisbon (Regensburg)
     and Leghorn (Livorno), even although Duncan is not quite
     consistent on the latter usage.

50   Letter, Pavia, 3 November 1795. Like many of the descriptions that
     Duncan provided for his father, this passage is an implicit
     comparison with similar activities in Edinburgh. Duncan supplied
     an interesting insight into the arrangements of clinical teaching in
     Edinburgh when he remarked: 'The royal stables are among the
     greatest curiosities in Hanover ... They are filled with the finest of
     horses, and at the stall of each is hung a board with its name and
     pedigree. It put me in mind of the patients' names in your clinical
     ward.' Letter, Göttingen, 6 July 1795.

51   Letter, Pavia, 3 November 1795.

52   Letter, *ibid.*

53   Letter, Pavia, 16 November 1795.

54   This is an implicit comparison with Edinburgh University where the
     professors did not receive salaries. Their income as teachers derived
     from the fees paid by students to attend their lectures, see J.B.
     Morrell, 'The University of Edinburgh in the late eighteenth

century: its scientific eminence and academic structure', *Isis*, lxii
(1971), 158-71.

55 Letter, Pavia, 1 December 1795.

56 The account of tourists' itineraries in J. Black, *The British Abroad:
The Grand Tour in the Eighteenth Century* (London: Alan Sutton,
1992) allows comparison to be made with Duncan's travels. Duncan
emerges, his interest in clinical medicine aside, as a very typical
tourist – as his attendance at the celebrations for Holy Week in
Rome and the Festa della Sensa in Venice exemplify.

57 Letter, Pavia, 31 December 1795. Description of hospitals is almost
a distinctive genre of eighteenth-century travel literature. The
paradigmatic text was John Howard, *An Account of the Principal
Lazarettos in Europe* (London: J. Johnston, 1791); see also V.C.P.,
'Matthew Baillie's Diary of Travel in 1788', *British Medical Journal*,
19 March (1927), 523-24.

58 Letter, Leghorn, 18 April 1796.

59 *Ibid.*

60 Letter, Venice, 2 May 1796.

61 Letter, Venice, 15 May 1796.

62 Letter, Vienna, 1 June 1796

63 Letter, Prague, 22 June 1796.

64 Letter, Pavia, 1 December 1795.

65 This was the brother of the Lord Daer that Robert Burns had been
so delighted to meet in 1786; see Kinsley, *op.cit.* (note 16), 239-40.

66 For the importance of Paris to Scottish medical students at the
beginning of the nineteenth century, see L. S. Jacyna, 'Robert
Carswell and William Thomson at the Hôtel-Dieu of Lyons:
Scottish views of French medicine', in R. French and A. Wear (eds),
British Medicine in an Age of Reform (London and New York:
Routledge, 1991), 110-35. Paris was, of course, an essential stop on
the Grand Tour for both medical and non-medical travellers alike;
see Black, *op.cit.* (note 56).

67 Letter, Florence, 10 November 1797.

68 *Ibid.*

69 Letter, Pisa, 12 December 1797.

70 *Ibid.*

71 Letter, Leghorn, 1 March 1797.

72 *Ibid.*

73 Letter, Florence, 10 November 1797.

74 *Ibid.*

75 Letter, Bremen, 6 June 1798.

76 A. Duncan, 'Letter containing Experiments and Observations on

Cinchona, tending particularly to shew that it does not contain Gelatine', *Nicholson's Journal,* vi (1803), 225-8.

77 For the impact of Continental pathological anatomy in Britain, see R.C. Maulitz, *Morbid Appearances: The Anatomy of Pathology in the Early Nineteenth Century* (Cambridge and New York: Cambridge University Press, 1987).

78 D.L. Cowen, 'The Edinburgh Pharmacopoeia', in R.G.W. Anderson and A.D.C. Simpson (eds), *The Early Years of the Edinburgh Medical School* (Edinburgh: Royal Scottish Museum, 1976). See also D.L. Cowen, 'The Edinburgh Pharmacopoeia', *Medical History,* i (1957), 123-39; D.L. Cowen, 'The Edinburgh Dispensatories', *Papers of the Bibliographical Society of America,* xlv (1951), 85-96; D.L. Cowen, 'The Influence of the Edinburgh Pharmacopoeia and the Edinburgh Dispensatories', *Pharmaceutical History,* xii (1982), 2-4.

79 Anon., 'Edinburgh New Dispensatory', *Nicholson's Journal,* vi (1803), 241.

80 Crowther and White, *op. cit.* (note 41).

81 A. Grant, *The Story of the University of Edinburgh,* 446. For the history of the Library, see J.R. Guild and A. Law (eds), *Edinburgh University Library, 1580-1980: A Collection of Historical Essays* (Edinburgh: The Library, University of Edinburgh, 1982).

82 Letter, Pavia, 17 December 1795.

83 Este, *op. cit.,* (note 32), 2.

84 *Ibid.*

85 *Ibid.* For an exemplary description of medical education in eighteenth-century London, see S. Lawrence, *Charitable Knowledge: Hospital Pupils and Practitioners in Eighteenth-century London* (Cambridge and New York: Cambridge University Press, 1996).

86 *Ibid.*

87 *Ibid.* 3.

88 *Ibid.,* 189-91.

89 As well as providing his son with an expensive education, Duncan senior was able, for example, to afford to run a hothouse and grow exotic fruit in it. His son remarked, à propos of Southern Germany: 'It appeared to me at first strange to see the lower classes drinking wine, but we got here wine at about twopence a bottle ... I bought a bunch of grapes weighing a pound and a half for a halfpenny, and grapes like which your hothouse produce nothing' (Letter, Vienna, 20 October 1795).

90 G. Risse, *Hospital Life in Enlightenment Scotland: Care and Teaching at the Royal Infirmary of Edinburgh* (Cambridge and New York: Cambridge University Press, 1986).

91 For example, L.S. Jacyna (ed.), *A Tale of Three Cities: The Correspondence of William Sharpey and Allen Thomson, Medical History Supplement,* ix (London: Wellcome Institute for the History of Medicine, 1989).

92 For Moore, see H.L. Fulton, 'John Moore, the Medical Profession and the Glasgow Enlightenment', in A. Hook and R.B. Sher (eds), *The Glasgow Enlightenment* (East Linton: Tuckwell, 1995), 176-89; also R. Anderson *The Life of John Moore, M.D. with Critical Observations on His Works* (Edinburgh: Stirling and Slade, 1820).

93 J. Moore, *A View of Society and Manners in Italy* (2 vols; London: Strahan and Cadell, 1781), ii, 217-8.

94 *Ibid.,* 486-95

95 Letter, Pavia, 3 November 1795.

96 See note 9 above.

97 Letter, Göttingen, 6 July 1795

98 Letter, Göttingen, May, no day given.

99 Letter, Leghorn, 2 October 1797.

3

Richard Jago's *Edge-Hill* Revisited:
A traveller's prospect of the health and disease of a
succession of national landscapes.

Matthew Craske

The majority of essays in this collection concern the effects of travel, shifting landscapes and climactic conditions, upon the health, both physical and mental, of the traveller. My concerns are somewhat the inverse; travellers' observations of the health of the landscape and the search in the topography of the landscape for visual indications of the state of the 'body politic'. The focus of my attention is not upon foreign travel, the subject which has preoccupied several of the other contributors, but upon indigenous tourism, in particular eighteenth-century English tourists' view of the landscape of their motherland.

My interpretation of the word 'disease' is, perhaps, a little broader than that encountered elsewhere in this volume. I extend it, as the material with which I deal necessitates, to the notion of 'dis-ease' or absence of ease. When considering the concept of a healthy or sick landscape in the eighteenth century it is, I contend, impossible to dissociate the imagery of war and violence from that of physical infection. Those human agencies which prevented travellers, labourers and livestock from experiencing a state of ease in the landscape were as much a feature of its sickness as 'bad air' or contaminated water. Thus, whilst my chief concern is with the imagery of physical illness and contamination, I shall also dwell on the imagery of highway crime, civil war and political corruption. It is by this circuitous route that an essay on the subject of pathology comes to focus upon the analysis of the imagery of politics, in particular travellers' perceptions of the corruption and improvement, degeneration and regeneration, of state.

This essay is based upon an analysis of the poetics of the landscape prospect. The rise of this tradition of versifying was strongly associated with the boom in indigenous leisure travel which occurred during the mid-eighteenth century, in particular the quest for fine views.[1] The practice of walking up to and viewing from such

121

vantages was considered to be part of the therapeutics of travel. The exercise of climbing, as long as not too extreme, was thought to be of constitutional benefit.[2] Views afforded a variety of sights; this variety was considered to refresh the mind and to provide the sort of stimulus which was necessary to mental well-being. Particularly in English intellectual culture, where the Lockean conception of the mind as a *tabula rasa* was most prevalent, the act of viewing from a prospect was associated with the natural and healthy quest of the mind to be bombarded and formed by outward stimulus. The very notion of looking out over a vista was associated with personal release. Views were, as we shall see, equated with liberty, in both the political and creative spheres of culture. The healthy release of the imagination was thought to have considerable therapeutic value in a society where conventional medical opinion gravitated towards the notion that excess of familiar sights sickened the fancy.[3] Hill tops, inevitably, became identified as the resort of men of particularly well-developed capacities for fancy. They were regarded, in poetic conception, as places of transcendent vision; places where an individual might attain a special insight into the workings of the world.

Prospect poems typically recorded the reveries experienced by the reflective traveller upon reaching some viewpoint from which a broad vision of the physical condition of the landscape could be attained. In many cases the achievement of a vantage point was regarded as an opportunity for political reflection, musings upon the state of body politic as manifested in the topography of the panorama. One of the most celebrated examples of this type of writing was Richard Jago's *Edge-Hill, or the Rural Prospect Delineated and Moralised.* Published in 1767, this long and turgid work is now, quite justifiably, excised from the canon of English literature. The poem does, however, remain an important historical testimony of how travellers, or tourists, were expected to envisage the world through which they passed. Although Jago's language is somewhat opaque, one can discern a mind behind the verse which is fully engaged in contemporary debates concerning the influence of human history upon the development of the landscape, the ethics of travel, and the philosophy of perception.

Before becoming embroiled in a discussion of the complex ideas developed within Jago's text, it seems prudent to introduce some basic historical context. I must ask patience, for a few pages, from those of my readers fixed firmly on the topic of pathologies. Those passages of the poem pertinent to the subject of health and disease can only be understood with some gloss on the poet and his patrons and their social and political affiliations.

Richard Jago was a gentleman cleric of quite humble means. He lived for some time in Birmingham and found celebrity as a poet by associating himself with the literary wit, William Shenstone. A frequent guest at Shenstone's estates at Leasowes in Worcestershire, he moved into the circle of Shenstone's most socially exalted friends.[4] One of this circle, though by no means the richest or most powerful, was Sanderson Miller, an Oxford-educated country gentleman who inherited from his father an estate at Radway in Warwickshire. On this estate was situated the important civil war battleground of Edge Hill. Here in 1642 Parliamentary troops and those of Charles I had first clashed with great loss of life on both sides. Inspired by contemporaries who had developed their gardens into attractions for genteel excursionists – Shenstone at Leasowes, George Lyttleton at Hagley and Lord Cobham at Stowe – Miller decided to landscape the battlefield with strategic planting and quasi-gothic buildings. His efforts to attract the public seem to have been successful. Edge Hill became a well-known site on the national tourist itinerary. It featured in some of the most celebrated published travel diaries such as those of Richard Pococke and the George Lipscombe.[5]

Miller's decision to develop the battlefield on which the political 'constitution' (a corporeal term initialy emerging from the language of pathology) of the nation had been temporally ruined relates directly to a well-established tradition of patriotic touring. Since the Restoration the idea of the excursion to form an 'idea of England', a nationalistic alternative to the cosmopolitan experience of the Grand Tour, had had a currency in English polite culture. The purpose of such travel, the literature of which has been recently reviewed by John Brewer, was to acquire a love of the English countryside and an appreciation of national antiquities.[6] As the introduction to Thomas Cox's once famous topographical compendium *Magna Britannia* (first published 1715) made clear, patriotic tourists were also expected to learn the history of the Constitution from visiting historic sites where constitutional liberties had been established or fought over. Thus, when he developed the battlefield and built paths for visitors, Miller could be considered to be performing a patriotic service in facilitating the education of the touring public.

Miller built a gothic tower as the central attraction of the Edge Hill gardens. This edifice was intended to appear in a state of dramatic ruin; its broken forms probably being intended to remind the spectator of the ruin of state which had occurred on this site and the violence of the struggle for constitutional liberties. Designed by

Miller himself, who was a leading amateur enthusiast for the Gothic tradition of building, the tower was placed at the supreme viewpoint on the site where, Miller believed, Charles I had set up his camp. The sham ruin was described in Jago's poem.[7] From the lawns around its base the poet took up his 'prospect'. It is the focal point of the poem, the place from which much of narrative proceeds.

Although the octagonal form of the tower was derived from the architecture of nearby Warwick Castle, the basic idea of erecting it was probably borrowed from Lord Cobham's garden at Stowe. Here, on the highest viewpoint available, Cobham had employed James Gibbs to design a Gothic structure known first as the Temple of Ancestral Liberty and secondly as the Temple of Saxon Liberty. The Temple probably changed its name in the 1740s when a group statues symbolic of Saxon Deities was placed in a ring around its base. The function of this iconography, as we shall see in more detail below, was to encourage visitors to the viewpoint that they might look out upon the world with historical eyes and remember the lessons of ancient history.

Building his tower in 1745-7, approximately the time the Saxon Deities were put into place at Stowe, Miller borrowed this idea. In the upper viewing room he had built four niches intended for statues symbolic of the British, Roman, Saxon and Danish inhabitants of the country in ancient times. Owing to structural weaknesses in the tower – for Miller had an unfortunate reputation for unsound building – only one of these statues, a figure of the British King Caractacus in chains, was actually made.[8] The idea, nevertheless, was to surround with a historical narrative the person who looked out onto the landscape, obliging that person to engage his historical imagination in the act of viewing. It was broadly in this spirit that Jago wrote his poem. He too used the vantage to envisage imaginatively the various phases of ancient rule that had shaped the topography of the scene before him.

The publication of Jago's *Edge-Hill* can be construed as part of Miller's broader attempt to publicise his battlefield garden. Miller was, in some respects, the patron of the poem. He not only subscribed but also was instrumental in gaining a high proportion of the most notable subscribers.[9] A few years before the publication Miller had employed a surveyor to make a map of the battlefield at Edge Hill which was engraved and published to elucidate the site. Jago's poem can be seen as an extension of this mapping process, a sort of literary map made for the traveller's delectation which incorporated not only the battlefield but also the great rolling landscape beyond.

The idea of the traveller's tendency to map – to find vistas from where he can develop a map-like image of the landscape – is central to Jago's narrative. The first edition of the poem includes, on the opening page, a fine little print by Wale and Grignion of the viewpoint at Edge Hill in which a pair of sightseers are seen to gaze out into the landscape with the aid of a telescope. The text has at its heart a philosophical debate on sight and the use of telescopes and lenses which were the essential tools of the cartographer. Jago writes of a view stretching out from the prospect point of Edge Hill in all directions, encompassing dozens of landscape features and estates, whose proprietors' names are extolled. This manner of looking at the world had much in common with contemporary conceptions of mapping.[10] In the mid-eighteenth century the great majority of maps of the English countryside depicted the landscape as a succession of estates; the traveller passing through the landscape was largely envisaged as travelling from the realm of one estate to another. Jago's intention, as stated in the preface, was to form a sort of three-dimensional and moving map of the landscape; he spoke enigmatically of inventing 'imaginary line(s)' which could transport the reader from estate to estate and simultaneously from one time of day or season to another.

Jago's concept of vision goes far beyond the obvious optical process of viewing. He is also concerned with historical vision, a capacity which is identified as the province of the inner eye or imagination. As Jago takes up his position upon an historic vantage point his poetic instinct is to look back in time as well as out into space. His poetic imagination wanders back to an ante-diluvian landscape informed by the deluge theories of Dr John Woodward and Alexander Catcott and thence through ancient history from Roman Britain to the Saxon world.[11] Thence he visits a 'gothic' world of the medieval barons, a world reduced by the yoke of a plethora of unspecified tyrants. At last, his imagination tarries long in the mid-seventeenth century and, in particular, upon the Battle of Edge Hill.

In the preface to the poem Jago compares the spatial to the historical prospect, depicting the former as agreeable and the latter as disturbing:

> The title is Edge-Hill, a place taken notice of by all topographical writers, who have had occasion to mention it for its extensive and agreeable prospect and further unhappily distinguished by being the scene of the first battle between the forces of King CHARLES and those of the parliament under the command of the Earl of Essex in the year 1642.[12]

In order to contrast the 'agreeable' modern prospect from the 'unhappy' historical scene Jago divides his poem into four books. In the first two books where Jago describes the modern prospect of 'healthy champain' the poetic narrative takes place in the favourable seasons of Spring or Summer.[13] The description of the seventeenth century in the final book is presaged by plunging the landscape into winter, a 'season of pain, sickness and old age' in which foul air harrows a formerly healthy scene. It is in his description of winter that Jago resorts to his most patently pathological imagery. The first frosts of that season, for instance, are compared to a 'sickness' which blights 'the Virgin's early bloom'.

A key concept of Jago's verse, particularly relevant to our theme of pathology, is that a landscape could, in the manner of a body, become prone to a general state of health or disease. The poem is suffused with images of elemental movement, both of air, water and beams of light. Free movement of these elements is habitually equated with health, whereas obstruction, turgidity or violent collision is associated with disease. Such perceptions of the health and sickness of the landscape relate directly to the contemporary understanding of the body as a fluid system which gravitated towards disease on account of obstructions or malfunctions in flow. Jago was by no means unusual in thinking of the landscape in this manner. In William Gilpin's *Dialogue* upon travel, printed as a tourist guide to Lord Cobham's garden at Stowe (1749), a conversation between two fictive visitors turns to the flow of water through the gardens:

> Water... it is observed... is of as much use to the landscape as blood in a body: without these essentials it is impossible that there can be life in either the one or the other.[14]

The writer goes on to suggest that it is impossible to conceive of a truly healthy landscape without free-running water. Such comments are testimony to the passage into common knowledge of Hervey's theories on the circulation of the blood and the impact of a basic medical education upon travellers' interpretation of the landscape through which they passed.

Jago does not consider that conditions of healthy flow, diseased obstruction or fevered collision are simply determined by natural occurrences such as exceptional weather conditions. Whilst storms and foul winds are discussed as the sources of disease in the landscape, he always makes clear that the impact of these conditions is largely determined by the quality of land management or national governance. Looking down from Edge Hill at the estate of Lord

Archer at Understade, for instance, Jago is moved to praise the peer's management of the system of streams which irrigate his land:

So shall your lawns with healthful verdure smile,
While others, sickening in the sultry blaze
A russet wild display, or the rank blade
And matted tufts the careless owners shade.[15]

On a number of occasions Jago describes the function of the genial landlord as the ministering hand that maintains the flow of life-giving water through the landscape.

These interpretations of the landscape cannot be dismissed as merely the effusive images that a sycophantic poet resorted to in the search of aristocratic subscribers. The most serious and prosaic of geographical and economic commentators were committed to similar interpretations of the landscape. In his *Political Survey of Great Britain* (first published 1774), for instance, John Campbell argued forcefully that natural geographical advantages alone did not determine the health and prosperity of a national landscape. He takes as his examples the present state of Italy and Spain, countries which, he maintained, had the favourable climate and geographical advantages to make them great in times past but had become ruined and depopulated by despotic government and poor land management. The corruption of the Spanish state, he suggests, meant that now 'the bulk of the people are lazy, poor and proud' and that the landscape of the country had become a 'desert' which was 'deformed as well as depopulated'.[16] Campbell's ultimate objective was to find firm geographical evidence to support patriotic rhetoric; to demonstrate that the respect for liberty in modern English government had allowed the country to become a strong, healthy and well-populated land.

The idea of portraying the 'prospect' as a vantage for poetic reflections on the health of the state was not of Jago's own invention. The most famous example of this poetic device was contained within Alexander Pope's *Windsor Forest* of 1712, a poem which Jago cites in the preface as one of his main sources of inspiration. In his *Windsor Forest* Pope looks down upon the verdant pastures of England under Queen Anne's rule and thence imagines a succession of past 'desert' landscapes, worlds of waste and dissolution created by gothic 'tyrants'. Creating this image of the healthy modern landscape famously gave Pope the opportunity to make a political point. He stressed his Tory allegiances to the Stuart monarchy, implying a distaste for the events of 1688 and the instalment of William of Orange:

See Pan with flocks, with fruits Pomona crown'd,
Here blushing Flora paints the enamel'd ground,
Here Ceres' gifts in waving prospect stand,
And nodding tempt the joyful reaper's Hand,
Rich Industry sits smiling upon the plains,
And Peace and plenty tell, a STUART reigns.[17]

One of Pope's models in the writing of *Windsor Forest* was Sir John
Denham's Cooper's Hill, an overtly political work. First published in
1642, a year before the battle of Edge Hill, the poem was the
acknowledged foundation work of the genre of English prospect
poetry. Denham took as his prospect a hill which looks down on the
Thames at Runymede, the place where the Magna Carta was signed
and national liberties established. The healthy and secure landscape
of the Thames valley was depicted as an emblem of the prosperous
rule of Charles I on the eve of the Civil War.

That Jago's poetic form had its roots in tributes to Stuart rule was
no coincidence. *Edge-Hill* was clearly penned in a pro-Caroline spirit,
parliamentarians are painted as the villains of the battle and Oliver
Cromwell as that of seventeenth-century history in general. The
possibility of a covert Jacobite agenda lurks unstated behind the
flights of vague pro-Caroline rhetoric. Indeed, a reading of the poem
as a piece of covert and tempered Jacobitism is justified by an
examination of the politics of the chief sponsor of the poem,
Sanderson Miller.

Although of a Parliamentarian family, Miller passed as a student
at Oxford into the circle of Dr William King, the Principal of St
Mary's Hall who was widely held to be Oxford's leading Jacobite
College man. King became a figure of national celebrity in 1749
when, in his speech to mark the opening of the Radcliffe Camera, he
repeatedly employed the word 'restore' (or 'return' depending on
one's translation of the Latin) which encouraged the supposition that
he was covertly calling for the restoration of Stuart rule.[18] This
supposition was not without some foundation. In High Church
Oxford circles the Laudian church's support of the Restoration was
still remembered with pride and inevitably linked to the aspiration to
'restore' the Stuart dynasty in the eighteenth century.

Throughout his life Miller continued to regard King as a mentor.
The owner of Edge Hill's pro-Stuart sympathies are charted in his
extensive correspondence which has been preserved for history and
now resides in Warwick Record Office.[19] Fortunately many letters
survive from Miller to his friends which date from the period of the

second Jacobite Rebellion of 1745. These show him to be treading the cautious path which many Tories sympathetic to Jacobite rule, but without the resolve to support rebellion, were obliged to take at this time. Miller was cautious never to be openly Jacobite in his correspondence but was equally never a declared supporter of Hanoverian rule.

It was shortly after leaving Oxford in the mid-forties where he had been immersed in high Tory society that Miller decided to build his gothic tower. The hero of Miller's terrain was unambiguously Charles I and the villain Cromwell. One of the prime uses of the tower, apart from acting as a tourist vantage point, was as a site where Miller and his friends could annually toast the anniversary of the death of Cromwell.[20] One cannot help but speculate that when placing a figure of Caractacus chained within the tower that began to be built in 1745 Miller, had some covert pro-Stuart meaning in mind. In the figure of the noble and just British King who was set in chains and dragged out of his native land by the force of foreign Roman rule, there may well have been some hint of an intended of comparison with the 'Pretender'.

The absence of any direct support for the Hanoverian replacement of Stuart rule was essential to the narrative of Jago's poem. By tradition, the political hero of prospect poetry was the Prince or his consort. It had been so for Denham and Pope. Jago, by contrast, attributed the health and prosperity of the modern landscape to a succession of landlords who, by no coincidence, appear as principal subscribers to the first edition of the work. The major landowners cited in the text were not generally men in great power at Westminster, rather they were 'country' magnates. This selection of local worthies conforms with Jago's rather enigmatic declaration in the preface to the first edition of the poem that he was writing in praise of the 'local'. Jago's vision of the modern political realm is bound by the limits of his sight at the summit of Edge Hill. London and Westminster are unseen and play no role in the system of power which he considers to shape the landscape. It is local governance which is seen to have brought health and prosperity to this landscape much as it was national disputes between crown and parliament which had brought devastation to it in the seventeenth century.

Jago, thus, resisted the strong tradition of setting up a single prince or head of state as the force of nature which was considered to bring health and fecundity to the landscape. As Martin Warnke has demonstrated in his survey of the *Political Landscape* in European artistic tradition, the notion that a prince or monarch could be compared to the sun which brought life and health to the national landscape was prevalent in early modern culture.[21] Despite the distrust of absolutist rhetoric in eighteenth-century England, such imagery was not unknown. A sycophantic prospect poem published in praise of Queen Caroline (consort of George II) in the *St James' Evening Post* of March 29, 1733 is, perhaps, the ultimate expression of this mode of thought. Taking the voice of a traveller enjoying the view from the Queen's Mount in Kensington, the anonymous poet compares the healthy breezes which ventilate the Kent and Surrey landscape to the soft inhalations and exhalations of the Queen. As the Queen breathes in the morning air she is seen to soften the landscape and ease the 'ruder winds' provided by mere mother nature. Caroline's nature is depicted as the unblemished nature of the world before the Fall. She is compared to an Eve destined never to succumb to the temptations of sin. A more fabulous image of the health of the Hanoverian body politic is difficult to imagine. For Richard Jago, with his somewhat subversive 'local' image of the body politic, the inhalations and exhalations of the inhabitants of the Court at Kensington were simply irrelevant. Jago's sun did not rise from an Hanoverian palace nor the did his healthy breezes emanate from Westminster.

Jago's vision is that of the traveller jaundiced with the metropolitan workings of state and seeking the true spirit of the nation in its localities. His 'prospect' allows him to explore the tensions between the search for the 'local' and the desire for an expansive vision. Whilst the poet's declared intention is to discover the properties of a local landscape, the purpose of reaching the viewpoint at Edge Hill is to gain a wide survey. The world he seeks has both a liberating sense of space and a comforting sense of the local and familiar. The local, he argues, gives the character to the general. It is through care for the details of local land management that Jago's generally healthy landscape atmosphere is generated. The majestic movement of the River Avon through the landscape, for instance, is depicted as encouraged on its way by the care of the wise landlords who maintain its banks. The hand of George Lucy of Charlecote is imagined as stimulating the Avon herself to 'exhilarate the meads'.[22] The rural landscape with its extensive and unencumbered views is seen as a liberation from the constraints of urban life, a scene of 'retirement' from the corruption of cities and courts. Liberation, however, is not achieved at the expense of becoming a stranger. Rather, the sensation of agreeable touring is achieved through finding a sense of feeling local, of positioning some seemingly familiar delight within a wide survey.

Jago, a Birmingham clergyman, could with justice feel a local within the landscape viewed from Edge Hill. It is, however, the poet's conviction that his landlord/subscribers offer him, and other gentlemen travellers, a hospitable welcome that is central to his sense of belonging. This is, Jago suggests, a landscape to which a gentleman away from his immediate hearth can expect a friendly welcome. Describing the estates of Charles Mordaunt at Walton, for instance, the poet refers to the 'smiling villa's ever open gate'. The poet's sense of the friendliness of the modern landscape is inseparable from the feeling of health and well-being it generates within him. That the landscape is dotted with genial, hospitable proprietors (genial, at least, to gentlemen in the circle of Sanderson Miller), sustains the poetic illusion that it is a healthy world for the tenants and livestock that are part of its natural scene.

Prosaic reality, of course, was a little more complex and dark. Sanderson Miller, though no draconian landlord, was responsible for some unpopular and controversial enclosure schemes in the acres that bordered Edge Hill.[23] It was the increased revenues of enclosure which allowed Miller, whose inherited estates were not in themselves the foundation of a substantial fortune, the luxury of indulging his dilettante pursuits as a landscape gardener. Thus, the site at which Miller generously provided lessons on liberty for genteel excursionists was formed at the expense of a policy of enclosure which was criticised as an infringement of popular liberties.[24]

Jago's eulogy of the modern landscape is built upon the constant association between the imagery of political liberty, spatial openness, unrestricted sight and health. His images of the savage past, by contrast, are suffused with the imagery of enclosure, visual obstruction and disease. The openness of a modern landscape of peace and plenty is strongly contrasted with a 'gothic' world where awesome and ugly boundaries mark the limits of man's trust of his fellow man. Referring to Lord Archer's estates, Jago indulges in a reverie on the subject of liberty:

What happy lot your cheerful walks attends!
By no scant boundary, nor obstructing fence
Immur'd or circumscribed; but spread at large
In open day; save what to cool recess
Is destin'd voluntary, not constrain'd
By sad necessity, and casual state

Of Sickly Peace! Such as the moated hall
With circumference of watery guard,
And pensile Bridge portends, or rear'd aloft
And inaccessible the massy towers,
And narrow circuit of embattled walls
Raised on a mountain-precipice![25]

Jago proceeds to claim that 'fair liberty and freedom's generous reign' can be surveyed in the 'open scenes and cultur'd fields' of Archer's estates. A nightmare vision of 'portcullis huge and moated fence' brings the reader back to 'savage times' when 'distrust, barbarity and gothic rule' were seen to scar the landscape.[26] The imagined gothic past once more supplied the contrast which was supposed to stimulate social gratitude for Archer's administration.

The idea that human barriers which blocked the flow of the landscape could be considered the central metaphors of the disease of state is most strongly expressed in Jago's claim that awesome gothic boundaries only declared a 'sickly peace'. By this the poet surely means to condemn those states of peace maintained by the instruments of tyranny and thus, by their nature, frail and impermanent. The association of turgid movement with sickness of state is most vivid in the final book of the poem where Jago describes his imaginative voyage back into the seventeenth century. His poetry here is little short of bizarre in its employment of pathological imagery. A state of winter is evoked to prepare our minds for the scene of civil war. The highly contemporary concern over cattle 'distemper', a disease which ruined English farmers' livelihoods throughout the mid-eighteenth century, is then triggered. The passage of dank winter air which transforms the landscape, is now the villain of the piece. Impending sickness in the state is compared to the disgusting dribbling of thick mucus from the cows' noses. The herds themselves are transformed from healthy props of the pastoral idyll into a 'dew-eyed race' distinguished by their 'plaintive lowing' whose:

... heavy eyes, confess'd the poisonous gale,
And drank infection in each breath they drew.
Quick through their veins the burning liquor ran
And from their nostrils streamed the putrid rheum,
Malignant our their limbs faint languor crept
And stupefaction, all senses bound.[27]

Shortly afterward Jago describes the sicknesses which the same climactic conditions afflicted upon sheep. Here he describes (unfortunately in rather contorted language) the way in which the sight of sick pastoral animals, metaphors of the sicknesses which afflict the political affairs of men, ruins the traveller's enjoyment of the landscape. The traveller is envisaged moving swiftly through the landscape holding his breath to guard him from the smell of putrid sheep flesh, trying not to look at the decayed corpses from which the stench emits:

> Nor seldom coughs, the watery Rheums afflict
> The woolly tribes, and on their vitals seize
> Thinning the folds; and, with their mangled limbs
> And tatter'd fleeces, the averted eye
> Disgusting, as the squeamish traveller
> With long-suspended breath, hies o'er the plain.[28]

In the first book of the poem Jago had constructed the notion of the healthy modern body politic around vivid images of transit through lush pastoral bliss. He was obliged, for the sake of balance, to search in the final book for exceedingly disgusting imagery to illustrate the blighting of this traveller's Eden.

As the disease of the mid-seventeenth-century state is summoned up with images of unhealthy melancholic viscosity, the alarm engendered by this disease is described in terms of manic rushing motion. One is reminded of the tendency in eighteenth-century medical thought to regard mania, a condition of fury and frenzy, as an inevitable pathological progression from states of excessive melancholic torpor.[29] When Jago comes to the description of the Battle of Edge Hill he employs imagery of licentious and wild movement, which is recalled in calculated contrast to the calm and healthy modern liberty of movement extolled in the first book. Death is seen to move through the fields on 'hostile wings'. The quiet breezes that accompanied the scenes of modern peace are transformed into winds that whip up the clouds into a 'wild encounter'. The savage and diseased face of nature is abroad.

In these passages Jago comes closest to his declared model, Pope's *Windsor Forest*. Immediately after declaring the healthy benefits of Stuart reign, Pope recalls historical eras of barbarity when unreason allied with tyrannical ambition caused suffering to gallop promiscuously through the land. Pope's imagery is that of hunting; 'despotick reign' is compared to a 'bloody chase' through the landscape in which the prey is the humble citizen. Such rulers, Pope declares, disease the landscape turning it into:

A dreary desert and a gloomy waste,
    To savage beasts and savage laws a prey...[30]

Pope, and Jago afterward, associate liberty with government of reason, and tyranny with government of unrestrained passion. The former is conceived as the source of rural abundance and health, the latter the source of galloping disease and, ultimately, of depopulation. Government led by the passions is the rule of the wild 'desert' where openness is mere savagery roaming without constraint. Jago's description of the battle of Edge Hill contains a forceful rail against the straying of the passions into the business of government:

Such are the fruits of passion, forward will,
    And unsubmitting pride! Worse storms than those
    Of elemental rage that waste our field.[31]

Jago's vision of history is organic, society passes cyclically from states of civilisation to barbarism as reason competes with the passions for control over the affairs of man and the landscape which he inhabits. The historical processes which influence the landscape are overtly compared to the cycles of the seasons. This is also a cycle of health and disease; the body politic is considered to respond naturally to the cycles in its affairs by flourishing and sickening. Modern England is envisaged on the ascending phase of this cyclical process.

Such ways of understanding the development of the landscape were much more familiar in the literary debate on the modern ruinous state of the once great Roman world. The notion of the organic cycle of civilisation was, of course, central to Edward Gibbon's *Decline and Fall*, a work first conceived in Rome, where the author was conducting his Grand Tour, a few years before Jago published his *Edge-Hill*. Much as travel to view the ruins of Rome was thought to act as a spur to philosophical reflection on the biological cycle of civilisation, the sight of Gothic ruins on the tour of England were considered in Jago's poem to encourage contemplations on the pathology of state.

The lessons of Roman and Gothic ruin may have been considered analogous; they were, however, by no means the same. Jago (and, as we shall see, a host of contemporary travel writers who theorised upon the didactic properties of 'gothic' ruins) believed that they spoke from the vantage of a society enjoying a high point of health and prosperity. This vantage had its symbol in the hilltop at Edge Hill. The 'gothic' past was by no means unworthy of nostalgia. It provided a forum for heroic worthies struggling for liberty: it was, however, when contrasted to the modern nation, considered to be an environment of hardship, waste and impending disease. This was a patent reversal of the classic Grand Tour view of the Roman *campagna*, in which modern ruin and agricultural waste was habitually compared to ancient grandeur and healthy productivity.[32] A gothic ruin in the English landscape, such as the tower at Edge Hill, could be held as a symbol of the progress of modern society whereas the ruins of the Roman world were unambiguous symbols of degeneration.

Behind Jago's poem lurked a debate on the relative merits of indigenous and foreign travel.[33] Jago, it would appear, was allying himself with the champions of indigenous travel who argued that there was as much to learn from the tour of the national landscape as from the more cosmopolitan experience of the Grand Tour. Hints as to the importance of comparisons between 'gothic' and 'classical' travel to the design of the garden's at Edge Hill and the narrative of the poem can be gleaned from Shenstone's surviving correspondence with Jago. In 1754, some years before the writing of the poem, Shenstone wrote to Jago about Miller's work on the battlefield at Edge Hill. He reports a conversation with Miller who had recently employed a surveyor to make a plan of the battlefield:

> This he proposes to enrich with a number of anecdotes gleaned from his neighbourhood; which must render it extremely entertaining; and surely the Edge Hill fight was never more unfortunate for the nation than it was lucky for Miller. He prints together with his plan, a sheet of Radway Castle. I approve his design. He will by these means turn every bank and hillock of his estate if not into classical at least into historical ground.[34]

Our understanding of the last sentence is much improved by comparing it to a passage in work entitled *Unconnected Thoughts on Gardening* published within Shenstone's *Essays on Men and Manners.* Here Shenstone discusses the merits of landlords improving the historical resonances of their land:

> What an advantage must some Italian seats derive from the circumstance of being situated on ground mentioned in the classics? And even in England wherever a path or garden happens to have been the scene of any event in history one should surely avail oneself of that circumstance to make it more interesting to the imagination. Mottoes should allude to it, columns record it, verses moralise upon it and curiosity receive its share of pleasure.[35]

It is reasonable to posit, on the basis of such thoughts being current in the circle of Miller and Jago, that the intention of their 'gothic' reflections on history was to inject into the English landscape similar levels of moral meaning as were held to exist in the landscapes of the Classical world. Jago's pathological imagery may well be understood as an attempt to aggrandise the debate on the English landscape by imitating the sort of majestic philosophical reflections on the biological cycles of Empires which characterised the literature of the Grand Tour. The narrative of English 'historical ground' might never truly equal to that of 'the classics' but it could, at least, emulate the grandeur of its historical processes.

In some respects travel in England was superior to that of the Grand Tour. Much as a decadent *campagna,* whose undrained marshes emitted 'bad air' and whose highways swarmed with violent *banditti,* was considered a danger to travellers, the modern English countryside cast up images, in Jago's literary fiction at least, of safety and prosperity.[36] The care of those patrons who owned such vantage points provided that essential state of physical security which enabled the tourist to indulge in patriotic reflections without looking over his shoulder. Wildness and violence were to be recalled in the historical imagination rather than experienced in modern reality. Jago, indeed, makes much of the fact that his journey to the top of Edge Hill, where he is to imagine frightening scenes of war and disease, is made easy by the provision of paths and banks of flowers by the landlord. The function of the flowers is considered to still with their fragrance 'every tumult in the breast'. That of the paths is 'to ease our winding steps', preventing the traveller from having to attempt the wild 'precipice(s)' of other routes of ascent.[37] Such smooth and easy experiences define the world of modern travel at Edge Hill from the violent and hostile scene of battle which would have been encountered a hundred years before.

Despite the fact that Jago appears to have been Tory in outlook, his general allegiance was to what we would now term a 'whig' conception of national history. The landscape viewed from Edge Hill is a more fecund and fertile environment than that of any other period which the poet chooses to recall. Jago was by no means the only poet to find in the contemplation of a monument on a rural historic site an opportunity for a verse evoking the traveller's sense of gratitude for the modern pastoral scene. Mark Akenside had written a verse *For a Column at Runymede* (the site of the signing of the Magna Charta) which starts with a call to the attention of the traveller 'who the verdant plain dost traverse' to remember that this state of verdure is the sacrificial gift of those who struggled for national liberties.[38] The very form of this verse imitated of that of Classical roadside memorials. The inscriptions on such memorials frequently began with an invocation to the traveller such as *siste viator*. Often the declared purpose was to strike the traveller through Arcadia with some shaft of sobering wisdom. Akenside, like Sanderson Miller when designing the tower at Edge Hill, was attempting to transfer to the world of 'gothic' history a tradition developed for travellers through the Roman *campagna*. The wisdom offered by these monuments in the English countryside was that of learning to be grateful to one's forbears for the peace and plenty that they had created.

A prospect poem entitled *Ode to Lansdowne Hill*, published some twenty years after Jago's *Edge-Hill*, and in obvious imitation of it, developed these ideas with a fresh set of vivid pathological images.[39] Lansdowne Hill was a natural site for poetic reflection on the health of the body politic. The Hill was scene of a bloody civil war battle and stood directly above the city of Bath, the nation's foremost health spa. A well-known area of constitutional walks and rides for those coming to Bath for cures, the hill offered the poet plenty of opportunity to play on the relationship between the concepts of national and physical constitution.

Lansdowne Hill became a place of public resort by courtesy of the heirs of Lord Lansdowne who owned the site and in the 1720s built a monument to the battle – in the form of an heraldic griffin perched upon a gigantic plinth – on the summit of the Hill.[40] Lansdowne was so keen to develop the hill as a resort for genteel excursionists, that he had employed an old lady who had as a child witnessed the battle to act as permanent guide to the site.[41] The monument was erected to the memory of Lansdowne's ancestor, Sir Bevile Granville, who had died in the Royalist cause. Despite its position at the summit of the local countryside, the monument on Lansdowne Hill was a subversive statement. Lord Lansdowne was a fairly open Jacobite and exiled as such.[42] The inscription on the monument with ample reference to blood sacrifice in the Stuart cause could be interpreted in many ways, but none of them was favourable to the Hanoverian Succession.

The author of *Ode to Lansdowne Hill*, like Jago, was passionately anti-Cromwellian and seems to find some 'gothic' romance in the lost cause of Stuart monarchy. His theme is also that of the modern travellers' Arcadia bought at the price of Royalist blood. The poem begins, in the manner of *Edge-Hill* with a eulogy on the pleasures of a peaceful constitutional walk to the summit which affords a view of modern peace and plenty. The Hill itself is regarded as a form of elevated reservoir which provides the waters for the landscape around:

> Hail Verdant Lansdowne! Health providing Hill!
> That o'er the thermal city, Bath presides;
> T''is from thy sources her warm lavers fill,
> And cheerful vigour reigns over all her rides.

It proceeds a few verses later with the question:

> And who can sum the population great
> Which thy broad eye contemplates all around?
> Fair token of our fair governed state,
> Now wasting war gives away to peace profound.

The poet goes on to heed the mournful message of history and attribute the modern peace to the blood which ran out upon this summit. The blood which ushered from these patriotic sacrifices in the cause of the national political constitution is compared to the water which springs from the hill's inner reservoir to the benefit of the constitutions of those who visit the city below. It is to the worthies who shed blood for the maintenance of the political constitution, the reader is told, that those who enjoy the modern scene of peace and plenty owe their pleasures.

There developed in English tourist literature of the second half of the eighteenth century a strong tradition of political digressions on the improvement of national society intended to make the reader feel gratitude for being born into the modern world. An encounter with a Gothic ruin was, for many writers of tour literature in this period, regarded as an ideal opportunity for making literary reflections on the good fortunes of the modern English citizen.[43] The most impassioned of these digressions appear in the travel writings of the Buckinghamshire antiquary George Lipscombe. Encountering Gothic ruins at Bury Pomeroy in his *A Journey to Cornwall* (published 1799), for instance, Lipscombe was moved to recall:

> My imagination hastened back to the era of feudal splendour, and contemplated, in these ruins, the pomp and solemnity of ancient day. But, the Age of Chivalry is gone! and while every patriot feeling beats in the remembrance of these 'generous virtues nursed in the schools of fortitude, honour and courtesy' we cannot forget that the magnificence of past ages was formed on the ruins of public freedom

and the usurpation of private property; and may console ourselves
for the loss of this splendid pageantry by the happy reflection that,
by that loss, we have also exchanged the savage manners and
ferocious customs of a gothic age, for the refined delights and softer
virtues of science and civilisation.

These type of digressions, which generally post-date Jago's poem,
communicate a broadly similar interplay between nostalgia and
progressivism as encountered in the verse of *Edge-Hill*. They can be
described as the prose equivalents of the poem.

There were also very important painted equivalents. An
instructive comparison can be drawn between Jago's poem and
Richard Wilson's paintings of ruined Gothic castles situated on the
mountainous crests of the Welsh landscape. In many of these
paintings peaceful rural scenes occur in the foreground contrasting
starkly with the warlike remains of the castle ramparts in the
distance.[44] The closest in spirit to Jago's poem is that of the landscape
around the primitive hilltop fort of Dinas Bran (1770-71). The
landscape depicted was the property of the Williams Wynn family of
Wynstay and the painting became a possession of this family. In the
foreground Wilson shows an attractive young woman chatting with
two agricultural labourers one of whom chops at a fallen tree. We
can, perhaps, see in this woman approaching two strong men with
axes the visual evidence of the security of modern times, for she has
nothing to fear of them. The Fort of Dinas Bran on the hilltop which
dominates the scene reminds the viewer of more violent times when
such an encounter would have been impossible. As in Jago's poetic
world, the safty of the potentially vulnerable individual is evidence of
the prosperity of the modern landscape.

Whilst this painting depicts a landscape geographically distant
from Jago's Warwickshire, it is not altogether unlinked. Dr King,
who was Sanderson Miller's mentor, was also a close acquaintance of
the high Tory Williams Wynn family.[45] Watkin Williams Wynn the
elder was a senior member of the Oxford Jacobite circle which
Sanderson Miller entered as a student. King, in fact, supplied the
inscription for the monument to Sir Watkin William Wynn the elder
(died 1749) which is in the church at Ruabon. The poetic and
painted images of modern rural peace existing in the shadow of
prospect points reminiscent of ancient wars share a Tory agenda. It is
a hospitable Tory peace which shades these lands. A conservative
tendency, not peculiar to Toryism but characteristic of it, has ensured
the preservation of the physical evidence of past conflict and

violence. The effect of preserving such war-like ruins was to provide a majestic contrast with the secure modern Arcadia which such landlords believed they had constructed within their estates.

There was a long tradition of the figure of the traveller in the landscape acting as a sort of indicator of health and prosperity of the scene. An early example of this convention can be found in Ambrogio Lorenzetti's frescoes of *Good and Bad Government* in Siena's Palazzo Publico (1344) in which the quality of rule is illustrated by four landscapes, two urban and two rural, demonstrating the effects of governance upon the physical environment. A road runs through the rural scene of good government where travellers wander safely through a scene of agricultural plenty: this road in the scene of bad government is largely deserted, except for a few poor souls who run from violence amongst a sea of rank weeds.

In eighteenth-century England, the experience of the traveller was conventionally considered to be the clearest indicator of the historical progress of the nation. Travellers in their passage through the landscape were the natural witnesses of the progress and decadence of the state. The speed, comfort and security of progress through the landscape was itself indicative of the progress of civilisation. One seldom turns to a piece of eighteenth-century tour literature – whether in manuscript or published form or concerning foreign or indigenous travel – that does not have something to say on the subject of social progress. Whilst this is no place to review the immense range of opinion, it will suffice to say that there were those, particularly individuals of nostalgic turn of mind caught up in the study of chivalry, heraldry and medieval remains, who saw little in their travels that did not remind them that national civilisation was not as grand as it used to be.[46] These were the objects of George Lipscombe's criticism when, in the quotation cited above, he exalted at the passing of an 'age of chivalry'.

Travellers such as Jago, and afterward Lipscombe, found in the very exercise of their freedom to roam and to view the landscape a sort of ritual reminder of their modern liberties. Improvements in the quality of paths and roadways enabled travel to become a pleasure and allowed curious citizens to take to the road to inspect for themselves the state of the body politic as manifested in its disparate geographical members. It is no coincidence that the genre of travel literature cast up two of the most enthusiastic polemics of national improvement produced in England in the eighteenth century. Daniel Defoe's *Tour Through the Whole Island of Great Britain* and Arthur Young's *A Six Months Tour*, rightly feature as classic works in the canon of European literature associated with the Enlightenment faith in progress. Part of the rationale for the therapeutics of travel through the supposedly 'improved' landscape of eighteenth-century England was that it instilled that sense of well-being which grew from the visual reassurance that the world was becoming a better place. It is that characteristic mid-eighteenth-century travellers' confidence in the 'smiling' and 'healthy' face of the modern world that dominates Jago's view of the pathology of the landscape as seen from Edge Hill.

Jago is at his clearest on the subject of national progress when, in the third book, he enters a substantial digression on mining and the iron industry of Birmingham, a town just visible on the horizon. At this point he anticipates the confidence of Lipscombe when he claimed that 'the softer virtues of science' laid the path of human progress. Jago's theme is how the toil and physical discomfort of industry lies behind the rural idyll of modern England. He cannot resist waxing lyrical on the steel ploughs of Birmingham turning the soil of the Warwickshire landscape. Alighting on the theme of mining, Jago returns to his pathological metaphors. In his main professional capacity as a Birmingham cleric the poet was moved by Christian compassion to dwell upon the sacrifice of the miners who tunnelled unseen, for the sake of others' prosperity, beneath the scene of rural plenty. The world beneath ground is the exact inverse of that above which is healthy by virtue of free circulation of air, and shafts of light. The miners, Jago reflects:

Of sun's cheering light, and genial warmth.
And oft, a chilling damp of unctuous rust,
Loos'd from the crumbling caverns, issues forth,
Stooping the spring of life.[47]

The poet's conscience concerning the prosperous modern world's debt to such subterranean miseries, is, however, quickly appeased by the reflection that new technology was easing conditions of labour. He turns exultantly to praise for the Queen's physician Dr Stephen Hales, described as 'illustrious Hales', who had invented ventilation machines which, although first intended to increase the flow of air through hospitals, were being put to use in mining. Hales, Jago claims, released miners from the 'foul imprisoned air' bringing 'charity to the sickening crowd' who formerly had been robbed of 'nature's balmy draughts'.[48]

That Jago should choose the ventilation machine as an emblem of human progress conformed with his general tendency to read the landscape as a bodily system sustained in health and condemned to

141

disease through the circulation of elements. By the ministrations of patriotic Englishmen – underground, Stephen Hales and, above ground, a host of supposedly genial landlords – the circulatory system of the modern nation was maintained. It was upon their schemes of social therapeutics that the progress of English state towards optimal health was founded.

Slightly earlier in the text Jago had extolled the virtues of another instrument of modern science, the telescope. This device, the poet maintains, assists mankind in achieving progress by liberating it from the constraints of its primitive passions. The discussion of the telescope is part of a wider discourse on the nature and politics of visual perception. In the second book of the poem Jago equated the view from a hilltop with a state of liberty. He describes the roaming of his 'unimprisoned eye' which surveys with 'pleasing freedom' so delighted by the variety of things to see as to be relieved from all constraints of 'dull satiety'.[49]

When debating these ideas further in book three, Jago turned his attention to the philosophic discourse on the relationship between the working of the inner vision or 'imagination' and the operations of the eye and of artificial lenses. The ideas expressed here were by no means original; they had been most fully elucidated in Mark Akenside's then famous poem *The Pleasures of the Imagination* (first published 1741). They are, none the less, interesting for the circumstances of their application. Jago talks of the imagination as a force which is difficult to constrain by reason. He describes it as a liminal condition of mind, a state between a sleeper's dream and wakeful thought. The imagination can, the poet argues, be affected by fever, bringing about a delirium, or 'frenzy', in which the sufferer oscilates uncontrollably between 'disease and health'.[50] The eyes, by contrast, are described as clarifying mechanisms which naturally seek out the steady truth of perception. The healthy eye, clear and watery, is itself depicted as a liberation from the fetid confusion that is likely to hang around in the far reaches of the human fancy. Jago reflects with wonder upon:

> The curious structure of these visual orbs,
> The windows of the mind, substance how clear,
> Aqueous, or crystalline; through which the soul,
> As thro' a glass all outward things survey.[51]

So it is that the poet proceeds to reflect with equal wonder upon the telescope, that most treasured instrument of the topographer, cartographer and view-seeking tourist. In the clear lenses of such devices he finds an even stronger impression of the truth of nature. The clear vision of the world seen through a telescope becomes the complete healthy alternative to the fevered illusions of the imagination. The telescope is considered the instrument of reason and of liberty. Looking through this clarifying mechanism is part of the healthy experience of tourism for it is seen as a curative to the rise of the licentious imagination which is held to signify diseased states of mind. The beauty of the telescope was that it sharpened a sense, the visual sense, at the expense of the passions which existed in dangerous alliance with the imagination.[52] To give free range to the passions and imagination was thought potentially hazardous to man and society; but giving free range to a sense such as sight could be considered only beneficial. By assuming a wide survey of the world, assisting his eye in its natural and healthy search for 'liberty', the citizen widened the scope of reason and in so doing brought about the progress of society.

The scene of a traveller dwelling upon conceptions of the liberty of the eye when finding himself at a vantage point is not unique to Jago's *Edge-Hill.* It also occurs in the aforementioned *Dialogue* on the subject of travel which was published along with William Gilpin's guide to Stowe gardens. In this text two visitors to Stowe who are engaged in a conversation on the philosophy of travel finally reach the highest point on the estate from which they resolve to reflect on the view. On this vantage point they find the 'gothic' Temple of Saxon Liberty which Cobham had erected some years before. This Temple, created in honour of the Ancient political liberties of the Englishman, is immediately recognised by the travellers as a natural place to debate the 'liberty' of vision. One of them observes that:

> The eye naturally loves liberty, and when it is in quest of prospects, will not rest content with the most beautiful dispositions of Art, confined within a narrow compass but (as soon as the novelty of sight is over), will begin to grow dissatisfied, till the whole limits of the horizon be given it to roam through.

The reference to the search of the eye for variety beyond the reach of art relates to an eighteenth-century debate which may need some elucidation. The debate between these fictive visitors to Stowe had its roots in Addison's reflections upon the mechanisms of taste, aired in his *Spectator* essays. In his essay for June 23 1723, Addison argued that the human drive for aesthetic satisfaction ultimately derived from the need to satiate a natural thirst for novel experience. In Addison's view, the healthy and natural mind was that which continually sought the stimulation of some object of art as yet not invented or sight beyond the immediate horizon:

> Our imagination loves to be filled with an object, or to grasp at anything that is too big for its capacity. We are flung into a pleasing astonishment at such unbounded views, and feel a delightful stillness and amazement in the soul at the apprehension of them. The mind of man naturally hates every thing that looks like a restraint upon it, and is apt to fancy itself at a sort of confinement, when the sight is pent up in a narrow compass, and shortened on every side by the neighbourhood of walls or mountains. On the contrary, a spacious horizon is an image of liberty, where the eye has room to expiate at large on the immensity of its views, and to lose itself amidst the variety of objects that offer themselves to its observation.

The search of the traveller for a point from which his eyes could exercise with liberty was, in the Addisonian tradition, considered a sign of that individual's healthy desire for aesthetic refreshment.[53] This process could be compared, and the construction of 'gothic' viewpoints certainly encouraged this comparison, to the natural search of the citizen for political liberty. The quest for the origins of political 'liberty', as Cobham implied in his decision to place his 'gothic' Temple of Liberty upon a view point, could be satisfied not simply by looking out into the modern world, but by looking back in time. It was in seeking out the lessons of history, in particular at Stowe the trials of the Saxon forbears, that the quest for liberty could be satiated. Finding the distant roots of liberty required a historical imagination as clear in its vision, and earnest in its curiosity, as a healthy and curious eye in search for beauty in the wide and various landscape. The search of the political mind for liberty was considered as natural and healthy as the search of the aesthetic sensibilities for beauty.

Eighteenth-century 'gothic' buildings situated on viewpoints are all too often described by architectural historians as 'follies', a word which implies an absence of meaning and purpose. It is, however, the interpretations of this architecture rather than the architecture itself that have been vacuous. It would be difficult to prove that every eighteenth-century 'gothic' viewpoint was designed by individuals cognizant of philosophic debates on the ethics of sight and processes of history; a number of such buildings, however, clearly have sophisticated meanings.

One function of such buildings may well have been to symbolise the political spirit of independence, an attribute commonly associated in mid-eighteenth-century political rhetoric with the concept of liberty. Independence was a virtue of mind exalted by 'country' politicians and landowners, proud of their ability to exist without falling into some faction at Westminster. It is not a coincidence that many of the earliest 'gothic' towers or temples on view points were erected on the estates of families accustomed to taking an oppositionist or independent line in national politics. One can cite as an introduction: Lord Strafford's ruined castle viewpoint at Stainborough on his estates of Wentworth Castle, George Lyttleton's 'gothic' ruin at Hagley (designed by Sanderson Miller); Lord Cobham's Temple of Liberty at Stowe, and, of course, Sanderson Miller's towers at Edge Hill.[54]

One can see in these rustic structures projecting out from high points in the landscape a rude sign to a world which would threaten this independence. Gothic architecture, criticised by the proponents of classicism as a rude (as in uncultivated) form of building, was a highly appropriate medium for such gestures. It is reported Sanderson Miller exhibited on his staircase at Radway a print of the 'gothic' tower of his own design which had been erected on a vantage point at Wimpole in Cambridgeshire.[55] The print bore the following inscription:

> On towers such as these Earl, Baron, Vavasour,
> Hung high their banners floating to the air.
> Free, hardy, proud they braved their feudal lord
> And tried their rights by ordeal of sword.
> Now the full board with Xmas plenty crowned
> Now ravaged and oppressed the country round.
> Yet freedom's cause once raised the civil broil
> And Magna Charta closed the glorious toil.

Miller implies that, when erecting 'towers such as these', modern landlords were imitating their forbears who dared to be independent for the sake of constitutional liberties. These towers can be construed as the watch towers of liberty. To those in the countryside looking up towards them they were a symbol of the local landlord's independence. For those looking out from them they were a vantage from which to inspect the degree to which respect for liberty and constitutional rights was manifested in the landscape.

Lines five and six of this poem are the most problematic. Here is discussed the Gothic 'baron's' dual reputation for having 'crowned' their tables with 'Xmas plenty' and having 'ravaged and oppressed the country round'. The anonymous poet seems to couple a reference to those aspects of the Gothic past which merited nostalgia with a reference those aspects which were to be deplored. The Gothic forbears are seen to be at once hospitable and savage. The passing of the tradition of civic violence was to be applauded as much as the decline of Gothic hospitality was to be lamented. What modern English society had gained in its achievement of civilised peace it had lost in the passing of that lusty, primitive, sense of community which was considered to define the Gothic world.

The appeal of Gothic hospitality to the eighteenth-century imagination, in particular the Tory imagination, relates directly to the English cultural preoccupation with luxury that has been documented by John Sekora.[56] Occasional feasting, piling the tables with Christmas plenty for a great community meal, could be regarded as a morally satisfying form of sensual celebration: it was an indulgence of the community rather than the individual: an alternative to the appetite for self-indulgence that characterised the increase of luxury. Whereas the personal pampering associated with luxury was the source of effeminacy and the diseases of excess, Gothic hospitality was virile and healthy. The legend of Gothic hospitality satisfied that tendency in the mid-eighteenth-century culture of sociability to regard the outward-looking man as healthy and natural. In the structuring a literary fiction of virile hospitable Gothic ancestors, the culture of sociability found a sort of 'origins myth' in which a primitive national tendency for hearty conviviality was celebrated.

Nostalgia amongst eighteenth-century landlords, in particular those of a Tory persuasion, for the tradition then known as 'old English hospitality' is of great importance to the study of tourism in this period. The understanding that there was an ancient tradition of this type which was part of the history of the English landscape was a spur to landlords to keep an open gate for travellers. It was modern landlords' respect for this traditional ideal of hospitality that lay behind Jago's sense of belonging to, and well-being within, the countryside around Edge Hill. Respect for this ideal of hospitality, in all probability, lay behind Miller's decision to build a welcoming path to his Gothic vantage point. It would have been a manifest travesty of the values of liberty and hospitality to which this Gothic landscape feature was dedicated had the land around not been publicly accessible.

The subject of public accessibility returns us to the debate on circulation and health. One way of understanding the function of a traveller in the landscape was as a kind of witness to good management of the land. Thus, it could be construed that the

circulation of genteel and patriotic travellers, like that of air, water
and light, had some therapeutic value for the landscape. Enabling the
movement of travellers through estates was, therefore, regarded by
many as a defining characteristic of good husbandry. The first Duke
of Montagu, an individual with a wide reputation for philanthropy,
went to great effort to fit out his estates at Boughton in
Northamptonshire with gates that could be opened from horseback
and paths which allowed for easy ridings through his estates. After his
death he received considerable public praise in a national newspaper
for so doing.[57]

By contrast, owners who were hostile to travellers, and tried to
prevent the world looking in at their land, were often regarded as
individuals who had something to hide. A certain amount of social
prejudice was brought to bear on this issue. There were some who
associated the closure of land to travellers with the ways of 'new men'
from the city who bought up estates without having any appreciation
of the traditions of old English hospitality of which the more
established landlords had a natural grasp. William Bray in his *Sketch
of a Tour of Derbyshire and Yorkshire* (published 1783) recalls a
comment by Arthur Young on Wentworth Castle:

> Mr Young concludes by properly acknowledging the true politeness
> of Lord and Lady Strafford in permitting strangers to have easy
> access to a sight of this place and execrates, as everyone must do, the
> insolent pride of nabobs and contractors; who accidentally
> becoming possessed of fine seats refuse that gratification to all those
> that are not of their present acquaintance.[58]

It is not a coincidence that Wentworth Castle had, on the summit of
its landscape gardens at Stainborough, a 'gothic' castle viewpoint
which had been built in the 1730s under the command of the first
Earl Strafford. The builder of Stainborough Castle was at the time of
its construction in the vanguard of the House of Lords' opposition to
the administration of Robert Walpole. Here also, therefore, the
notion of liberty of viewing and the architecture of the ancient
struggle for liberty seems to have been combined. Members of
ancient families, who could be expected to understand the traditions
of 'old English hospitality', were also those who saw the benefits in
giving 'liberty' to the public eye.

The association of ancient country families with hospitable
freedom of viewing is most strongly expressed in a monument in the
'gothic' style erected at Lullingstone Castle in Kent at approximately
the same time as Miller was designing his gardens at Edge Hill. The

monument, which is constructed of stucco and probably designed by
Henry Keene, was erected against the east wall of the monumental
chapel of Lullingstone church (Fig. 1).[59] The church itself stands
approximately a hundred yards from the door of the house. In order
to gothicise its general atmosphere the name of the house was, at
about the same time as the erection of the monument, changed to
'Lullingstone Castle'. The probable date of the monument is
c.1755.[60] Like the tower at Edge Hill, this monument is certainly an
expression of Tory values and probably an emblem of Jacobitism.
Under the ownership of the principal person commemorated in the
monument, Sir Percyvall Harte (died November 1738), a 'sub-rosa'
room was made in the house in honour of the last Stuart monarch,
Queen Anne, in which secret toasts to the Pretender were made.[61]

The monument commemorated not only an individual but also
a dynasty. Percyvall Harte died without male heir leaving his estates
to the heirs of his son-in-law, Sir Thomas Dyke. It was the
representatives of the Dykes who, in honour to the ancient family
that had become extinct in the direct male line, erected what is
effectively a wall of heraldic devices in a 'gothic' frame. These devices

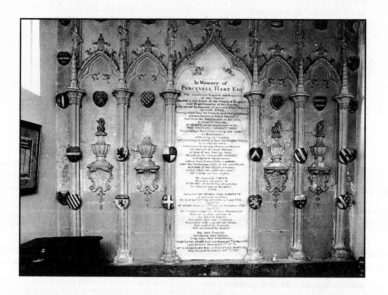

Figure 1.
Stucco monument to the Harte family,
Lullingstone Castle, Kent, c. 1755

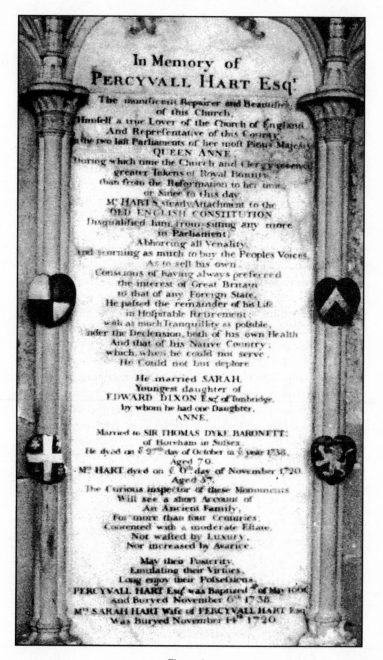

Figure 2.
Detail.

and the 'gothic' architecture were witness to the antiquity of the family in an era when, it was widely supposed, 'new men' with no claim to family or tradition were overtaking the countryside within a day's ride of London. The monument can be interpreted as a symbol of resistance to a threatening world not dissimilar to that of Sanderson Miller's imagined 'gothic' towers with their heraldic banners declaring abroad the independence and ancient traditions of their owners. The continuing health of the 'family tree' may well be symbolised in the curling tendrils of growth which can be observed in one of the upper sections of the monument. Gothic architecture was derived, according to architectural theorists of the day, from primitive imitations of linking arches of arboreal foliage. This was but one example of many 'gothic' designs of the era which were intended to emphasis the robust grandeur of this primitive style.[62] The imagery of this monument is one of virile primitive abundance; a phenomenon which was intended to contrast starkly with the notion of modern luxury, the degenerative origin of the sickness of civilisation.

Ancient virility, as preserved in the tradition of hearty English hospitality, is the main theme of the monument at Lullingstone. Virile Gothic architectural members act as a frame for a eulogy upon the traditional vigour of the body politic as enshrined in the primitive 'constitution'. At the centre of the inscription is the claim that Harte died in enforced retirement from public politics where he resolved, in 'hospitable retirement', to support the values of the 'OLD ENGLISH CONSTITUTION'. The final passage of the inscription is a direct address to the traveller or 'curious inspector':

> The curious inspector of this monument
> Will see a short account of
> An Ancient family
> For more than for centuries
> Contented with a moderate estate
> Nor wasted by luxury
> Nor increased by Avarice
>
> May their posterity
> Emulating their virtues
> Long enjoy their possessions

Part of the wit of this monument is that, although it is Gothic in style, it borrows directly from classical tradition. The whole idea of erecting an inscription in the countryside with a direct evocation to the passer-by was, as we have already seen, Roman. This inscription, like that composed by Mark Akenside for a column at Runymede, seems to gothicise the classical tradition of using roadside monuments to bring sobering philosophy to the traveller. The traveller, however, is called upon to do more than learn from his experience. He is invited to act as mobile witness to the good management of the estates.

The 'curious inspector' of these Kent estates, as the witness to the 'hospitable' traditions of the family, has a role in ensuring the healthy moderation which, it was believed, guaranteed the long life of a dynasty on the land. The traveller is asked to inspect, like a doctor ensuring that his patient keeps a healthy diet, the physical condition of the family lands for signs of whether they are being 'wasted' or 'increased'.[63] As hospitality was conceived as a sort of antidote to luxury, the very presence of the traveller in the landscape was thought of as a check to excess. Much as Jago in his view of the landscape is the admirer of all that is moderate, the patriotic 'inspector' of Lullingstone is considered a force of moderation within the scene of rural life.

The patriotic traveller could be expected not only to observe the state of the body politic in its localities but also to act as a form of guarantor of the continued health of the landscape. Theirs was a therapeutic as well as observatory role, shaping as well as monitoring the condition of the landscape. The construction of view points such as Edge Hill allowed the body politic to be observed. Through being observed, the prospects of this body remaining healthy were improved. Landlords such as Miller and Cobham who actively encouraged travellers to exert the liberty of their eyes were the declared inverse of those 'tyrants', ancient and modern, who closed up the land to the patriotic gaze. Since the very idea of the prospect was emblematic of liberty and health, it was reasonable to assume that the building of such view points could be considered a patriotic as well as a philanthropic act. Constitutional walks to the summits of hills were considered to have benefits for the public as well as the personal constitution. The image of the patriotic traveller taking up his vantage in a state of ease and security was, in itself, a powerful emblem of the health of the landscape.

If Jago's *Edge-Hill* can be said to have a single prevailing theme it is that of the moral virtues of properties of outwardness and openness. These properties are, of course, symbolically enshrined in the idea of the wide view. Open hospitality, political liberty, unencumbered sight, free passage of elements, and the poet's healthy passage through the scented paths of Edge Hill are the symbols of ultimate well-being. The sickness of the landscape is manifest in all that is inverse to these properties. The traveller's tendency to pathologise the world through which he passes is a central idea, if not *the* central idea, of Jago's poetic narrative.

Notes

1. A useful introduction to the expansion of indigenous tourism within England is Ian Ousby's *The Englishman's England: Taste, Travel and the Rise of Tourism* (Cambridge: 1990).

2. Notions of the health benefits of ascending hills have been preserved through the fame of Constitution Hill, a prospect point on the outskirts of London from which the city was traditionally viewed. The Hill had acquired its name by the mid-eighteenth century.

3. For a further discussion of these issues see Jonathan Andrews' article in this volume.

4. Many of the letters exchanged by Jago and Shenstone are printed in D. Mallam (ed.), *The Letters of William Shenstone* (University of Minesota Press: 1939).

5. J.J. Cartwright (ed.), *The Travels Through England of Dr Richard Pococke*, Camden Soc. new ser. 42-44 (Edinburgh: 1888); and G. Lipscombe, *A Journey into South Wales* (London: 1802) (Lipscombe visited Edge Hill on his way home).

6. J. Brewer, *The Pleasures of the Imagination* (London: 1997), Chapter sixteen, *Culture, Nature and Nation*, in particular, 632-4.

7. Jago, *Edge-Hill*, Book 1, lines 31-5.

8. Miller's tower to the parish church of Wroxton which was designed for Lord North collapsed in 1748, within a year of its initial construction, to the detriment of his reputation as a builder.

9. A letter from Charles Lyttleton to Sanderson Miller reveals the latter's role in gathering subscriptions for the poem: see L. Dickins and M. Stanton, *An Eighteenth-century Correspondence* (London: 1910), 178.

10. The great majority of mid-eighteenth-century maps and travel routes place strong emphasis on marking boundaries between estates and naming the owners of major tracts of property.

11. Jago explicitly cites Alexander Calcott's, *A Treatise on the Deluge* (London: 1768); many of his other ideas on geology are directly borrowed from Dr Woodward without direct reference.

12. Jago, *op. cit.*, vi.

13. Jago, *ibid.*, Book 1, line 430.

14. W. Gilpin, *A Dialogue upon the Gardens of the Right Honourable the*

Lord Viscount Cobham at Stowe in Buckinghamshire (Buckingham: 1749). (The dialogue has no page numbers).

15 Jago, *op. cit.*, Book 1, Lines 441-5.

16 These comments appear in the introduction to Campbell's book, 8-9.

17 A. Pope, *Windsor Forest*, lines 37-43.

18 The political controversy concerning Dr King's speech is best studied through a publication entitled, *A Translation of a celebrated oration (on the dedication of the Radcliffe Library by William King) Occasioned by a libel (by J. Burton) entiled Remarks on Dr K-g's speech, with a seasonable introduction* (London: 1750).

19 A printed edition of the letters was produced by Lilian Dickins and Mary Stanton entitled *An Eighteenth-century Correspondence,* (London: 1910). This is unfortunately a heavily edited text and many surviving letters in the collection are not printed. Those interested in the political and artistic career of Sanderson Miller are advised to consult the original letters and papers in Warwickshire Record Office.

20 For details of these ceremonies see L. Dickins, *The History of Radway* (Shipston-on-Stour: 1937), 174.

21 M. Warnke, *Political Landscape, the art history of nature* (London: 1994), chapter six, 'Political Nature Imagery'.

22 Jago, *op. cit.*, Book 1, Lines 57-8.

23 For Miller's policy of enclosure, see A.C. Wood, *Sanderson Miller of Radway and his Work at Wroxton* (Banbury: 1969).

24 Miller's will (PCC. 1780, 326) states that his 'old tenents' should 'have such good bargains as may be sufficient encouragement to manage the land in an husbandlike manner, being well convinced that the racking of land tenents too hard is as great a prejudice to the landlord as it is to the tenent.'

25 Jago, *op. cit.*, Book 1, Lines 365-77.

26 *Ibid.,* Book 1, lines 384-421.

27 *Ibid.,* Book 4, lines 279-85.

28 *Ibid.,* Book 4, lines 290-6.

29 The close relationship between conditions of mania and melancholia is discussed in R. Porter, *Mind Forged Manacles* (London: 1990), 46.

30 Pope, *op. cit.*, lines 44-5.

31 Jago, *op. cit.*, Book 4, lines 570-3.

32 The classic texts concerning British views on the state of the Roman countryside are J. Moore, *A View of the Society and Manners of Italy* (2 vols, London: 1795), in particular vol. 1, 333, and S. Sharp, *Letters from Italy describing the Customs and Manners of that Country in the Year 1765 and 1766* (London: 1766), in particular 44-5 & 69.

33 The movement to promote indigenous travel as a rival to the Grand
    Tour was well progressed by the 1720s when William Stukeley in his
    *Itinerarium Curiousum: An Account of the Antiquitys and Remarkable
    Curiousitys in Nature and Art, Observ'd in Travels thro' Great Brittan*
    (London: 1724) complained that 'our country lies neglected' as
    noblemen flocked to the Continent to complete their educations.
34 Shenstone to Jago, June 10, 1754 printed in Mallam., *op. cit.*, 98.
35 W. Shenstone, *Essays on Men and Manners* (London: 1884), Essay
    XXIII.
36 For my own introduction to the topic of *banditti* and highway crime
    in European Art see M. Craske, *Art in Europe,* (London: 1997),
    chapter two. For a defence of Italian culture against the accusation
    that it was a world ruled by assassins see Baretti's, *An Account of the
    Manners and Customs of Italy* (2 vols, London: 1768), i, 52-3.
37 Jago, *op. cit.*, Book 1, lines 23-4.
38 A complete text of this poem appears in M. Akenside, *The Poems of
    Mark Akenside MD* (London: 1772), 297-8.
39 Anon., *Ode to Lansdowne Hill* (London: 1786). The only extant
    copy of this verse is preserved in Cambridge University Library.
40 A description of this monument including a full transcript of
    inscriptions can be found in the *Gentleman's Magazine*, 1752, 257.
41 The death of this guide is recorded in the *London Evening Post*,
    October 20, 1737.
42 An introduction to the career of Lord Lansdowne may be had in E.
    Handysyde, *Granville the Polite, the Life of George Granville Lord
    Lansdowne 1666-1735* (London: 1933)
43 Good examples of this genre of political digression can be found in
    R. Warner, *A Companion in a Tour to Lymington* (London: 1789),
    221, and George Lipscombe's *A Journey into South Wales* (London:
    1802), 257-61.
44 Wilson's paintings of this type include: *Pembroke Castle and Town &
    Carnaervon Castle*, National Museum of Wales.
45 Watkin Williams Wynn, the father of the purchaser of this painting,
    was one of the executors of Dr Radcliffe. Dying before the opening
    of the Camera, he was eulogised by Dr King in his great 'restore'
    speech.
46 For travel literature stressing reactions against progress see R.
    Warner, *A Walk through Wales* (London: 1792).
47 Jago, *op. cit.*, Book 3, lines 438-43.
48 *Ibid.*, Book 3, lines 444-58.
49 *Ibid.*, Book 1, lines 455-8.
50 *Ibid.*, Book 3, line 24.

51 *Ibid.*, Book 3, lines 29-33.

52 *Ibid.,* Book 3, lines 70-82.

53 Jago, significantly, placed a quotation from Addison's commentaries on vision and variety, drawn from the *Spectator* essays, on the fly leaf of the first edition of the poem.

54 The first Earl Strafford was a regular voter against Walpolian policies in the House of Lords during the 1730s. Lord Cobham was, of course, a major figure in the opposition. George Lyttleton was part of Cobham's opposition faction and noted for his oppositionist publications, in particular the *Persian Letters.* After the fall of Walpole he oscillated in and out of opposition.

55 This print and verse are recorded in Dickins and Stanton, *op. cit.*, 273.

56 J. Sekora, *Luxury: the Concept in Western Thought* (Baltimore: 1977).

57 *The London Chronicle*, 1765, February 15, 180.

58 W. Bray, *Sketch of a Tour of Derbyshire and Yorkshire* (London: 1783), 256.

59 I consider that this monument was constructed by Keene on the basis of a strong similarity of the workmanship and that of 'gothic' stucco monuments within Hartwell church in Buckinghamshire, the latter being designed for the Lee family into which the Dyke family married during this period.

60 Stained glass in the church can be accurately dated to 1754, the period in which work was in progress at Hartwell. Restorations were conducted under the direction of Sir Thomas Dyke who died in August 1756. Antiquarian commentators much admired the restorations. See E. Hasted, *The History and Topographical Survey of the County of Kent* (4 vols, Canterbury: 1778-99), i, 314 & J. Thorpe, *Registrum Rofense* (London: 1769), 1042-4.

61 Relics of Jacobite toasting rituals still exist in the house, as well as a fine stucco portrait of Queen Anne, the last Stuart monarch, above the fireplace of the room where 'sub-rosa' drinking rituals were held. This stucco portrait was probably made by the same team who constructed the monument from the same material. Thomas Dyke was considered as a Tory candidate for Oxford in 1737 and was an opposition candidate for the Free and Independant Electors of Westminster.

62 A useful compendium of fascinating designs on the theme of the primitive in Gothic architecture appear in T. Wright, *Universal Architecture, Book I, Six Original Designs for Arbours* (London: 1755) ills. D & C, and T. Wright, *Universal Architecture, Book II, Six Original Designs for Grottos* (London: 1758), ills. I & M.

63 Regimes of abstemious dieting were a common eighteenth-century

remedy recommended by many highly respected physicians. The popularity of such diets was, in part, based upon the supposition that rich foods were a main enemy to health in a society bombarded by new luxuries. The most notable advocate of dieting was George Cheyne, who in his *English Malady* (London: 1733), makes firm connections between luxury and modern disease. The particular concern of the 'luxury debate' within this family relates to the first marriage of Lady Anne Harte, later Dyke, to John Bluett, the author of a notable attack on Mandeville's *The Fable of the Bees*, the central philosophical defence of luxury.

4

'The Rime of the Ancient Mariner', a Ballad of the Scurvy

Jonathan Lamb

There have been roughly four eras in the reception of 'The Rime of the Ancient Mariner.'[1] In the first the poem was thought unintelligible, a cock and bull story in verse. The second saw the elaboration of various allegorical readings that traced the original sin of the birdslayer through the phases of its forgiveness. The third arose from applying post-Freudian and poststructuralist theories of the uncanny to the poem, and produced a mariner in the grip of the compulsion to repeat his unteachable tale. The last is the postcolonial reading which, following William Empson's hint ('It is about adventure and discovery; it celebrates and epitomises the maritime expansion of the Europeans'[2]), is still investigating the mariner's complicity in the slave trade. The purpose of this essay is to avoid allegory altogether, and to combine elements of the third and fourth readings into an explanation of the first.

Of the first edition of the *Lyrical Ballads* Coleridge believed the greater part 'had been sold to seafaring men, who having heard of the Ancient Mariner, concluded that it was a naval song-book, or, at all events, that it had some relation to nautical matters'.[3] If this wasn't an example of disingenuous retrospection, and Coleridge really believed there was something in the ballad that might appeal to sailors, the nautical matters of the 'Rime' would fall, as Empson points out, into the categories of adventure and discovery rather than of trade and settlement. Although the mariner may anticipate the means by which 'Western European society has sought to imprint its imperial and slave-owning image on the New World',[4] in the course of his voyage he makes no landfall and he does not traffic. He appears to have gone on a journey for no definite purpose, rather like William Dampier and Woodes Rogers in their privateering cruises through the Pacific, where a treasure ship was to be hoped for but not relied upon. Indeed it is on such a cruise that the poem was loosely based, George Shelvocke's *A Voyage round the World by way of the Great South Sea*

(1726). According to Wordsworth, who remembered how he and Coleridge were short of money for a projected walking tour, and how they planned to write some verse for a quick sale, including a ballad of a sailor who kills a bird, the hint was taken directly from Shelvocke's account: 'I had been reading in Shelvocke's *Voyages* a day or two before that, while doubling Cape Horn, they frequently saw albatrosses in that latitude, the largest sort of sea-fowl, some extending their wings twelve or thirteen feet. "Suppose", said I, "you represent him as having killed one of these birds on entering the South Sea, and that the tutelary spirits of these regions take upon them to avenge the crime."'[5]

As it happens Wordsworth was indebted to Shelvocke for the whole idea. His entry into the Pacific Ocean was remembered like this:

> In short, one would think it impossible that any thing living could subsist in so rigid a climate; and, indeed, we all observed, that we had not had the sight of one fish of any kind, since we were come to the Southward of the streights of Le Mair, no one sea-bird, except a disconsolate black Albitross, who accompanied us for several days, hovering us as if he had lost himself, till Hatley, (my second Captain) observing, in one of his melancholy fits, that this bird was always hovering near us, imagin'd, from his colour, that it might be some ill omen. That which, I suppose, induced him the more to encourage his superstition, was the continued series of contrary tempestuous winds, which oppress'd us ever since we had got into this sea. But be that as it would, he, after some fruitless attempts, at length, shot the Albitross, not doubting (perhaps) that we would have a fair wind after it. I must own, that this navigation is truly melancholy, and was the more so to us, who were by ourselves without a companion.[6]

The dejection of the crew, Simon Hatley in particular, was well known on this run. Johann Reinhold Forster, who also shot an albatross in these Antarctic waters (*diomedea palpebrata*, or the sooty albatross), told of the mood in which he did it, a gloom unrelieved by the tedium of 'water, Ice & Sky': 'I put on a good face, & wanted to shew a mind superior to all these inconveniences ... but had my Shipmates had a Sight of my most private thoughts, they would have me found widely different, from what I wanted to appear.'[7] At the same point in the voyage Forster reports: 'We now have several people, that have some scorbutic symptoms, which prove a Scurvy that is gone pretty far viz. Bad Gums, livid Spots, Eruptions, difficult breathing, contracted limbs, & a greenish greasy Scum on the

Urine'.[8] Among the symptoms of scurvy he could have listed his feelings of private woe, as it was a well-known accompaniment of the disease. Scurvy was no doubt responsible for the melancholy that reached such extremes on Shelvocke's ship that it caused Dodd, his lieutenant of marines, 'to act the mad-man' in a fit of real or feigned lunacy.[9] Although Shelvocke never talks about scurvy, it was rife on his ship, the *Speedwell*, and on his consort, the *Success*, whose provisions he was carrying but with whom he refused to rendez-vous, they were desperate with the disease, and the mariners cursed him as they died of it.[10]

There were two routes carrying Coleridge towards a knowledge of scurvy and the composition of a ballad that might have had at least symptomatic appeal to sailors. The first was his interest in maritime literature, especially accounts of the South Seas; the second was his friendship with Thomas Beddoes. The circumnavigations of the Elizabathan mariners, Drake and Hawkins, which Coleridge found in Purchas, provided him with images for his poem, including the iridescence of the watersnakes, as John Livingston Lowes has pointed out in *The Road to Xanadu* (1927). Lowes also traces the extensive contributions made by Cook's second voyage to the imagery of the poem, particularly the accounts of phosphorescence and the *aurora australis* given in Cook's *A Voyage to the Pacific Ocean* (1784) and in George Forster's *A Voyage Round the World* (1777). In an article of 1956, recently republished in his *Imagining the Pacific* (1992), Bernard Smith has refined Lowes' insight into the importance of Cook's second voyage to Coleridge.[11] Beginning with the fact that the young poet was taught mathematics at Christ's Hospital by William Wales, the astronomer on the *Resolution*, Smith brings a good deal of evidence to bear on the likelihood that Wales' interest in atmospheric phenomena sensitised the young poet to the beauty of clouds and stars. He also supposes that Wales would have told vivid stories of the search for the Great Southern Continent, when Cook took his ship as close as he could to the icefloes of Antarctica to find this mysterious land, and the crew could hear the thunder of the icebergs splitting, and notice the unearthly sheen of their fantastic shapes. Smith closes the circle opened by Lowes when he shows that the 'rotting deep' first observed by Hawkins was noted also by Wales and Johann Reinhold Forster, who both argued that phosphorescence owes its beauty to the state of high putridity of an ocean affected by a long period of calm weather.[12]

Omitted from these detailed inspections of the traces of Coleridge's ideas of the South Seas is scurvy, and yet it is tangential to almost all the examples cited. It was the peril of all South Seas voyages because of the distances ships had to travel between landfalls, where, without a means of calculating the longitude, it was hard to find even those islands which had been mapped. The hostility of the Spanish sometimes made the mainland and the larger archipelagos inacessible even when they were located. 'The plague of the Sea, and the spoyle of Mariners', as Hawkins called it, scurvy was rife in the Pacific.[13] 'A Ship grows foul fast in these Seas', Woodes Rogers noted soon after he doubled the Horn, alluding to the complex of material and temperamental problems which made his cruise so difficult.[14] It is in fact a scorbutic condition of the ocean itself that Hawkins identifies as 'loathesome sloathfulnesse', a taint that affects everything in its vicinity: 'The experience I saw in Anno 1590 lying with a Fleete ... about the Islands of the Azores almost six moneths, the greatest part of the time we were becalmed: with which all the Sea became so replenished with severall sorts of gellys, and formes of Serpents, Adders, and Snakes, as seemed wonderfull: some greene, some blacke, some yellow, some white, some of divers colours, and many of them had life'.[15] William Empson supposes that the smaller sooty albatross (which he identifies as *diomedea fuliginosa*), the same species Forster shot and probably Hatley too, might have been destined for an anti-scorbutic soup.[16] Although Cook was credited with having beaten scurvy by a battery of preventive measures, including portable soup, spruce beer, good ventilation, dry clothes and keeping three watches instead of two, his second voyage was marred by outbreaks during the long runs in the high southern latitudes, as Forster and Wales testify. Sir James Watt calculates that the six weeks spent at Dusky Bay were needed to recover from scurvy contracted on the trip from the Cape to New Zealand. On 20 December 1772 Cook was distributing malt wort to 'such People as had symptoms of the Scurvy', and William Wales adds rather querulously, 'I suppose I shall be believed when I say that I am unhappy in being one of them.'[17] It is Watt, of course, who has earned derision for his thesis that Captain Cook's uncertain temper, especially volatile on his third and last voyage, was owing to an infestation of roundworm; but the point he makes is that intestinal worms reduce the body's capacity to absorb vitamins, and that Cook's strange behaviour may have been owing to a chronic deficiency.[18]

Apart from accidents and war, the majority of deaths occurring on all ships in passage were owing to scurvy. But in the Pacific the mortality curve became very steep. Thirteen hundred out of the two thousand who made up the complement of Anson's squadron perished from the disease.[19] The shipmates of the mariner, dropping down one by one, 'With heavy thump, a lifeless lump' to the number of two hundred are dying not of thirst, as he seems to imply, or yellow fever, as has recently been suggested,[20] but more likely scurvy, exactly the same number as died of it aboard the *Centurion*, Anson's flagship in the British expedition of 1740 to the South Seas. By the time he sighted land, only eight of the original complement were capable of working the vessel.[21] The threat of a ghost ship, with its crew all dead on the deck, had been a nightmare of Pacific navigation ever since de Quiros told of the prostration of his crew off Vanuatu ('The Ships were like a town hospital with the plague, and none could stand on their feet').[22] On the *Gloucester*, the *Centurion's* consort, the captain reported: 'We had but 10 Men and the 3 Lieuts; Master, Purser, Surgeon and myself, and seven small Boys that could stand the Deck, and those weak.'[23] The story of Anson's distresses was widely known in the eighteenth century – Cowper, Smollett, and Rousseau used it as a source. It was also on this narrative, admired as much for its accuracy as its elegance, that experts on scurvy such as James Lind and John Clark relied for data. No matter where you turn from 'The Rime of the Ancient Mariner' to actual naval history, there is a trace of scurvy.

Even among invented histories of the sea there is a scorbutic thread linking the poem to the disease. In *The Farther Adventures of Robinson Crusoe* (1719) Defore includes an account of a Bristol ship so short of provisions that everyone on board was close to death. It is told in the first person by a maidservant to the supercargo: 'This was her own Relation,' Crusoe says, 'and is such a distinct account of starving to Death as I confess, I never met with, and was exceedingly entertaining to me ... so distinct and so feelingly [given].'[24] She talks about the vividness of her dreams of eating, 'a kind of earnest Wishing or Longing for Food; something like, as I suppose, the Longing of a Woman with Child', and she describes the bitter disappointment of waking: 'I was exceedingly sunk in my Spirits, to find my self in the extremity of Famine... I fell into a violent Passion of Crying.' Here the psychological as well as physiological effects of starvation of overlap with those of scurvy, which was remarkable for the same alternation between fantasy and despair, and they contribute to a particularly lurid sequence in which the narrator is diverted from biting the flesh of her arm by drinking a bowl of her own blood, still standing from a nosebleed the day before; and shortly after quaffing it she hears the sailors cry out, 'A Sail, a Sail'.[26] Telescoped into a single gesture, it introduces the scorbutic climax of Coleridge's ballad: 'I bit my arm and sucked the blood,/ And cried, A sail!, a sail!'

Thomas Beddoes, Coleridge's friend, was an expert on scurvy. In his *Observations on Sea-Scurvy* (1793), he developed the theory that it is immediately 'owing to a gradual abstraction of oxygene from the whole system'.[27] A predisposing cause of this exhaustion is bad food, and Beddoes was well known for his interest in diet. His *Letter to William Pitt, on the Means of ... preventing the Diseases that arise from meagre Food* (1796), in which he pursues a theme of his earlier work concerning land-scurvy, was reviewed by Coleridge in *The Watchman*, where he weighs the advantages of a broth-machine, designed to supply 'a palatable and nutritious soup' for the poor.[28] For the idea that a poor diet causes the fluids of the body to lose oxygen, Beddoes was indebted to the most interesting writer on scurvy, Thomas Trotter, who had argued that 'dephlogisticated air' thickens and blackens the blood to produce scurvy's most legible symptom.[29] Beddoes' estimate of the temperature of inanition, 'the cool and relaxed condition of hungry poverty',[30] combined with Trotter's idea of blood suffocating into sludge, are represented in the effects of the spectre bark, whose female passenger 'makes the still air cold' (1798) and 'thicks man's blood with cold' (1817). Trotter may have formed another link in the mind of Coleridge the ardent abolitionist, for some of his most telling descriptions of scurvy were garnered from his experience as a surgeon aboard a slave-ship. Observing the rapid onset of the disease among the African prisoners, he became convinced that it resulted from a reciprocal action of the mind and the body in which despair and physical corruption were interchangeably causes and effects, and it led him to emphasise 'idiosyncrasy, or peculiarity of temperament' as a factor as important to the prognosis as the physical circumstances of the victims.[31] The spanned material and mental attributes of scorbutic decay are evident in Coleridge's picture of the spectre bark, piloted by Death and the figure of Life in Death, who personifies the mood of dying, a combination he found expressive of 'the Being of the Sea.'[32] The skeletal remains of the vessel, 'a plankless Thing/ A rare Anatomy!/ A plankless Spectre', has been related by Empson and more recently by Deirdre Coleman to Coleridge's belief that a slaver's decks would not last more than ten voyages, for the 'heat and stench arising from ... diseased bodies ... rot the very planks'.[33] A contagion that spreads from flesh to wood is confirmed in De Quiro's account of the disastrous end of Mendana's expedition, where the effects of scurvy ('ulcers coming out on feet and legs the sick rabid from the effluvia of mud and filth that was in the ship') are matched by the parlous condition of the vessel which, like the spectre bark, has lost its planking ('The ship was so open in the dead wood that the water ran in and out ... when we sailed on a bowline').[34] In both cases scurvy seems to cause the division between animate and inanimate substance to be as permeable as that between the mind and the body. Thus ships (like the ocean itself) can catch scurvy; and in the two eldritch figures on a rotten hulk, Coleridge builds a montage of these transposed infections. Certainly the broad and burning face of the sun, the blackness of Death's bones, edged with purple and green, and his sterterous breathing are typical of the disease Trotter and Beddoes had observed: the bloated and discoloured face, the blackening of the blood under the skin, the high colour and greenish scum of the urine, the asthmatic working of the lungs.[35] As for Death's partner, she exhibits not only an extravagant flow of spirits incident to certain stages of scurvy and starvation ('They are taken light-headed, and fall a-joking and laughing; and in this Humour they expire?'[36] but also the terrible whiteness of leprosy, a cutaneous degeneration sometimes confounded with scurvy.[37] Nor would it have escaped Coleridge that opium was recommended as a palliative for its wild swings of mood.[38]

The image of a ship whose putrescence infects and is in turn infected by its contents serves to introduce the putrefying ocean, described by Hawkins as a sea 'so replenished with severall sorts of gellys, and formes of Serpents, Adders, and Snakes, as seemed wonderfull: some greene, some blacke, some yellow, some white, some of divers colours, and many of them had life'.[39] Coleridge blends these colours into the picture of the spectre ship before having the mariner turn to look at the rotting sea, where he is appalled at the slimy things that live in it. But the same colours reappear in the delightful vision of the water-snakes, now crisply self-illuminated, 'whose elfish light/ Fell off in hoary flakes', so exquisite that 'I bless'd them unaware.' Forster, who described the effects of phosphorescence with great detail ('nay, the very bosom of this immense element seemed to be pregnant with this shining appearance') nevertheless believed their beauty to be owing to the putrefaction of marine creatures.[40] Intense disgust and exquisite pleasure alternate, perhaps even merge, in the presence of rottenness, and for no demonstrable reason. What was loathesome in Hawkins' account suddenly 'seemed wonderful'; Forster speaks of the effects of phosphorescent decay as 'a wonder which fills the mind with greater astonishment and revential awe, than it is in my power justly and properly to describe'.[41]

Why these images of scurvy should have clustered in Coleridge's ballad and provoked such opposite feelings is a problem that is not solved, but certainly more surely posed, if the oddities of the affliction are consulted. Scurvy is not a simple illness, and if the poem is read symptomatically it yields a complexity that is primarily aesthetic, rather than spiritual or ethical. I want to argue that in his scorbutic plight the mariner dramatises the problem of taste as it was formulated and experienced in the eighteenth century, a problem rendered especially acute by the growing demand for voyage literature, as well as by debates over slavery and sugar.

There are three aspects of scurvy important to note: first, its dramatic symptoms of physical corruption; second, its puzzling etiology; and third, its effect on the mind. In its later stages, the symptoms of scurvy were peculiarly gruesome, for the body seemed to rot while it was still alive. John Woodall said it 'oft offendeth the mouth and gummes of the diseased, and causeth the flesh thereof to rot and stink ... [and] the issuing of much filthy bloud and other stinking corruption thence'.[42] Richard Walter, the narrator Anson's voyage, reported that the legs of the victims 'were subject to ulcers of the worst kind, attended with rotten bones, and such a luxuriancy of fungous flesh, as yielded to no remedy' (102). 'A person so affected,' says James Rymer at the end of the century, 'is really in a state of actual dissolution and decomposition.'[43] Eventually, the legs would stiffen, as if in the rigour of death, and the skin would blacken, as if putrefying.[44] Anthony Addington concluded, 'Corruption seems to be the Essence of this Disorder'.[45] I have suggested that the view of the spectre bark presents a collocation of symptoms so faithful to the disease that the figures of Death and Life-in-Death reproduce between them the objective and subjective appearances of the malady. Scurvy presents in its most literal and material form is the corruption of the seagoing self which had been lamented in ancient days by Horace and Claudian, and more recently by Raynal and Diderot in the *History of the two Indies* (1783) where they had arraigned somewhat querulously 'this change in character in the European who quits his country ... a phenomenon of so extraordinary a nature, the imagination is so deeply affected with it, that while it attends to it with astonishment, reflection tortures itself in endeavouring to find out the principle of it, whether it exist in human nature in general, or in the peculiarities of navigators, or in the circumstances preceding or posterior to the event.'[46] The change is visible both in the mutation of the personality, the inexplicable savagery of allegedly civil beings, and in the ghastly rottenness of the bones and flesh, a medical enigma that resulted from spending too much time at sea.

If Raynal and Diderot could find no cause for the extraordinary degeneration of voyagers, neither could the surgeons account for the putrefaction of a living body. Walter called the disease 'the most singular and unaccountable ... its symptoms inconstant and innumerable ... its progress and effects extremely irregular'.[47] Pascoe Thomas aboard Anson's *Centurion* observed the embarrassment of the surgeon, Henry Ettrick, when he was forced to admit in the face of its multiform and confusing appearances, 'that though some of the concurrent helps of this disease were plain enough, yet that the grand centre was certainly the long continuance at sea, or an entire secret; and that no cure but the shore would ever take place.'[48] James Lind, who made a life's work of the study of scorbutic disorders, was never sure what caused it and what alleviated it. He admitted, 'There are frequent occurrences in this disease, which I think very difficult to account for.'[49] The mystery provokes a degree of enthusiasm in those who contemplate it. 'The effects of this disease were in almost every instance wonderful', exclaims Walter.[50] 'Throughout the whole symptoms of this disease', Trotter notes with awe, 'there is something so peculiar to itself, that no description, however accurate it may be, can convey to the reader a proper idea of its nature'.[51] 'The debility of Scurvy', he goes on, 'is of so singular a nature, that nothing seems analogous to it: certain it is, that no disease is related to it ... [it] is attended by a train of symptoms peculiar to itself, and which the genius of the distemper has rendered extremely difficult to explain'.[52] John Woodall concedes, 'But truly the causes of this disease are so infinite and unsearchable, as they farre pass my capacity to search them all out.'[53] Scurvy is a miracle, then, almost the print of the hand of God ('infinite and unsearchable'); or an object of intense curiosity whose symptoms are accumulated with the same mixture of wonder and obsession as a cabinet of exotic specimens. Lind observed, 'After the publication of the Right Honourable Lord Anson's voyage, by the Reverend Mr Walter, the lively and elegant picture there exhibited of the distress occasioned by this disease ... excited the curiosity of many to enquire into the nature of a malady accompanied with such extraordinary appearances.'[54] As curiosity was strongly excited, but undisciplined by reasons and demonstrations, it could do nothing but collect evidence of scurvy's multifarious appearances. These accumulated peculiarities denied both its victims and its observers a coherent narrative of its progress. Southey is identifying the scorbutic element of the poem when he says, 'the stanzas are laboriously beautiful, but in connection they are absurd or unintelligible'.[55] Coleridge posted off some doggerel to the *Morning Post* in which he told himself that his poem was 'incomprehensible/ And without a head or tail'.[56]

Owing to the lack of any clear cause of scurvy, and to the horrible circumstances in which it generally came about, it was frequently associated with non-physiological factors, such as mood. Dr Willis placed sorrow high on the list of causes.[57] John Clark maintained that dejection, and whatever might cause lowness of spirits, such as harsh discipline or bullying, were to blame for outbreaks of scurvy, and recommends, 'Officers should therefore carefully prevent every kind of oppression on board of ships'.[58] 'It attacks the discontented, the repining; whilst persons of more chearful dispositions escape.'[59] In this respect voyages of discovery, where the mind was constantly alert, were thought to be healthier than naval station-duty, where boredom was a problem. Trotter suggests that the pangs of homesickness precipitated the huge loss of life on slave-ships,[60] and before him Joseph Banks argued that scurvy was closely allied to a yearning for home.[61] But besides these contributory factors of mood, students of scurvy noticed in the victims an extraordinary susceptibility to sensation as they came to their crisis. Richard Walter had observed that then there develops 'a disposition to be seized with the most dreadful terrors on the slightest accident'.[62] Thomas Trotter found homesickness intensifying into a yearnings so keen and irresistible he named it 'scorbutic Nostalgia': 'I consider these longings as the first symptom and the constant attendants of the disease in all its stages. The cravings of appetite, not only amuse their waking hours, with thoughts on green fields, and streams of pure water; but in dreams they are tantalized by the favourite idea; and on waking, the mortifying disappointment is expressed with the utmost regret, with groans, and weeping, altogether childish'.[63]

In that distinct and feeling amount of starvation at sea given by Defoe in the *Farther Adventures*, the victim specifies the extravagance of this disappointment, well-known at sea. This fierce longing is commemorated on a dinner service presented to Anson at Canton, after his voyage was over, where scenes of Juan Fernandez and Tinian are blended with images of dogs, sheep, the Eddystone Light and Plymouth Sound, 'betraying the nostalgia which commonly accompanied vitamin deficiency'.[64]

'So in a Calenture, the Seaman fancies/ Green Fields and flowry Meadows on the Ocean'.[65] George Robertson, sailing with Samuel Wallis towards the discovery of Tahiti, reported men down with scurvy, longing for 'wild Game, gold, Silver, Diamonds Pearls & some for Girls'.[66] When a happy landfall allowed the victims to grapple with the exquisite things they had been imagining, then 'the spirits are exhilarated, by the taste itself, and the juice [of fruits] is swallowed, with emotions of the most voluptuous luxury'.[67] Herman Melville reports a mariner so scorbutic that the very smell of flowers wafting from the shore caused him to cry out in agony.[68] Anson told Richard Mead of one of his men at Juan Fernandez, almost dead of scurvy: 'When landed the poor man desired his mates, that they would cut a piece of turf out of the soft ground, and put his mouth to the hole: upon doing this, he came to himself, and grew afterwards quite well.'[69]

The slide from loneliness and disgust to an intense pleasure taken in shapes and colours commences what, in the allegorical era of Coleridge's poem, was construed as the moral regeneration of the mariner. A morbid sense of his repulsive situation yields to a spring of love as he looks at the colours successively thrown off the backs of the iridescent creatures. All navigators touched by scurvy go in the same cycle of disgust and wonder. Hawkins and Forster are at first repelled ('loathesome' 'stinking and putrid') and then fascinated by the rotting sea. De Quiros nearly died of famine and plague in a paradise he called the New Jerusalem. In the first Pacific voyage of 1520, Magellan found himself alternately loathing and loving what he found there. Walter tries to describe the crossing from dismay to voluptuous delight that occurred when the *Centurion* reached Juan Fernandez. On the boat everyone was awash in their own filth and in the grip of scorbutic nostalgia: 'In our distressed situation, languishing as we were for the land and its vegetable productions, (an inclination constantly attending every stage of the sea-scurvy) it is scarcely credible with what eagerness and transport we viewed the shore'.[70] When they land, it is like Satan's removal from Hell to Eden: 'Some particular spots occurred in these valleys, where the shade and fragrance of the contiguous woods, the loftiness of the overhanging rocks, and the transparency and frequent falls of the neighbouring streams, presented scenes of such elegance and dignity, as would will difficulty be rivalled in any other part of the globe. It is in this place, perhaps, that the simple productions of unassisted nature may be said to excel all the fictitious descriptions of the most animated imagination ... I despair of conveying an adequate idea of its beauty'.[71] Under the same stress Bougainville believed he had come across Cythera, and his colleague Commerson thought he had arrived at Utopia, when they made landfall at Tahiti and saw an apparition of Venus rise upon the deck. Irresistible voluptuous sensations were the only explanation Bligh could offer for the mutiny on the *Bounty*: his men were prepared to risk death for the prospect of 'allurements of dissipation beyone any thing that can be conceived'.[72]

There is no doubt that the intensity was experienced and that they were partly the result of sense perceptions altered by scurvy; but as the cause and tendency of the disease were unknown, and the sensations associated with it impossible to convey in all their richness, it is hard to extract an historic or moral significance from moments of sheer aesthesis that interspersed Pacific navigations. The reason that the terra incognita was so often represented as a utopia or a paradise was owing not only to a long literary tradition which had located immortal commonwealths in the South Seas, but also no doubt to this pathological state of the nerves, keyed up to overreact to any stimulus, especially after long voyages. Colours and birds loom largely as the objects of these unreasonable sensations. As he succumbed to scurvy, Forster became susceptible to the colours of the ice and the Southern Lights, just as Hawkins had reacted to the the green, black, yellow and white of the serpents in the scorbutic sea: 'as blue as Ultramarine, the shades were all blueish, even to the very sumits [sic]; the sea when washing it looked as a tincture of verdigrease'.[73]

His son's painting *Ice Island with ice-blink* (1772-73) gives full range to this palette, where vibrant blues lighten into sulphur yellows, and thicken into bruised purples and greens, all framing the surreal shapes of the ice.[74] Presumably sight is prone to the same morbid sensitivity as the palate and the nose. The result in this case is an image that glows so strangely because it is copied from a scurvied retina. Something of the same effect in reverse is given in the lines of the poem, 'Day after day, day after day,/ We stuck, nor breath nor motion,/ As idle as a painted Ship,/ Upon a painted Ocean,' where the ship is projected as the fantasm of a sick sea, daubed from the colours of the 'witch oils' which burn in it 'green and blue and white'. In his own experience Coleridge found that a mood of dejection made him extraordinarily sensitive to colours, such as the 'peculiar tint of yellow green' he spotted during a summer when, as he told Thomas Poole, he had suffered much from a want of vegetables.[75]

Sick and starving de Quiros listened with 'marvellous pleasure and contentation' to the birdsong in Vanuatu, and Walter saw a bird on Juan Fernandez, surpassing 'all Description, Imitation, or even Imagination'.[76] In Indonesia, Pigafetta discovered a bird more brightly coloured than he had ever seen before, perpetually on the wing, and he called it the bird of paradise. As for the albatross, it is produced (as Hatley produced his) as a focus of strong and contradictory feelings, an occasion of morbid intensities, not of the sort of moral lesson Mrs Barbauld was prone to draw from stories of cruelty to birds.[77] In locating a parallel for the death of albatross in Anders Sparrman's narrative of the landing at Dusky Bay, Bernard Smith provides a fine example not of moral evil but of scorbutic pleasure. The lengthy spell in New Zealand was taken to recover the scurvy caused by the fierce exposure to the ice. It was during this period that Sparrman remembers shooting ducks, and how 'the blood from these warm birds which were dying in my hands, running over my fingers, excited me to a degree I had never previously experienced.... . This filled me with amazement, but the next moment I felt frightened'.[78] Paul Carter has identified the same sinister lining of a voluptuous delight in an early nineteenth-century drawing of an Australasian specimen, 'something cruel about its exquisite lingering attention over every detail ... something deeply voluptuous about the blood-red pigments congealing into the wing of *Trichoglossus haematodus moluccanus*'.[79] Who is to say that on these unregulated moments of pure sensation, verging equally on terror and enchantment, the great divisions between the ignoble and the noble were not fantastically reared, so that ever since the orderly divisions of a universal taxonomy have obscured the 'chinks of excitement' they originally served to fringe?[80] These strange scenes of passion, ranging from mild curiosity to violent frenzy, fit Coleridge's judgment of Robinson Crusoe, Selkirk's fictional self, as a man inhabiting 'the vision of a happy night-mair'.[81] To locate the wonder of things otherwise disgusting is to inhabit the paradox of coincident extremes that Coleridge thought so pregnant as to 'constitute and exhaust all philosophy'.[82]

It has been noticeable that the alternation between horror and pleasure among the victims of scurvy extends to students of the disease, who are so curious in tracing its puzzling variety that they can't help calling its most gruesome effects wonderful, or referring to the mysterious agency of the disease as its genius. It is an affliction that suspends its observers amidst its variegations, incapable of making a judgment, just as the mariner is suspended in his own story, unsure what to make of it. It prompts one to wonder how many of its students were also victims. Thomas Trotter, who wrote so vividly about it, had probably suffered from it too. But even among the largely shore-based experts like Lind, there is a kind of contagion caught merely from meditating on an ailment that is an engine of the unique, capable of making all discourse about its symptoms itself symptomatic: peculiar, singular, extraordinary, distinct, and beyond the power of words to describe. Having compared the study of scorbutic symptoms to the collection of artificial curiosities, I would add that the analogy holds also in respect of this tautologous relation between the mode and object of representation; for if the discourse of scurvy is itself scurvied, so rarities are collected, as Shaftesbury complained, for rareness' sake: one is curious about that which is itself curious. Philip Saumarez of the *Centurion* said of its 'scarcely credible' symptoms: "'Tis not my province to account for what the most learned only perplex, but I could plainly observe that there is a Je ne sais quoi in the frame of the human system that cannot be renewed, cannot be preserved, without the assistance of certain earthly particles'.[83] Saumurez resorts to the language of aesthetics as many commentators in the eighteenth century are prone to do when the connexion between a feeling and a cause is not disclosed or not demonstrable. He evinces the primacy of the language of taste in situations where the reason is embarrassed, and he establishes a link not only between the undemonstrable causes of the disease and the equally undemonstrable nature of sensual pleasure, but also, as Howard Caygill has shown, with all the other mysterious connexions between the private appetite and the public good which dogged discussions of commerce and patriotism as well as of taste in the eighteenth century. Caygill observes, 'the theory of civil society was haunted by the problem of taste ... the British development of the theory of taste was ... distinguished by its revaluation of the je ne sais quoi into the necessary ignorance of the workings of providence'.[84] In a similar vein, Nicholas Thomas has argued recently that the practice of taste among South Seas collectors operated outside any satisfactory model of tabulation or theodicy: 'There was in this period nothing like Linnean classification that could be applied to artificial curiosities: they were not drawn into any comparative study of technology or craft; they played no significant part in the ethnographic project of discriminating and assessing the advancement of. the various peoples encountered ... they were specimens because they were treated as such, and their display in the space of the specimen ... was part of an expressive work that evoked the science of men like Banks and licensed their curiosity.'[85]

Outside the ambit of Kant's third *Critique*, where empirical anthropology and consensus were still the basis of aesthetic judgments, the slave trade introduced an extra element of instability into judgments of taste. Burke had argued that the difference between sweetness and bitterness is universally understood: 'A sour temper, bitter expressions, bitter curses, a bitter fate, are terms well and strongly understood by all. And we are altogether as well understood when we say, a sweet disposition, a sweet person, a sweet condition, and the like.'[86] Along with other abolitionists, such as Southey, who advised tea-sweeteners to 'reflect on the bitterness at the bottom of the cup', and Cowper, whose best anti-slave trade poem is called 'Sweet Meat has sour Sauce',[87] Coleridge was helping to undermine precisely this distinction: 'A part of that food among most of you, is sweetened with Brother's Blood'.[88] He was taking judgments of taste back to the indeterminate proposition ('the same object may be both sweet and bitter') from which Hume had tried to redeem it.[89] While trying to make a breach in common understanding for a political purpose, Coleridge entered through another door into the powerful ambivalence of his ballad, patterned according to symptoms of a disease closely associated with the 'unhallowed trade' he and Trotter deplored. For his part, Captain Cook had already found a novel blend of sweet and sour in the correction of scurvy, recommending the 'acid and fermenting' qualities of sugar as an antiscorbutic whose use 'will greatly contribute to rectify the putrescence of the salt food'.[90]

Those whose alibis for expressive work were less authoritative than Joseph Banks, and who had to content themselves with the matter of fact way of delivering marvels, ran into a problem of the voyage narrative which Coleridge's schoolmaster William Wales pithily stated as follows: 'If he tells nothing which is uncommon, he must be a stupid fellow to have gone so far, and brought home so little; and if he does, why – it is hm – aye, a toss of the Chin, and, – he's a Traveller!'[91] So many stories of the South Seas in the eighteenth century are defined by that desperate self-isolating egoism which is the signature of the eyewitness: 'Such confusion as cannot be imagined by any who were not Eye-witnesses of it'; 'It is impossible for the Tongue or Pen of Man to give a perfect Description of the prodigious Sufferings'; 'I cannot explain by any possible Energy of Words, what a strange longing or hankering of Desires I felt.' This is the rhetoric of scurvy too, whether delivered from the inside or the outside: 'A wonder which fills the mind with greater astonsihment than it is my power justly and properly to describe'. It is scarcely credible with what eagerness and transport we viewed the shore',[92] 'No description, however accurate it may be, can convey to the reader a proper idea of its nature'.[93] They are all variations played on the theme of the *je ne sais quoi*. A gulf opens between witnesses of these destabilising moments of wonder and the public that wishes to fit novelties into the scheme of things; and it can be bridged only by those local and particularised buttonholings the mariner is skilled at. By no stretch of the imagination can such an eyewitness be thought to occupy that broad field of vision which Mary Louise Pratt assigns the Imperial I, or to command the powers of appropriation which Stephen Greenblatt accords to Europeans in a state of wonder, or to exhibit the sentimental self-control Peter Hulme finds in stories like Yarico and Inkle. The narrative of these moments of astonishment never corresponds to a moral economy like Mrs Barbauld's, and least of all to Humboldt's programme for reports from remote regions, where 'every other consideration ought to be subservient to those of instruction and utility';[94] nor does it consolidate the scientific self as the subject of a universal history in the manner suggested by Foucault. When Hatley killed the albatross, when Sparrman felt excited by the blood on his hands, when a dying sailor sucked his life back through a hole dug in the soil of a desert island, and when Banks and Solander found that their first specimens in New Zealand were four Maori corpses, they did things they could not hope to justify or explain. They experienced sensations they could not hope to communicate. They had things on their hands and a sickness in their bones they could not possibly trace or categorise. 'The Rime of the Ancient Mariner' reminds its reader that this the predominant characteristic of narratives of voyages in the eighteenth century. If the mariner is an epitome, he epitomises the incommunicability of experiences gathered at the limit of the world and at the end of one's tether.

Notes

1 I want to thank Alan Bewell, Ted Underwood and Susan Wolfson for their help in getting this essay into its present form.

2 *Selected Poems*, William Empson (ed.), (London: Faber, 1972), 28.

3 *Table Talk*, Carl Woodring (ed.), (2 vols; Princeton: Princeton University Press, 1990), ii, 375.

4 Warren Stevenson, 'The Rime of the Ancient Mariner as Epic Symbol', in Harold Bloom (ed.), *Samuel Taylor Coleridge's The Rime of the Ancient Mariner* (New York: Chelsea House, 1986), 54.

5 *Letters of William and Dorothy Wordsworth: The Early Years 1787-1805*, Ernest de Selincourt (ed.), (Oxford: Clarendon Press, 1967), 211.

6   George Shelvocke, *A Voyage round the World by Way of the Great South Sea* (London: J. Senex, 1726), 72-3.

7   *The Resolution Journal of Johann Reinhold Forster 1772-75*, Michael E. Hoare (ed.), 4 vols; (London: The Hakluyt Society, 1982), ii, 214, 234.

8   Forster, *op. cit.*, 235.

9   Shelvocke, *op. cit.*, 218.

10 William Betagh, *A Voyage round the World*, 2 edn (London: J. Clarke, 1757), 221, 88.

11 'Coleridge's *Ancient Mariner* and Cook's Second Voyage', *Journal of the Warburg and Courtauld Institutes* 1-2 (1956).

12 Johann-Reinhold Forster, *Observations made during a Voyage round the World*, Nicholas Thomas, Harriet Guest and Michael Dettelbach (eds), (Honolulu: University of Hawaii Press, 1996), 58.

13 'Sir Richard Hawkins's Voyage into the South Seas', in Samuel Purchas, *Hakluytus Posthumus; or, Purchas his Pilgrimes* (20 vols; Glasgow: James Maclehose, 1906), xvii, 77.

14 Woodes Rogers, *A Cruising Voyage round the World* (London: A. Bell, 1712), 146.

15 Purchas, *op. cit.*, 76.

16 See *Selected Poems*, 36; John Livingston Lowes, *The Road to Xanadu* (London: Constable, 1927), 226; George Shelvocke, *A Voyage round the World by way of the Great South Sea* (London: J. Senex, 1726), 73.

17 James Cook, *Journal of the Voyage of the Resolution*, J.C. Beaglehole (ed.), (Cambridge: Hakluyt Society 1961), 64 n. 3.

18 Sir James Watt, 'Medical Aspects and Consequences of Cook's Voyages', in Robin Fisher and Hugh Johnston, *Captain James Cook and his Times* (Canberra: ANU Press, 1979), 130-4; 155. See also Christine Holmes, *Captain Cook's Second Voyage* (Hampstead: Caliban, 1984), 67 n. 1; and Marshall Sahlins, *Islands of History* (Chicago: University of Chicago Press, 1985), 108-9.

19 See Eleanora C. Gordon, 'Scurvy and Anson's Voyage', *The American Neptune*, xliv: 3 (1984), 155-66.

20 Debbie Lee, 'Yellow Fever and the Slave Trade: Coleridge's 'Rime of the Ancient Mariner', *English Literary History*, lxv (1998), 675-700.

21 Richard Walter, *A Voyage round the World in the Years 1740-44* (London: W. Bowyer, 1776), 105.

22 *The Voyages of Pedro Fernandez de Quiros*, Sir Clements Markham (ed.), (2 vols; London: Hakluyt Society, 1904), ii, 447.

23 Mathew Michell, 'A Journal of the proceedings on board his Majesties Ship the Gloucester 1740-42', PRO ADM 51/42; 20 June - 27 July, 1741.

24 Daniel Defoe, *The Farther Adventures of Robinson Crusoe*, 3 vols (Oxford: Basil Blackwell, 1927), iii, 69.
25 *Ibid.*, iii, 66, 67.
26 *Ibid.*, iii, 68.
27 Thomas Beddoes, *Observations on Sea-Scurvy* (London: J. Murray, 1793), 45.
28 Beddoes, *op. cit.*, 100-1.
29 Thomas Trotter, *Observations of the Scurvy* (London: T. Longman, 1792), 128.
30 Coleridge *op. cit.*, 102.
31 Trotter *op. cit.*, 67.
32 Unless specified quotations are from the 1798 edition, in Martin Wallen (ed.), *Coleridge's Ancient Mariner: An Experimental Edition of Texts and Revisions 1798-1828* (New York: Station Hill, 1993).
33 Lewis Patton (ed.), *The Watchman* (London: Routledge and Kegan Paul and Princeton University Press, 1970), 138 (No. III, March 1796), quoted in Empson 1972, 29; see Deirdre Coleman, 'Conspicuous Consumption: White Abolitionism and English Women's Protest Writing in the 1790s,' *English Literary History*, lxi (1994), 345.
34 De Quiros, *op. cit.*, 105-7.
35 Beddoes, *op. cit.*, 82; Trotter, *op. cit.*, 91, 122, 128.
36 John Bulkeley, *A Voyage to the South Seas 1740-44* (London: R. Walker, 1745), 158.
37 See William Jervey, *Practical Thoughts on the Prevention and Cure of Scurvy* (London: J. Nourse and J. Murdoch, 1769).
38 R. T. Crosfield, *Remarks on the Scurvy... with an Account of the Effects of Opium in their Disease* (London: for the author, 1797), 13-34.
39 Purchas *op. cit.*, 76.
40 Forster *op. cit.*, 58-9.
41 Forster *op. cit.*, 59 [see note 10].
42 John Woodall, *The Surgeon's Mate* (London: 1617), 161-2.
43 James Rymer, *An Essay upon the Scurvy* (London: J. Rymer, 1793), 36.
44 William Cockburn, *An Account of the Distempers of Seafaring People*, (2 vols; London: Hugh Newman, 1696), i, 9.
45 Anthony Addington, *An Essay on the Sea-Scurvy* (Reading: C. Micklewright, 1753), 3.
46 Guillaume Raynal, *A Philosophical and Political History of the Settlements and Trade of the Europeans in the East and West Indies*, (8 vols; London: W. Strahan and T. Cadell, 1783), v, 2. See also Anthony Pagden, *Lords of all the World* (New Haven and London: Yale University Press, 1995), 18, 61.

47 Walter, *op. cit.*, 101-2.
48 Glyndwr Williams, *Documents relating to Anson's Voyage round the World 1740-44* (London: Navy Records Society, 1967), cix, 86-7.
49 James Lind, *A Treatise of the Scurvy* (1773), 540; quoted in Kenneth J. Carpenter *The History of Scurvy* (Cambridge: Cambridge University Press, 1986), 70.
50 Walter, *op. cit.*, 102.
51 Trotter, *op. cit.*, 71.
52 Trotter, *op. cit.*, 106.
53 John Woodall, *The Surgeon's Mate* (London: 1617), 161.
54 James Lind, *A Treatise of the Scurvy*, second edn (London: A. Millar, 1757), vii.
55 Robert Southey, *Critical Review*, 24 (1798), 197.
56 Quoted in Maggie Kilgour, *From Communism to Cannibalism* (Princton: Princeton University Press, 1990), 193.
57 *Free Observations on the Scurvy* (Rochester: T. Fisher, 1785), 26.
58 *Observations on the Diseases which prevail in long Voyages* (London: J. Murray, 1792), 531.
59 Francis Milman, *An Enquiry into the Scurvy* (London: J. Dodsley, 1782), 14.
60 Trotter, *op. cit.*, 63.
61 *The Endeavour Journal of Joseph Banks*, J.C. Beaglehole (ed.), 2 vols; Sydney: Public Library of New South Wales and Angus & Robertson, 1962), ii, 152.
62 Walter, *op. cit.*, 101.
63 Trotter, *op. cit.*, 44.
64 Sir James Watt, 'The Medical Bequest of disaster at sea: Commodore Anson's circumnavigation', in *Journal of the Royal College of Physicians* 32:6 (Nov.-Dec. 1998), 577.
65 Nicholas Rowe, *The Ambitious Step-mother* (London: J. Derby, 1720), 41.
66 *Journal of the second voyage of the Dolphin*, Hugh Carrington (ed.), (London: Hakluyt Society No. 98, 1948) 113.
67 Trotter *op. cit.*, 141-2.
68 Herman Melville, Omoo (1968) 64
69 Richard Mead, 'A Discussion on the Scurvy', in Samuel Sutton, *'A New Method for extracting the foul Air out of Ships* (London: J. Brindley, 1794), 119.
70 Walter, *op. cit.*, 111.
71 *Ibid.*, 120.
72 William Bligh, *A Narrative of the Mutiny* (London: G. Nicol, 1790), 10.

73 Forster, *op. cit.*, 227 [see note 7].
74 See Smith, *op. cit.*, 152.
75 *Collected Letters*, Earl Lisle Griggs (ed.), (Oxford: Clarendon Press, 1958), i, 328.
76 Quoted in John Livingston Lowes, *The Road to Xanadu* (London: Constable: 1927), 316.
77 See Frances Ferguson, 'Coleridge and the Deluded Reader', in Bloom, *op. cit.*, 61.
78 Smith, *op. cit.*, 138 [see note 9].
79 Paul Carter, 'Strange Seas of Thought,' *Australian Review of Books* (June 1998), 20.
80 James Boon, 'Anthropology and Degeneration: Birds, Words and Orangutans', in J. Edward Chamberlain and Saner L. Gilman (eds), *Degeneration: The Dark Side of Progress* (New York: Columbia University Press, 1985), 42.
81 Quoted in John Livingston Lowes, *The Road to Xanadu* (London: Constable, 1927), 318.
82 *The Friend*, Barbara Rooke (ed.), (Princeton: Princeton University Press, 1969), i, 110; quoted in Kilgour (1990), 186.
83 Williams, *op. cit.*, 166 [see note 42].
84 Howard Caygill, *Art of Judgment* (Oxford: Basil Blackwell, 1989), 37-9.
85 *In Oceania* (Durham: Duke University Press, 1997), 113.
86 Edmund Burke, *A Philosophical Enquiry into the Origin of our Ideas of the Sublime and Beautiful*, James T. Boulton (ed.) (Oxford: Basil Blackwell, 1987), 14.
87 Quoted in Charlotte Sussman, 'Women and the Politics of Sugar', *Representations*, 48 (1994), 56.
88 Coleridge, 139, [see note 30].
89 David Hume, 'Of the Standard of Taste', in *Selected Essays*, Stephen Copley and Andrew Edgar (eds) (Oxford: Oxford University Press), 137.
90 J. K. Forster, *Observations made during a voyage round the world*, Nicholas Thomas, Harriet Guest and Michael Delfelbach (eds), (Honolulu: University of Hawaii Press, 1996), 368.
91 'Journal', in *Journal of the Voyage of the Resolution 1772-75* , 839.
92 Walter, *op. cit.*, 111.
93 Trotter *op. cit.*, 71.
94 Alexander von Humboldt, *Personal Narrative of Travels to the Equinoctial Regions of America* (3 vols; London: George Bell, 1907), i, 105. See also Mary Louise Pratt, *Imperial Eyes: Travel Writing and Transculturation* (London: Routledge, 1992); Stephen Greenblatt,

Marvellous Possessions (Chicago: University of Chicago Press, 1991); Peter Hulme, *Colonial Encounters* (London: Methuen, 1991); Michel Foucault, *The Archeology of Knowledge*, trans. A. M. Sheridan Smith (New York: Pantheon, 1972).

5

Lassitude and Revival in the Warm South: Relaxing and Exciting Travel, 1750-1830

Chloe Chard

'Indolent delicious reverie' and 'superflu de vie'

At the beginning of her *Diary of an Ennuyée* (an account of travels through France and Italy, published anonymously in 1826), Anna Jameson indicates that she is travelling through France and Italy in the hope of soothing her 'torn and upset' mind (upset, she repeatedly hints, as a result of an unhappy love affair): 'Who knows but this dark cloud may pass away. Continual motion, continual activity, continual novelty, the absolute necessity for self-command may do something for me.' The traveller then minutely calibrates the therapeutic or destructive effects of each place that she visits. In Venice: 'Pleasure and wonder are tinged with a melancholy interest; and while the imagination is excited, the spirits are depressed.' At some points, her own sorrows completely displace the scenes around her: she declares: 'I will say nothing of Bologna; – for the few days I have spent here have been to me days of acute suffering.' Once Jameson sets out for Naples, her responses become more complex, and the reader is almost encouraged to feel that she might recover: ' – my senses and my imagination have been so enchanted, my heart so very heavy – where shall I begin?' After leaving Genoa, on the return journey, she inserts in her narrative a 'Farewell to Italy', in verse, that includes the lines:

> In every kindling pulse
> I felt the genial air,
> For life is *life* in that sunny clime,
> - 'Tis *death* of life elsewhere.[1]

At Autun, an editorial note informs the reader – mendaciously – that the writer has died 'in her 26th year'. Just before this melancholy conclusion to Jameson's Grand Tour, the traveller suggests that she would rather have died earlier, while still in the 'sunny clime' of Italy:

'there it was "*luxury to be*" – there I would willingly have died, it so it might have pleased God.'[2]

While still enjoying the effects of the warm South, however, Jameson registers a desire not precisely for death itself, but for a less absolute dissolution of the sense of self and the bounds of selfhood. Her accounts of the climate of Naples express very strongly the wish for an extinction of burdensome individuality and the 'effort to reduce, to keep constant or to remove internal tension due to stimuli' that have since come to be associated with the Nirvana principle.[3] She describes one scene that gratifies such a wish:

> I know not whether it be incipient illness, or the enervating effects of this soft climate, but I feel unusually weak, and the least exertion or excitement is not only disagreeable but painful. While the rest were at Capo di Monte, I stood upon my balcony looking out upon the lovely scene before me, with a kind of pensive dreamy rapture, which if not quite pleasure, had at least a power to banish pain…
>
> All my activity of mind, all my faculties of thought and feeling, and suffering, seemed lost and swallowed up in an indolent delicious reverie, a sort of vague and languid enjoyment, the true '*dolce far niente*' of this enchanting climate.[4]

Such an account of 'vague and languid enjoyment' might seem distinctly at odds with Jameson's declaration of faith in 'continual motion, continual activity, continual novelty' at the beginning of her narrative. Her descriptions of Naples and the South do in fact name other therapeutic properties of the climate, more in keeping with this initial emphasis on movement and novelty: alongside her accounts of 'pensive dreamy rapture', she also charts the reviving effects of 'excitement' – the quality that the reference to 'every kindling pulse' in her poem serves to recall:

> To stand upon my balcony, looking out upon the sunshine, and the glorious bay; the blue sea, and the pure skies – and to feel that indefinite sensation of excitement, that *superflu de vie*, quickening every pulse and thrilling through every nerve, is a pleasure peculiar to this climate, where the mere consciousnesss of existence is happiness enough.[5]

Change of air

Another travel narrative of the same decade – in this case, an overtly fictionalized Grand Tour – tells the story of a traveller who, like

Jameson, dies in the course of his travels. The Marquis of Normanby's collection of sketches, *The English in Italy* (1825), includes a narrative entitled 'Change of Air', in which the narrator begins, unsurprisingly, by reflecting upon 'the practice of ordering patients to the South for "change of air"'. He comments:

> Many of the physicians who issue this mandate must entertain a very erroneous idea of what the South is. No doubt they imagine it the land of eternal zephyrs, of never varying summer, sunshine, and fragrant vegetation. I fear few of them take into account the Bisc or the Siroc, or that the "land of the South, the clime of the sun," is the most variable of all climes, and that perhaps in which most precaution is necessary, even on the part of the strong and healthy.[6]

Lord Normanby then recounts the experiences of a 'victim' of this belief in the healing powers of the South. 'Over-exertion in his last studies at Oxford', we are told, 'had enfeebled the health of young Bouverie to an alarming degree. He languished even in the leisure of his paternal home'. After a physican has recommended foreign travel as a source of reviving 'variety', Bouverie sets off for Paris, and experiences 'very strong momentary excitements, awakened at intervals, and at first perhaps of some duration, but gradually and in a little time of a very passing kind'. He is overcome by unexpected 'languor and ennui' in his solitary journey through France and northern Italy, but nonetheless proceeds from Florence to Rome in a state of 'restless desire and anxiety':

> Before poor Augustus reached the hotel where he was to stop, he paid the strongest tribute that perhaps ever pilgrim paid to the overpowering grandeur of Roman greatness. He had felt ill on approaching the gate; he supported himself during the continuance of the motion; but no sooner had the carriage rolled under the portal, and stopped for the inspection of the officers of police and customs stationed there, than the youth fainted utterly.[7]

A visit to Naples aggravates his condition: 'The unequalled variability of this boasted climate he found more insufferable, more of harm, and oppressive to him, than any he had as yet visited'. On his return to Rome, 'Augustus Bouverie, alone and exiled from his family, sunk gradually through all the melancholy stages of his disease, tended by the careless hands of strangers, and at last expired'.[8]

What, then, are the arguments and assumptions that supply the preconditions for these two narratives of dying abroad, and for the diverse observations that are appended to them, as the narrators turn their attention to the effects of climate, atmosphere, and the practice of travel itself? In attempting to chart such preconditions, this essay is concerned primarily with the discursive regularities that can be traced within travel writings: more specifically, within writings that delimit their objects with reference to the imaginative topography mapped out by the Grand Tour, as a practice of travel that traces out a movement from the cold North to the warm South. The medical discourses of the time will only enter into this analysis obliquely, as discourses on which travellers sometimes draw in order to formulate observations about travel and health.

During the late eighteenth and early nineteenth centuries, travel writings often discuss whether or not travel in general – and travel to Italy in particular – has any therapeutic effects. Jameson's *Diary of an Ennuyée* and Normanby's 'Change of Air' are not the only travel narratives of the period to proclaim a preoccupation with such effects – or with the traveller's need for them – in their titles: Henry Matthews' *Diary of an Invalid* (1820) and James Johnson's *Change of Air* (1831) are among other works that encourage the reader to expect some discussion of medical matters, amid commentaries on the sights of Europe. Travellers often note the mental and physical benefits of Italian air, climate and atmosphere. Matthews, in Rome in the month of April, declares: 'There is something so soft and balmy in the air, that I feel every mouthful revive and invigorate me.'⁹ Sydney, Lady Morgan, in *Italy* (1821), remarks on 'the descent into the Valley of the Arno':

> In hours so fresh as these, in scenes so lovely, and in airs so pure, there is a sort of intoxication in existence, which raises the spirit so far above the sad regions of "low-thoughted care", that "the ills which flesh is heir to" are as much forgotten as its crimes.¹⁰

At the same time, many travel books emphasize, as Normanby does, that the healing powers of the Italian climate are open to attack. Sydney Morgan's husband, Sir T. Charles Morgan, M.D., in his appendix 'On the State of Medicine in Italy, with Brief Notices of some of the Universities and Hospitals', at the end of the first volume of his wife's travel narrative, notes: 'Upon the slightest suspicion of pulmonary disease, it is our custom in England to hurry the patient off to Italy; and the public papers abound with that bitter sarcasm on the practice, "died in Italy, where he went for the recovery of his health."' Charles Morgan himself pronounces: 'From the experience which a rather extensive journey has afforded me, I should think no climate less adapted to an invalid.' Like Lord Normanby, he cites extremes of heat and cold in support of this judgement. (He notes, too, such 'social deficiencies' as 'the absence of chimneys, of carpets, and of doors and windows that exclude the air'.)[11] The option of stoutly denying that Rome and Naples have a warm delicious climate is very frequently adopted in travel writing: Matthews describes himself in Naples, 'shivering, with a bleak easterly wind', and, during the Sirocco, suffering from 'that leaden oppressive dejection of spirits, which is the most intolerable of diseases'.[12] James Johnson, in *Change of Air*, describes the effects of the Roman and Neapolitan climates in yet more alarming terms: 'The air of the Campagna, at all times, has a depressing effect on the animal spirits – and the enervating SIROCCO is infinitely more suicidal in its tendency, than the November fogs of an English atmosphere.'[13]

Bracing and relaxing travel

Johnson nonetheless endorses the belief in the healing or reviving powers of 'continual motion' voiced by Jameson – a belief that Lord Normanby attacks when he denies that eager movement onwards is of benefit to the unfortunate Bouverie. After a long, gloomy account of the dangers of Italy for those suffering from a range of different afflictions, mental and physical, he declares, more cheerfully:

> Finally, I would say that the dyspeptic, nervous, or hypochondriacal invalid, cannot adopt a more salutary maxim or principle, in Italy, than that which the Home Secretary has laid down for the guidance of the New Police in England – 'KEEP MOVING.'[14]

The view that 'motion' might help to revive an invalid is stated more explicitly – and in more technical terms – by Tobias Smollett, in a much earlier travel book, *Travels through France and Italy* (1766):

> Thus have I given you a circumstantial detail of my Italian expedition, during which I was exposed to a great number of hardships, which I thought my weakened constitution could not have bore; as well as to violent fits of passion, chequered, however, with transports of a more agreeable nature; insomuch that I may say I was for two months continually agitated either in mind or body, and very often in both at the same time. As my disorder at first arose from a sedentary life, producing a relaxation of the fibres, which naturally brought on a listlessness, indolence, and dejection of the spirits, I am convinced that this hard exercise of mind and body, co-operated with the change of air and objects, to brace up the relaxed constitution, and promote a more vigorous circulation of the juices, which had long languished even almost to stagnation.[15]

183

Smollett himself, in this passage, implicitly invokes Edmund Burke's explanation, in his *Philosophical Enquiry into the Origin of our Ideas of the Sublime and Beautiful* (1757), of 'how pain can be a cause of delight':

> Providence has so ordered it, that a state of rest and inaction, however it may flatter our indolence, should be productive of many inconveniences; that it should generate such disorders, as may force us to have recourse to some labour, as a thing absolutely requisite to make us pass our lives with tolerable satisfaction; for the nature of rest is to suffer all the parts of our bodies to fall into a relaxation... At the same time, that in this languid inactive state, the nerves are more liable to the most horrid convulsions, than when they are sufficiently braced and strengthened. Melancholy, dejection, despair, and often self-murder, is the consequence of the gloomy view we take of things in this relaxed state of body.[16]

The sublime, in Burke's account, serves to dissipate such lamentable effects:

> As common labour, which is a mode of pain, is the exercise of the grosser, a mode of terror is the exercise of the finer parts of the system... if the pain and terror are so modified as not to be actually noxious..., as these emotions clear the parts, whether fine, or gross, of an dangerous and troublesome incumbrance, they are capable of producing delight; not pleasure, but a sort of delightful horror...[17]

In defining the bracing effects of the sublime, Burke draws on part of Montesquieu's explanation, in *De l'esprit des lois* (1748), of 'combien les hommes sont différents dans les divers climats'. On the one hand, his references to 'labour' and 'exercise' invoke the industry that Montesquieu defines as characteristic of the North. On the other hand, his allusion to the 'relaxed state of body' that induces 'melancholy, dejection, despair, and often self-murder' draws upon another chapter of *De l'esprit des lois*, in which Montesquieu focuses on the specifically English penchant for suicide. This inclination results from 'un défaut de filtration du suc nerveux': in the suicidal inhabitant of England, 'la machine, dont les forces motrices se trouvent à tout moment sans action, est lasse d'elle-même; l'âme ne sent point de douleur, mais une certaine difficulté de l'existence.'[18]

The strategy of locating the benefits of travel in such bracing and throwing into movement is taken up by James Johnson not only in the context already cited, but also at another point in his survey and narrative of European travel, when he explicitly elides an endorsement of the beneficial effect of hardship upon a 'relaxed constitution' with an analysis of the physiological effects of the sublime. Johnson, in other words, grasps the incipient continuities between the arguments about 'bracing' exercise and agitation put forward by Smollett and by Burke:

> In the greater number of nervous and hypochondriacal complaints, the attention of the individual is kept so steadily fixed on his own morbid feelings as to require strong and unusual impressions to divert it from that point. The monotony of domestic scenes and circumstances is quite inadequate to this object; and arguments not only fail, but absolutely increase the malady, by exciting irritation in the mind of the sufferer, who thinks his counsellors are either unfeeling or incredulous towards his complaints. In such cases, the majestic scenery of Switzerland, the romantic and beautiful views in Italy and the Rheingau, or the keen mountain air of the Highlands of Scotland or Wales, combined with the novelty, variety, and succession of manners and customs of the countries through which he passes, abstract the attention of the dyspeptic and hypochondriacal traveller (if any thing can) from the hourly habit of dwelling on, if not exaggerating, his own real or imaginary sensations, and thus help to break the chain of morbid association by which he is bound to the never-ending detail of his own sufferings.[19]

Such a journey, 'in which mental excitement and bodily exercise are skilfully combined', Johnson asserts, could actually 'prevent many a hypochondriac and dyspeptic from lifting his hand against his own existence', and 'would unquestionably preserve many an individual from mental derangement'. He then tells the story of an ascent of Mont Blanc beset by extremes of temperature: 'one Hypochondriac nearly threw me over a precipice, while rushing past me', he claims, explaining that the party view the glacier with their clothes, drenched from a storm, drying on their bodies. Such hardships, however, merely confirm 'in a most striking manner, the acquisition of strength which travelling confers on the invalid': 'Even the Hypochondriac above-mentioned regained his courage over a bottle of Champagne in the evening..., and mounted his mule next morning to cross the Col de Balme.'[20]

Jameson, in crossing the Alps, says nothing of the vicissitudes of travel, but does acknowledge that the sublime has, for a while, revived her. At Geneva, she declares:

> Now I feel the value of my own enthusiasm: now am I repaid in part

for many pains and sorrows and errours it has cost me. Though the natural expression of that enthusiasm be now repressed and restrained, and my spirits subdued by long illness, what but enthusiasm could elevate my mind to a level with the sublime objects round me, and excite me to pour out my whole heart in admiration as I do now, how deeply they have penetrated into my imagination![21]

When Jameson notes the advantages of 'pure elastic air' in Naples, on the other hand, her account of delightful enervation has more in common with Burke's definition of the quality that he sets in symmetrical opposition to that of sublimity: the beautiful.[22] Section 19 of Burke's *Philosophical Enquiry*, entitled 'The physical cause of LOVE', begins by defining the response to 'such objects as excite love and complacency' as a reaction 'accompanied with an inward sense of melting and languor'. He then embarks on an explantion of such a marked physical effect:

> From this description it is almost impossible not to conclude, that beauty acts by relaxing the solids of the whole system. There are all the appearances of such a relaxation; and a relaxation somewhat below the natural tone seems to me to be the cause of all positive pleasure. Who is a stranger to that manner of expression so common in all times and in all countries, of being softened, relaxed, enervated, dissolved, melted away by pleasure?[23]

The *Philosophical Enquiry* does not itself draw any explicit parallel between this effect of relaxation and the relaxing effects of a warm climate. In his account of being 'melted away by pleasure', however, Burke obliquely invokes one of the most renowned eighteenth-century accounts of bodily relaxation: Montesquieu's contrast between North and South, in which the physical state of the inhabitants of the warm South is defined by opposition to the vigour of those of the North:

> L'air froid resserre les extrémités des fibres extérieures de notre corps; cela augmente leur ressort, et favorise le retour du sang des extrémités vers le cœur. Il diminue la longueur de ces mêmes fibres; il augmente donc encore par là leur force. L'air chaud, au contraire, relâche les extrémités des fibres, et les allonge; il diminue donc leur force et leur ressort.
>
> On a donc plus de vigueur dans les climats froids.[24]

Montesquieu then relates his famous account of his experiment of

186

freezing one half of a sheep's tongue, and discovering that the little pyramids with brush-like tips upon it, which appear to be 'le principal organe du goût', contract and disappear as a result of this process, and begin to reappear as the tongue thaws. This experiment leads him to conclude that in cold climates the sensations are less lively, and the inhabitants will have 'peu de sensibilité pour les plaisirs'. In warmer climates, on the other hand, receptiveness to pleasure will be greater, up to the point where the heat becomes so great that 'la paresse y sera le bonheur'.[25] (In travel writings, as in Burke's account of beauty, these two stages of sensibility to pleasure, on the one hand, and passive indolence, on the other, are in fact constantly elided: Charles Dupaty, for example, in his *Lettres sur l'Italie* (1788), remarks, in the Bay of Naples, that he feels his thoughts softening – 'Je sens mes pensées s'amollir' – at the awareness of gentle and alluring nature around him, and recalls to mind the scenes of both indolence and more active self-indulgence by which such spots would have been distinguished in antiquity.)[26]

Where travel writings debate the therapeutic effects of travel, then, they draw on at least two quite distinct clusters of arguments and assumptions: first, the arguments that assign beneficent powers to travel itself, and sometimes to sublime regions, such as the Alps, as a result of the bracing effects of motion or of sublimity, and, secondly, the arguments that assign beneficient powers to the warm South, as a result of its relaxing effects. Such views are usually summarized in terms that disguise the physiological specificity of such effects of bracing and relaxing, and thereby allow travellers to avoid any explicit recognition of a contradiction between the two sets of assumptions. Anna Jameson endorses, at different junctures, the view that travel and the sublime have supplied a beneficent excitement, and the view that 'vague and languid enjoyment' in a warm climate might prove efficacious in countering pain and sorrow. Lord Normanby, on the other hand, strives to establish that neither the excitement of travel nor the 'eternal zephyrs' of the South are quite as therapeutic as his readers may imagine.

Danger and destabilization

Accounts both of relaxation and of motion and agitation, moreover, are also determined by two new options which travellers begin to follow, around the end of the eighteenth century and the beginning of the nineteenth, in defining the kinds of experience that their journeys encompass. The eighteenth-century view of travel as an occasion for gathering and ordering knowledge of the world is supplemented, at this period, and partially displaced, by a view of travel as an adventure of the self, in which the traveller crosses symbolic boundaries as the same time as he or she traverses geographical limits. Travel of this kind – which can, for convenience, be termed *Romantic travel* – is seen as holding out possibilities of self-realization and self-discovery, but also as placing the self at risk, and bringing in its wake various forms of danger and destabilization.[27] Where travellers adopt this Romantic approach, and view the experience of alterity as potentially destabilizing, illness and disease supply convenient metaphors for the more generalized threat to stability and identity posed by the encounter with the foreign. One of the main strategies deployed by early nineteenth-century travellers, in dismissing the claim that the tour of Italy is beneficial to health, is to emphasize the physical and mental afflictions that beset the Italians themselves, and to point out that not only the Italians, but foreigners too, may be susceptible to these complaints. Enervation, in many travel writings, is presented as an affliction of both mind and body, exemplifying the dangers of the South. James Johnson observes darkly:

> It is not for me, in this place, to predicate the influence of frequent travels or protracted sojourns in a climate so celebrated, in all ages, for its enervating effects on the minds and bodies of the inhabitants – a climate which unmanned not only the conquering Romans but the conquerors of Rome.[28]

Malaria, above all, provides an occasion for conjuring up visions of hidden peril. James Johnson, in one of his many observations on the disease, notes that even travellers who keep to 'elevated positions' are 'not exempt from danger': 'They may escape fevers and agues, the more prominent features of malarious maladies, but they run the risk of imbibing the taint of a poison which will evince its deleterious influence for years afterwards, in forms anomalous and unsuspected, but more destructive of health and happiness than the undisguised attacks of remittent and intermittent fevers'. He later returns to the 'gloomy horror or despondency' that, he claims, malaria sometimes generates, and again emphasizes the tendency of malaria to recur periodically:

> This is peculiarly the case when it produces, or contributes to produce, through the instrumentality of dyspepsia, that terrible mental despondency – or, as I have heard it emphatically termed by some of its victims, that 'utter desolation of heart,' which suddenly overcasts the sunshine of the soul – prostrates the most energetic

intellect – and converts, with magic wand, the smiling landscape of
hope into the gloomy desert of despair.[29]

The insidious character that malaria assumes, in such writings, is
derived not only from uncertainty as to its cause, but also from its
role as a danger that erupts in the midst of pleasure. John
MacCulloch, formulating a sternly admonistory account of the
dangers of malarial 'misery and death' in his treatise *On Malaria*
(1827), acknowledges the fascination of the pleasures that ensnare
travellers to malarial regions by the very effect of irony through
which he attempts to dismiss such pleasures: 'he who, in the language
of the poets, wooes the balmy zephyr of the evening, finds death in
its blandishments.'[30] Sydney Morgan, in Rome, describing the Villa
Albani, the home of Cardinal Albani, begins by elaborating
rapturously on the delights of the spot:

> Its walls are encrusted with basso-rilievos – its corridors grouped
> with fauns and nymphs – its ceilings all azure and gold – its salons
> perfumed by breezes, loaded with the odours of orange-flowers. Its
> gardens, studded with temples, command a view, terminated by a
> waving line of acclivities, whose very names are poetry. When I
> visited it, a distant blue mist veiled the intervening wastes of the
> Campagna, and the dews and lights of morning lent their freshness
> and lustre to a scene and fabric, such as Love might have chosen for
> his Psyche when he bore her from the wrath of Venus.[31]

In the midst of this vision of pleasure, however, Lady Morgan
introduces malarial danger through an effect of sudden bathos: 'But,
when the first glimpse of this vision faded, the true character of the
Roman villa came forth; for artichokes and cabbages were flourishing
amidst fauns and satyrs, that seemed chiselled by a Praxiteles!' The
villa, she reveals, is only rarely visited by the current Cardinal Albani,
and its gardens are hired out to a market gardener 'to raise vegetables
during the spring and winter', while 'in summer even the custode
vacates his hovel, and the Villa Albani is left in the undisputed
possession of that terrible scourge of Roman policy and Roman
crimes – the Mal-aria'.[32]

In Germaine de Staël's novel *Corinne; ou, l'Italie* (1807), Lord
Nelvil, a Scotsman on the Grand Tour, embarking on a romantic
relationship with the eponymous heroine, visits the Campagna with
her, and suggests that danger not only erupts insidiously amid the
'blandishments' of the Italian climate, but actually imparts an added
allure to such blandishments: 'J'aime... ce danger mystérieux,

invisible, ce danger sous la forme des impressions les plus douces.'[33] (This sense of a danger that itself assumes the alluring quality of the delights that accompany it provides the reader with a metaphor for Nelvil's own entanglement with Corinne.) Other travellers forge a yet closer link between pleasure and danger, toying with the possibility that death amid the delights of the South might positively be welcome – the possibility recognized by Jameson when she comments: 'there it was "*luxury to be*" – there I would willingly have died.'[34] Shelley, in the preface to *Adonais* (1821): describing the Protestant cemetary in Rome, where Keats is buried, declares: 'It might make one in love with death, to think that one should be buried in so sweet a place.'[35]

The rhetorical usefulness of disease in general, and malaria in particular, in indicating the pleasurable but destructive destabilization that may befall the traveller to Italy, is recognized in a passsage of William Hazlitt's essay on 'English Students at Rome'. Hazlitt comments on the visitor to this city: 'if ever he wishes to do anything, he should fly from it *as he would from the plague.*' He continues:

> There is a *species of malaria* hanging over it, which infects both the mind and the body. It has been the seat of too much activity and luxury formerly, not to have produced a corresponding torpor and stagnation (both in the physical and moral world) as the natural consequence at present. If necessity is the mother of invention it must be stifled in the birth here, where everything is already done and provided to your hand that you could possibly wish for or think of. You have no stimulus to exertion, for you have but to open your eyes and see, in order to live in a continued round of delight and admiration.[36]

Tourism and the *dolce far niente*: relaxing pleasures

At the same time that the view of travel as a destabilizing activity is formulated, however, another approach to the encounter with the foreign is mapped out, in implicit opposition to Romantic travel. This approach – which may helpfully be termed *tourism* – recognizes the possibility that travel might entail putting the self at risk, but incorporates an assumption that the main aim of the traveller, in managing the pleasures of the foreign, will be to keep danger and destabilization at bay.[37] From the very end of the eighteenth century onwards, travellers constantly oscillate between Romantic and touristic stances. Like the view of travel as a destabilizing activity,

190

tourism generates a range of new concepts, themes, arguments and rhetorical strategies, which play a part in determining accounts of enervation and excitement.

One of these concepts is the idea of travel as leisure: in other words, travel as an activity that, far from consolidating the personal and cultural identity of the traveller, in the manner of seventeenth-century and eighteenth-century travel on the Grand Tour, actually suspends identity, and allows the traveller to enjoy a brief rest from duty and responsibility. (The contrast between such a concept and the earlier view of travel may be indicated, for example, by quoting from the preface of Richard Lassels's *Voyage of Italy* (1670), which unequivocally defines the Grand Tour as a *rite de passage* initiating the traveller into adulthood, and confirming his [*sic*] identity as an English gentleman: 'traveling preserves my yong [*sic*] nobleman from surfeiting of his parents, and weanes him from the dangerous fondness of his mother.')[38] William Hazlitt, in his essay 'On Going a Journey' (1822), argues explicitly that the pleasure of travel is situated in the lifting of the responsibility of socially imposed identity:

> The *incognito* of an inn is one of its striking privileges – 'lord of one's self, uncumbered with a name.' Oh! It is great to shake off the trammels of the world and of public opinion – to lose our importunate, tormenting, everlasting personal identity in the elements of nature, and become the creature of the moment, clear of all ties – to hold to the universe only by a dish of sweetbreads, and to owe nothing but the score of the evening – and no longer seeking for applause and meeting with contempt, to be known by no other title than *the Gentleman in the parlour!*[39]

The idea that travel might actually provide a temporary escape from identity, rather than a consolidation of it, is emphasized yet more strongly in a discussion of the pleasures of travelling in a prose section of Samuel Rogers' poem *Italy* (1822). Rogers observes: 'Almost all men are over-anxious. No sooner do they enter the world, than they lose that taste for natural and simple pleasures, so remarkable in early life.' A temporary escape from the relentless 'pursuit of wealth and honour' is nonetheless available to them: an escape that leads them away from wearisome adult existence and back towards 'the golden time of their childhood':

> Now travel, and foreign travel more particularly, restores to us in a great degree what we have lost. When the anchor is heaved, we

double down the leaf; and for a while at least all effort is over. The old cares are left clustering round the old objects, and at every step, as we proceed, the slightest circumstance amuses and interests. All is new and strange. We surrender ourselves, and feel once again as children. Like them, we enjoy eagerly; like them, when we fret, we fret only for the moment.[40]

This new option of defining travel as a temporary release from anxiety, responsibility and 'effort' makes it possible for travellers to classify the delights of enervation in the warm South as therapeutic rather than dangerous – in other words, to follow the option chosen by Anna Jameson, as opposed to that followed by James Johnson. The destabilized approach remains in use, but is now open to oblique challenge from accounts of happy irresponsibility in southern Europe. If indolence is seen as the product merely of a provisional sense that 'for a while at least all effort is over', it can be removed from the category of dangerous pleasures, and viewed as one of the forms of trivial, innocent gratification that suits the needs of the tourist. During the early nineteenth century, travel books begin to present southern languor as promoting a capacity for reposefulness that is worthy of investigation and even perhaps of imitation. Jameson, in her account of drifting into 'an indolent delicious reverie, a sort of vague and languid enjoyment' in Naples, describes this reverie as 'the true "*dolce far niente*" of this enchanting climate'. References to the *dolce far niente* proliferate in commentaries on Italy during this period.[41] Stendhal, in *Rome, Naples et Florence*, offers a definition of the concept that allows the reader to see it as a harmless delight, providing an entirely appropriate model for the traveller committed to temporary abandonment of responsibility and anxiety:

> Par ces mots célèbres, *dolce far niente*, entendez toujours le plaisir de rêver voluptueusement aux impressions qui remplissent son cœur. Otez le loisir à l'Italie, donnez-lui le travail anglais, et vous lui ravissez la moitié de son bonheur.[42]

The aquatic sublime

In early nineteenth-century accounts of Naples and other coastal regions of Italy, moreover, the pleasures of a melting away of care, in a setting where, as Jameson puts it, 'the mere consciousness of existence is happiness enough', are endorsed through descriptions that merge the relaxing effects of the beautiful with an awareness of sublime infinitude and indeterminacy, prompting a joyous sense of freedom from constraining bounds and limits. Jameson, after describing her 'enthusiasm' in the face of natural sublimity at Geneva earlier in her Grand Tour, presents the Alpine sublime as too overwhelming for her rapture to continue: 'by degrees the vastness and the huge gigantic features of the scene, pressed like a weight upon "my amazed sprite;" and the feeling of its immense extent, fatigued my imagination, till my spirits gave way in tears.' In their accounts of 'the blue sea, and the pure skies' (as Jameson terms them) of coastal regions of Italy, early nineteenth-century travellers manage to suggest that the mixture of beauty, on the one hand – soft, balmy air, the soothing effects of which are reinforced by gentle visual gradations – and sublime boundlessness, on the other, produce an effect of modified sublimity that entails a less dramatic and destabilizing experience than the Alpine sublime. Jameson herself, on her way from Rome to Naples, reflects upon the difference between the two versions of the sublime:

> In some of the scenes of to-day – at Terracina particularly, there was beauty beyond what I ever beheld or imagined: the scenery of Switzerland is of a different character, and on a different scale: it is beyond comparison grander, more gigantic, more overpowering, but it is not so poetical. Switzerland is not Italy – is not the enchanting south. This soft balmy air, these myrtles, orange groves, palm trees; these cloudless skies, this bright blue sea, and sunny hills, all breathe of an enchanted land; "a land of Faery."[43]

When describing the Bay of Naples as viewed from her balcony, Jameson again emphasizes 'the enchantment of the earth, air, and skies', and charts the gently reviving effect of 'the atmosphere without a single cloud', in which 'every breeze visits the senses, as if laden with a renovating spirit of life, and wafted from Elysium'. While the 'overpowering' qualities of the sublime are absent from the scene, however, the ability of nature to revive the traveller is located not simply in the 'bland luxurious airs' of the South (as Jameson terms them in her poem 'The Song of the Syren Parthenope', which she inserts in her narrative), but also in the removal of boundedness. The contrast between the sense of freedom induced by extent of sea and sky and the awareness of limitation induced by the climate of northern Europe is all the sharper for Jameson's suggestion that she can only reluctantly induce herself to suggest that anything might be lacking amid the domestic comforts of the 'vapoury' North (comforts which, tellingly, are mapped out in terms of repeated enclosure and spatial limitation):

> Then evening comes on, lighted by a moon and starry heavens,
> whose softness, richness, and splendour, are not to be conceived by
> those who have lived always in the vapoury atmosphere of England
> – dear England! I love, like an Englishwoman, its fire-side
> enjoyments, and home-felt delights: an English drawing-room with
> all its luxurious comforts – carpets and hearth rugs, curtains let
> down, sofas wheeled round, and a group of family faces round a
> blazing fire, is a delightful picture; but for the languid frame, and the
> sick heart, give me this pure elastic air 'redolent of spring;' this
> reviving sun shine and all the witchery of these deep blue skies.[44]

Mary Shelley, in her journal of 1824, following her return to England
some time after her husband's death, is more straightforward in
voicing her view that the 'vapoury atmosphere' of the country has a
depressing effect upon the spirits: after 'the imprisonment attendant
on a succession of rainy days' in London, she remembers the sea and
sky at Genoa, and exclaims: 'I can hardly tell but it seems to me as if
the lovely and sublime objects of nature had been my best inspirers
& wanting these I am lost'. 'The sunny deep' and 'the starry heavens',
she suggests, prompted an imaginative freedom that corresponded to
the freedom from spatial 'imprisonment' supplied by a milder
climate:

> Then I could think – and my imagination could invent and
> combine, and self become absorbed in the grandeur of the universe
> I created – Now my mind is a blank – a gulph filled with formless
> mist.[45]

In similar reflections a few months earlier, Shelley, like Jameson,
emphasizes 'the blue expanse of the tranquil sea', and presents this
'blue expanse' as encompassing both the 'balmy air' of a relaxing
climate and the power of the sublime to prompt a transcendence of
bounds: 'Then my solitary walks and my reveries – They *were*
magnificent, deep, pathetic, wild and exalted – I sounded the depths
of my own nature'.[46]

In enjoying an escape from the depressing effects of constraint
and limitation, the traveller inclines towards a Romantic rather than
a touristic attitude towards the foreign, acknowledging that he or she
is crossing symbolic as well as geographical boundaries, while
nonetheless defining these symbolic traversals as leading to self-
realization rather than danger. At the same time, however, such
accounts of a sublime disregard of limits reinforce the suggestion, put
forward in descriptions of the pleasures of relaxation and enervation,

that the warm South, with its blue sea and sky, might prove therapeutic rather than dangerous.

Excitement and novelty

Another concept that plays a part in narratives of revival and relapse, over this period, complicates still further the equivocations between Romantic and touristic stances that govern early nineteenth-century travel writing: the concept of novelty. Jameson mentions 'continual novelty' at the outset as one of the aspects of travel that may restore her to health and well-being. When she experiences a 'sudden renovation of health' at Gaeta, contemplating 'the azure sea', and viewing it as part of a scene of sublimity mingled with 'the most wonderful and luxuriant beauty', she explicitly mentions a sense of novelty as one element in her delight in nature that rescues her from 'dejection, lassitude, and sickness': 'The impression made upon my mind at that instant I can only compare to the rolling away of a palpable and suffocating cloud: every thing on which I looked had the freshness and brightness of novelty'.[47]

Such a consciousness of nature as new and reviving would seem readily compatible with Rogers' outline of a safely touristic experience of travel, in which 'all is new and strange', and we can 'surrender ourselves, and feel once again as children'. Novelty, however, together with the excitement that it generates and the curiosity that drives travellers to pursue it, is also easily incorporated into accounts of travel as a destabilizing activity. Burke, in his *Philosophical Enquiry*, defines curiosity – or 'whatever pleasure we take in novelty' – as restless and addictive:

> We see children perpetually running from place to place to hunt out something new; they catch with great eagerness, and with very little choice, at whatever comes before them; their attention is engaged by every thing, because every thing has, in that stage of life, the charm of novelty to recommend it. But as those things which engage us merely by their novelty, cannot attach us for any length of time, curiosity is the most superficial of all the affections; it changes its object perpetually; it has an appetite which is very sharp, but very easily satisfied; and it has always an appearance of giddiness, restlessness and anxiety. Curiosity from its nature is a very active principle; it quickly runs over the greatest part of its objects, and soon exhausts the variety which is commonly to be met with in nature; the same things make frequent returns, and they return with less and less of any agreeable effect.[48]

When Anna Jameson offers her accounts of 'excitement' – of a sense of inner renewal amid scenes of novelty – she carefully avoids any implication that this excitement might be giddy, restless and anxious, by repeatedly eliding the experience of a '*superflu de vie*' with the more relaxing and enervating physical and psychological effects of a warm climate: when tempered by the 'bland luxurious airs' of the South, such elisions seek to persuade the reader, excitement is never too dangerously exciting. In an extended account of the therapeutic effects of a region where nature 'lays forth all her charms', both upon those afflicted by 'pale disease' and upon sufferers from 'want | Or grief', Jameson's 'Song of the Syren Parthenope' moves imperceptibly from the animation of 'dancing spirits' to soothing 'balm':

> There is a power in these entrancing skies
> And murmuring waters and delicious airs,
> Felt in the dancing spirits and the blood,
> And falling on the lacerated heart
> Like balm, until that life becomes a boon,
> Which elsewhere is a burden and a curse.[49]

At one point, however, Jameson questions the benefits of 'continual motion', and of a constant search for the excitement of the new. On setting out for Naples, she remarks: 'I left Rome this morning exceedingly depressed', and adds: 'Madame de Staël may well call travelling *un triste plaisir*: my depression did not arise from the feeling that I left behind me any thing or any person to regret, but from mixed and melancholy emotions.'[50] The passage from *Corinne* that she invokes is one in which de Staël, charting Lord Nelvil's progress through northern Italy, implies that the urge to move on is something that takes hold of us against our better judgement, and is beyond our conscious control:

> Voyager est, quoi qu'on en puisse dire, un des plus tristes plaisirs de la vie. Lorsque vous vous trouvez bien dans quelque ville étrangère, c'est que vous commencez à vous y faire une patrie; mais traverser des pays inconnus, entendre parler un langage que vous comprenez à peine, voir des visages humains sans relation avec votre passé ni avec votre avenir, c'est de la solitude et de l'isolement sans repos et sans dignité; car cet empressement, cette hâte pour arriver là où personne ne vous attend, cette agitation dont la curiosité est la seule cause, vous inspirent peu d'estime pour vous-même, jusqu'au moment où les objets nouveaux deviennent un peu anciens, et créent autour de vous quelques doux liens de sentiment et d'habitude.[51]

The Marquis of Normanby's attack on the contention that travel is in itself reviving implicitly invokes this description of travelling as 'cette hâte pour arriver là où personne ne vous attend'. Lord Normanby begins with a long analysis of the mistaken decision of 'young Bouverie' to travel alone:

> Young Bouverie, in forming this resolution, over-rated considerably the sources of pleasure, which foreign scenes prove to the traveller; or rather he considered falsely such enjoyment to be like a fresh ray of sunshine evenly spread over the whole of one's thoughts and time. On the contrary, he experienced the delights of foreign travels to consist in very strong momentary excitements, awakened at intervals, and at first perhaps of some duration, but gradually and in a little time of a very passing kind.[52]

Such stimulation, it is emphasized, is positively harmful to the traveller: 'for the purposes of restoring health and relieving languor, I need not say, that the delights and amusements, which instead of being equal and continuous, are of excitement, and consequently are succeeded by a stare of depression proportionate to the degree of elation, must be far more pernicious than beneficial.' The narrator, in other words, implies that pleasures of a 'strong momentary' kind will prove to be unsatisfactory for precisely the same reason that Burke decries the pleasures of novelty. Once 'poor Augustus' embarks on his journey to Rome, the reader is told that it is 'the very enthusiasm of excitement' that is 'pernicious to his feeble health'. While conceding that 'the mind and body are linked together certainly, and in most cases the disorder of one occasions the derangement of the other', he classifies young Bouverie as an instance of an exception to this rule: the case of 'the decay of the body gradually and without pain, by the withdrawing or pining away of the vital principle':

> It is then, that as the bodily powers sink in utter languor and prostration, the spirit still retains not only its wonted vigour, but seems to exert itself with more than usual power, to shine with unearthly splendour, and to anticipate, as it were, by the loftiness of its views and conceptions, the pure state of being which it then approaches.[53]

In Bouverie's case, this exertion of the spirit assumes the form of an obsessive preoccupation with ancient history:

> It was not the wanness of the cheek of Augustus that struck me with forebodings of his fate, but some of those eccentric flights of fancy,

seldom indulged in by those who have a strong hold of life. For his own part, he seemed to lose sight altogether of his precarious state of health: one idea alone occupied his mind; and his sole wonder was, how he could have tarried so long in that dull Lombardy and trifling Tuscany, instead of having hurried by a bird's path at once to the scenes where all associations of past greatness centred. His day was one long, though interrupted, monologue of raving; from which he sunk, at intervals, to a dreary lethargy, and started thence again each moment to some anticipation of the immortal city, or some recollection of its story.[54]

Excitement, then, in this account, is an effect in which the established itinerary of the Grand Tour plays a major part. The Tour is mapped out, in travel writings from the early seventeenth century onwards, as a sequence of sights and wonders, which proclaim themselves as singular and exceptional objects of attention. Stephen Greenblatt, in his essay 'Resonance and Wonder', emphasizes the status of the wonder as a localized exception when he notes its power 'to stop the viewer in his tracks, to convey an arresting sense of uniqueness, to evoke an exalted attention'.[55] Wonders, on the one hand, play a useful part in the touristic approach: by virtue of their singularity, they provide the traveller with sharply delimited objects of contemplation, which it is possible to enjoy without becoming absorbed in the topography of potentially dangerous and destabilizing foreignness that surrounds them. On the other hand, this very 'arresting sense of uniqueness' that they convey invests them with an intensity that can itself be classified as a source of incipient danger. For Bouverie, the ruins of Rome are a generalized wonder, full of dangerous intensity. Charlotte Eaton explores the idea that just one of the wonders of the city might unsettle the susceptible traveller. In *Rome in the Nineteenth Century* (1820), Eaton presents herself as so enraptured by the *Apollo Belvedere* that she teeters on the brink of derangement; as though anticipating incredulity, she then cites another traveller more unquestionably unhinged than herself:

> You will think me mad – and it were vain to deny it – but I am not the first person who has gone mad about the Apollo. Another, and a far more unfortunate damsel, a native of France, it is related, at the sight of this matchless statue, lost at once her heart and her reason. Day after day, and hour after hour, the fair enthusiast gazed and wept, and sighed her soul away, till she became, like the marble, pale, but not like the marble, cold. Nor, like the lost Eloisa, nor the idol of her love, could she 'forget herself to stone,' till death at last closed

the ill-fated passion, and the life, of the maid of France.[56]

The most famous account of the incipient intensity and danger of encountering the great sights of Italy is, of course, Stendhal's description of his visit to Santa Croce in *Rome, Naples et Florence* (1826):

> J'étais arrivé à ce point d'émotion où se rencontrent les sensations célestes données par les beaux-arts et les sentiments passionnés. En sortant de Santa Croce, j'avais un battement de cœur, ce qu'on appelle des nerfs à Berlin; la vie était épuisée chez moi, je marchais avec la crainte de tomber.[57]

The eagerness with which travellers seek out sights and wonders, moreover, is often seen as inducing a fatigue which, in itself, is dangerous to health. James Johnson specifically warns that 'residentiary invalids' in Italy 'should beware of... fatigue in sight-seeing'.[58] Anna Jameson, after attending High Mass at St Peter's during Holy Week, declares: 'for the whole universe, I would not undergo such another day of fatigue, anxiety, and feverish excitement'.[59] Stendhal, in his *Promenades dans Rome* (1830), expresses his awareness of the ease with which viewing art and architecture can tip the traveller into a state of destabilized restlessness: 'Malgré l'extrême chaleur, nous sommes toujours en mouvement, nous sommes comme affamés de tout voir, et rentrons, chaque soir, horriblement fatigués.'[60]

Jameson, in Italy, tries hard to contest the idea that viewing the great sights and wonders of the country need necessarily have a destabilizing effect. She presents her desire to concentrate on art and nature as part of a touristic programme of carefully limited experience of the foreign, defining her aim as that of maintaining 'that state of *calm benevolence* towards all around me, which leaves me *undisturbed* to enjoy, admire, observe, reflect, remember, with pleasure, if not with profit':

> I am not come to spy out the nakedness of the land, but to implore from her healing airs and lucid skies the health and peace I have lost, and to worship as a pilgrim at the tomb of her departed glories. I have not many opportunities of studying the national character; I have no dealings with the lower classes, little intercourse with the higher. No tradesmen cheat me, no hired menials irritate me, no innkeepers fleece me, no postmasters abuse me. I love these rich delicious skies; I love this genial sunshine, which, even in December, sends the spirits dancing through the veins; this pure elastic

atmosphere, which not only brings the distant landscape, but almost Heaven itself nearer to the eye; and all the treasures of art and nature, which are poured forth around me; and over which my own mind, teeming with images, recollections, and associations, can fling a beauty even beyond their own.[61]

At one point, in Florence, Jameson implicitly recognizes that viewing works of art might send the spirits dancing slightly too excitedly through the veins. Before her account of 'the gallery' – the Uffizi – she notes ominously: 'All that I see, I feel – all that I feel, sinks so deep into my heart and my memory! the deeper because I suffer.' The effect of an initial visit is overwhelming and confusing: 'I came away with my eyes and imagination so dazzled with excellence, and so distracted with variety, that I retained no distinct recollection of any particular object except the Venus.' Jameson concludes, however, by stoutly maintaining that, for a discerning traveller such as herself, art can be experienced as reviving rather than dangerously exciting:

> This morning was much more delightful: my powers of discrimination returned, and my power of enjoyment was not diminished. New perceptions of beauty and excellence seemed to open upon my mind; and faculties long dormant, were roused to pleasurable activity.
>
> I came away untired, unsated; and with a delightful and distinct impression of all I had seen. I leave to catalogues to particularise; and am content to admire and to remember.[62]

One conclusion that might be drawn, then, from this exploration of some of the arguments and assumptions that play a part in Jameson's *Diary of an Ennuyée* and Normanby's 'Change of Air', is that arguments about health and disease readily become entangled with theoretical options and rhetorical strategies that initially appear to be formulated in response to quite different concerns: the aesthetic experience of landscape, for example, and the experience of viewing works of art. A precondition for the ease with which late eighteenth-century and early nineteenth-century travellers move between commentary on health and commentary on other domains of objects is, perhaps, the assumption that the practice of travel on the Grand Tour includes at least two elements that can always be defined in physiological terms, however swiftly and imperceptibly travellers' discussion of them is transmuted into the language of emotion, or of aesthetic responsiveness. The first of these is the 'bracing' or 'exciting' experience of pursuing novelty, experiencing travel as motion, and encountering the sublime (particularly on the Alps, where the dramatic effect of witnessing natural sublimity is reinforced by the excitement of crossing the major symbolic boundary between North and South). The second such element is the experience of the relaxing forms of enjoyment offered by a warm climate.

Notes

1   Anna Jameson, *Diary of an Ennuyée* (London: 1826), 4 (on p.351, Jameson tells the reader that 'like a true woman, I did but stake my all of happiness upon one cast – and lost!'); 5, 65, 84, 208, 348.

2   *Ibid.*, 353, 354.

3   Sigmund Freud, 'Beyond the Pleasure Principle', in *On Metapsychology: The Theory of Psychoanalysis*, translated from the German under the editorship of James Strachey, edited by Angela Richards, The Penguin Freud Library, xi (Harmondsworth: Penguin, 1985), 269-338, 329, with reference to Barbara Low, *Psycho-Analysis: A Brief Account of the Freudian Theory* (London: George Allen & Unwin Ltd, 1920), 73-4. See the account of the Nirvana principle in Jean Laplanche and J.-B. Pontalis, *Vocabulaire de la psychanalyse*, edited by Daniel Lagache (Paris: Presses Universitaires de France, 1967), 331-2.

4   *Diary of an Ennuyée*, 261-2. See also Jameson's account of 'most luxurious indolence' and 'a kind of vague but delightful reverie' in Rome, 272-3.

5   *Ibid.*, 265-6, 239; see also, for example, 294 (in Rome): 'I love this genial sunshine, which, even in December, sends the spirits dancing through the veins.'

6   [Constantine Henry Phipps,] Marquis of Normanby, *The English in Italy*, 3 vols (London: 1825), ii, 114, quoting, in adapted form, Byron, *The Bride of Abydos*, Canto I, Section I, lines 16-17.

7   *Ibid.*, ii, 116, 119, 114, 129, 132.

8   *Ibid.*, ii, 130, 135.

9   Henry Matthews, *The Diary of an Invalid, Being the Journal of a Tour in Pursuit of Health in Portugal, Italy, Switzerland and France in the Years 1817, 1818 and 1819*, second edition (London, 1820), 228.

10   Lady Morgan, Italy, 2 vols (London: 1821), ii, 4.

11   Lady Morgan, Italy, ii, 4, i, 345.

12   *Op. cit.*, 172 (see also 187, 224), 206.

13   James Johnson, *Change of Air; or, the Pursuit of Health; an Autumnal Excursion through France, Switzerland and Italy, in the Year 1829, with Observations and Reflections on the Moral, Physical, and Medical Influence of Travelling-Exercise, Change of Scene, Foreign Skies, and*

Voluntary Expatriation, fourth edition (London: 1831), 300.

14   *Ibid.*, 301.

15   Tobias Smollett, *Travels through France and Italy*, edited by Frank
     Felsenstein (Oxford: Oxford University Press, 1981), 294.

16   Edmund Burke, *Philosophical Enquiry into the Origin of our Ideas of
     the Sublime and Beautiful*, edited by James Boulton (Oxford:
     Blackwell, 1987), 134-5.

17   *Ibid.*, 136.

18   [Charles Louis de Secondat, Baron de] Montesquieu, *De l'esprit des
     lois*, edited by Victor Goldschmidt, 2 vols (Paris: Garnier
     Flammarion, 1979), i, 373, 385 (Book XIV, Chapter 2, Chapter
     13). Smollett's account of travel also invokes Montesquieu's
     classification of travel as one of the stimulants sought out by the
     inhabitants of the North (together with hunting, war and wine), in
     order to set in motion 'une machine saine et bien constituée, mais
     lourde' – in other words, a constitution unreceptive to pleasure
     (*Ibid.*, i, 376; Book XIV, Chapter 2). For Montesquieu's account of
     the industry of the North and the indolence of the South, see *ibid.*,
     ii, 28-9 (Book XXI, Chapter 3).

19   *Op. cit.*, 19-20.

20   *Ibid.*, 20-1.

21   *Op. cit.*, 32-3.

22   *Ibid.*, 239.

23   *Op. cit.*, 149-50.

24   *Op. cit.*, i, 373 (Book XIV, Chapter 2).

25   *Ibid.*, i, 375, 376 (Book XIV, Chapter 2).

26   *Lettres sur l'Italie en 1785*, 2 vols (Rome: 1788), ii, 308.

27   For a more extended account of this approach to the foreign, see my
     *Pleasure and Guilt on the Grand Tour: Travel Writing and Imaginative
     Geography, 1600-1830* (Manchester: Manchester University Press,
     1999), Chapter 4, 'Destabilized Travel' (173-208).

28   *Op. cit.*, 293.

29   *Ibid.*, 138, 139, 300. In contesting the view that Italy is a country of
     benefit to invalids, Jameson also (298-9) invokes the susceptibility of
     the Romans themselves to 'sudden death – or, as it is cooly termed,
     ACCIDENTE', as well as to nervous disorders: in Rome, he
     observes, women 'often faint, or go into convulsions, on perceiving
     the odour of the most pleasant flower', while 'not females only, but
     effeminate males evince the same morbid sensibility to odoriferous
     emanations'. See also Hester Lynch Piozzi, *Observations and
     Reflections Made in the Course of a Journey through France, Italy, and
     Germany*, 2 vols (London: 1789), i, 417-18, for an account of this

same sensitivity to agreeable smells.

30 *On Malaria: an Essay on the Production and Propagation of this Poison, and on the Nature and Localities of the Places by which it is Produced; with an Examination of the Diseases Caused by it, and of the Means of Preventing or Diminishing them, both at Home and in the Naval and Military Service* (London: 1827), 381.

31 *Op. cit.*, ii, 224-5.

32 *Ibid.*, ii, 225.

33 [Germaine] de Staël [Anne Louise Germaine de Staël-Holstein], *Corinne; ou, l'Italie* (1807), edited by Claudine Herrmann, 2 vols (Paris: Éditions des Femmes, 1979), i, 132-3 (Book V, Chapter 3).

34 *Op. cit.*, 240, 353.

35 [Percy Bysshe] Shelley, *Poetical Works*, edited by Thomas Hutchinson, corrected by G.M. Matthews (Oxford: Oxford University Press, 1988), 431.

36 *Criticisms on Art: and Sketches of the Picture Galleries of England*, edited by William Hazlitt Junior, 2 vols (London: 1843-4), ii, 203-4; emphasis is added.

37 See my account of the touristic approach to the foreign in *Pleasure and Guilt on the Grand Tour* (Manchester: Manchester University Press, 1999), Chapter 5, 'Tourism' (209-48).

38 Richard Lassels, *The Voyage of Italy*, 2 parts (Paris, 1670), i, unpaginated preface.

39 'On Going a Journey', in *The Essays of William Hazlitt: A Selection*, introduced by Catherine Macdonald Maclean (London: Macdonald, 1949), 29-40; 34.

40 Samuel Rogers, *Italy, A Poem* (London: 1830), 171.

41 See, for example, Sydney, Lady Morgan, op. cit, ii, 393, Normanby, *op. cit.*, i, 178-9, 179, iii, 178, Jameson, *op. cit.*, 262 (quoted above), Stendhal [Henri Beyle], *Promenades dans Rome*, edited by Armand Caraccio, 3 vols (Paris: Champion, 1938), i, 179, Louis Simond, *Voyage en Italie et en Sicile*, 2 vols (Paris: 1828), ii, 355.

42 Stendhal [Henri Beyle], *Rome, Naples et Florence*, edited by Pierre Brunel (Paris: Gallimard, [1817; revised edition first published in 1826] 1987), 188. The respectability with which Italian languor is invested by the early twentieth century is demonstrated in E.M. Forster's 'Story of a Panic' (1902), when the narrator (a testy Englishman, given to remarks such as 'those miserable Italians have no stamina', equably observes that, after a picnic lunch, 'we reclined, and took a *dolce far niente*' (in Forster, *Collected Short Stories* (London: Penguin, 1954), 9-33; 33, 12.

43 *Op. cit.*, 239, 33-4, 208-9.

44 *Ibid.*, 239, 224, 239-40.

45 *The Journals of Mary Shelley, 1814-1844*, edited by Paula R. Feldman and Diana Scott-Kilvert, 2 vols, continuous pagination (Oxford: Oxford University Press, 1987), ii, 476; journal entry for 14 May.

46 *Ibid.*, ii, 471.

47 *Op. cit.*, 5, 265-7.

48 *Op. cit.*, 31.

49 *Op. cit.*, 224-5.

50 *Ibid.*, 5, 206.

51 *Op. cit.*, i, 25 (Book 1, Chapter 2).

52 *Op. cit.*, ii, 119.

53 *Ibid.*, ii, 129-130.

54 *Ibid.*, ii, 130.

55 Stephen Greenblatt, 'Resonance and Wonder', in *Learning to Curse: Essays in Early Modern Culture* (London: Routledge, 1990), 161-183; 170.

56 Charlotte Eaton, *Rome in the Nineteenth Century*, 3 vols (London: 1820), i, 169-70. (In the text, the inverted commas begin just before the words 'nor the idol of her love...')

57 Stendhal [Henri Beyle], *Rome, Naples et Florence*, edited by Pierre Brunel (Paris: Gallimard, 1987 first published in 1817; revised edition published in 1826), 272. ·

58 *Op. cit.*, 301.

59 *Op. cit.*, 304.

60 *Op. cit.*, i, 13; see also 40, 41, 42, 120, 121. Richard Wrigley, in 'Infectious Enthusiasms: Influence, Contagion and the Experience of Rome' (in *Transports: Travel, Pleasure and Imaginative Geography, 1600-1830*, edited by Chloe Chard and Helen Langdon; New Haven and London: Yale University Press, 1996, 75-116), discusses some of the more extreme reactions evinced by French artists on embarking on sightseeing tours of Rome. The perils of sightseeing have been recognized, too, by twentieth-century travellers. Evelyn Waugh, in *Labels: A Mediterranean Journal* (Harmondsworth: Penguin, 1985; first published in 1930), 36, describes 'those pitiable droves of Middle West school teachers whom one encounters suddenly at street corners and in public buildings, baffled, breathless'; he notes their 'haggard and uncomprehending eyes, mildly resentful, like those of animals in pain, eloquent of that world-weariness we all feel at the dead weight of European culture'. Larry Keevil, in Elaine Dundy's novel *The Dud Avocado* (London: Virago, 1993; first published in 1958), 11, evokes the figure of the 'Eager-Beaver-Culture-Vulture' who all but 'collapses of aesthetic

indigestion each night and has to be carried back to her hotel'.

61   *Op. cit.*, 293-4.
62   *Ibid.*, 89.

6

Pathological Topographies and Cultural Itineraries: mapping 'mal'aria' in 18th- and 19th-century Rome.

Richard Wrigley

The word malaria was introduced into popular English usage by the geologist John Macculloch (1775-1835) in his 1827 book *On Malaria: an essay on the production and localities of the places by which it is produced: with an enunciation of the diseases caused by it, and the means of preventing or diminishing them, both at home and in the naval and military service.*[1] Macculloch's anglicised usage derives from the generic Italian term 'mal'aria', sometimes known as 'aria cattiva', which referred to the bad air which was believed to be the prime cause of a variety of diseases. Macculloch's study reviews existing opinion regarding the causes, incidence and international locations of 'mal'aria'; Rome, however, recurs throughout the book as one of the most notorious and persistent sites of malarial blight. He believed that any progress in identifying the essential nature of the phenomenon would only emerge out of a synthesis of empirical obervations, yet he continually draws attention to the apparent incompatibility between findings in different locales. Indeed, he repeatedly emphasises that the provisional and fragmentary conclusions he was able to offer were an accurate reflection of the lack of reliable information available. The fruits of Macculloch's endeavours were expressed in the form of a call for more systematic keeping of medical records, but this did nothing to conceal his sense of frustration at 'mal'aria's elusive ubiquity. Little concerning 'mal'aria' was certain beyond the enormous extent and devasting nature of its effects. Thus, it is perhaps not surprising to find that, at both the outset of his book and in its conclusions, he resorts to a compilation of ironical metaphor:

> This must suffice for the pure, the bright, the fragrant, the classical air of Italy, the Paradise of Europe. To such a pesthouse are its blue skies the canopy – and where its brightness holds out the promise of life and joy, it is but to inflict misery, and death. ... To him who knows what this land is, the sweetest breeze of summer is attended

207

by an unavoidable sense of fear – and he who, in the language of the poets, wooes the balmy Zephyr of the evening, finds death in its blandishments.[2]

Macculloch's remarks are, in fact, typical of the eclectic language employed in commentaries on Rome in order to characterise its climate and the specific phenomenon of 'mala'ria' or bad air. Such rhetorical circumlocutions were justified – and necessitated – by the general admission that medical understanding of the problematic nature of Rome's climate was extremely limited. Where medical knowledge ended, the language of the poets began. This paper is concerned with aspects of the language and knowledge *in between* medicine and literary texts – shared vocabulary and borrowings in both directions – more particularly with ways in which this language and knowledge inform travel narratives devoted to Rome, and the interplay between its hygienic and cultural identity.

As well as looking in to changing ideas on the nature and causes of 'mal'aria', this study will explore how these impinged on the practices of cultural tourism in Rome during the eighteenth and nineteenth centuries. My principal focus is the interplay between advice on the avoidance of 'mal'aria' in regard to its location, and how this affected the encounter with Rome as a 'museum city'.[3] The pathological dimension to commentaries on Rome is, in fact, remarkably frequent, but has been obscured by the extraordinary power of the city's primary reputation as a centre of artistic creativity and regeneration. The superlative artistic achievements to which the city had been host, were believed to have been caused by the all-pervasive qualities and properties of Roman air, which were understood to have impregnated the city's fabric and atmosphere, and still had an almost magical effect on travellers. For Creuzé de Lesser, even skeptical newcomers found themselves transformed as the result of breathing in the special air of Rome:

> ce qu'il y a de singulier, c'est qu'on respire dans cette ville le goût des arts, et que l'homme qui y est arrivé avec le plus grand éloignement pour eux finit assez promptement par en devenir très amateur.[4]

This was in tension with, though often outweighed by, awareness that the same climate that had fostered cultural inspiration was also responsible for the curse of indigenous diseases.[5]

We find remarkable contrasts in the language used to characterise Roman air. In texts like Macculloch's, bad air is referred to as a malevolent, invisible predator; yet Henry Matthews, in his *The Diary of an Invalid* (London: 1820) compared 'the genial air of Rome' to deliciously sweet cowslip wine.[6] Behind this ambivalence in terminology was the scientific cul de sac produced by the chemical analysis of air in different places using the eudiometer. Rather than identifying any pathogenic elements, this merely served to demonstrate that air's constitution was exactly the same everywhere.[7]

In considering the relations between ideas about the likelihood of contracting diseases in Rome and how this impinged on the experience of the city as a cultural spectacle, the notion of mapping provides a useful link. My use of mapping here is primarily analogical, rather than strictly cartographic (though I will refer to some maps later). In so far as mapping is both a conceptual and a practical activity, it connects, on the one hand, those medical topographical initiatives which it was hoped would reveal certain underlying empirical facts about the nature of diseases through the identification of their distribution, and on the other hand, the construction of cultural itineraries by means of which the excess of Rome's incomparable resources could be negotiated. The notion of mapping can also be extended to a more general level, in so far as this paper offers a case study in historicising the interrelation between art and science, which in eighteenth-century terms are categories as flexible or amorphous as, in modern usage, they are supposedly mutually exclusive. We will see how, as applied to Rome in the later eighteenth and early nineteenth centuries, contrary to modern expectations, it was cultural phenomena which, broadly speaking, provided the certainties. By contrast, in medical science, the commitment to empirical analysis of problems resulted less in confident progressive assertions than apologias that such initiatives had been inconclusive, and the recognition that the answer to manifold medical problems was, as yet, beyond the grasp of existing techniques of diagnostic assay.[8] The language by means of which such incomplete knowledge was conveyed pulls in a variety of political, ethnographic and poetic ingredients through a kind of rhetorical osmosis, which ultimately tells us less about the nature of 'mal'aria' than it does about the intellectual contexts of medical thinking and theorizing.

Interchange between travel and medical literature was likely because the experience of Rome had a perplexingly multiple aspect. On the one hand, Rome's character changed according to season – winters were claimed to be so benign and healthy as to restore invalids, the summers were associated with high risk of disease. On the other hand, the elusive nature of the causes of 'mal'aria' led medical commentators to seek evidence beyond the domain of scientific enquiry; the experiences of travellers, both written up and observed, and also local customs and sayings, were valuable raw material in this respect.

Location came to the fore in eighteenth- and nineteenth-century explanations of the nature and causes of the diseases clustered under or dependent on the notion of 'mal'aria', because of a reliance on essentially Hippocratic principles according to which environment and climate were primordial factors in determining the prevailing degree of salubrity. During the eighteenth century, these beliefs were translated into studies of the physical and pathological characteristics of specific locations. Enquiries into the particularities of the Italian climate in general, and that of Rome in particular, are examples of the deployment across Europe of the type of essentially empirical, statistical study that constituted medical topography.[9] One outcome of this approach was maps. In the case of 'mal'aria', graphic specification was a highly promising way of trying to pin down and get hold of what was a notoriously elusive phenomenon.

Early maps rely on fundamental Hippocratic co-ordinates: latitude and prevailing winds. In his *De Romani aeris salubritate* (*On the Salubrity of Roman Air*) (Rome, 1599), Marsilio Cagnati includes two maps. Firstly, one locating Rome in terms of longitude and latitude. Secondly, a simple but, in his own terms, perfectly effective map showing a city bounded by its historic hills and the city walls, framed by personifications of the prevailing winds.[10] In the early eighteenth century, Giovanni Maria Lancisi (1654-1720), an influential Roman medical figure, relied on a broad environmental picture to account for both general conditions of salubrity and outbreaks of particular diseases.[11] In his study of marshes and their relation to the incidence of disease, he acknowledged, like Cagnati, the crucial role of winds, but with a more precise focus, noting the way that their course had been altered by the felling of ancient woods. This reflected his belief in the importance of airborne pathogenic matter as a key dimension to the impact of disease. At the same time, he ascribed great importance to telluric influence. The map included in his study identified areas of 'black' and 'red' soil as influential in determining the salubrity of particular locations.[12] According to the Hippocratic theory of disease, a crucial factor – symptomatic of the specific combination of local earth with air and water – was the presence of invisible, vaporous miasmata, released into the atmosphere. In extreme cases, as occurred with marsh gas, they were credited with emerging in tangible form. Different kinds of soil released more or less noxious emanations, causing particular locations to be healthy or hazardous. In relation to the environs of Rome in the eighteenth and nineteenth centuries, this latter factor could be related to lack of cultivation. More skeptical, pragmatic commentators saw this rather as reprehensible evidence of the failings of an outdated and iniquitous system of government.[13] Traversing the *campagna* en route for Rome was the *locus classicus* for such remarks. The preponderant impression of barren emptiness was described in travel narratives of the encounter with Rome as a sombre prelude to the revelation of a mass of cultural treasures that awaited pilgrims to the Eternal City.

The most elaborate kind of pathological topography of Rome I have so far come across for the early nineteenth century is that in Jean-Baptiste Michel's *Recherches médico-topographiques sur Rome et l'Agro Romano* (Rome: 1813).[14] Michel was the doctor in charge of the French military garrison. His study was primarily intended for the expatriot French audience, but also contains opinions on the state of the local population's health. He produced two maps relating to the distribution of disease across the city. One map serves as a frontispiece, 'Plan géométral de la ville de Rome dans son état actuel en l'an 1814'. This combines hospitals and local topography in the form of *rioni*, with a historic dimension, for Michel also notes the sites of Ancient Roman temples to the goddess of Fever and to Minerva Medica, thus reinforcing the recognition that the city's health problems had a long-term history. Michel's other map was more extensive, taking in the environs of Rome, incuding the Agro Romano, and identifying three types of location in the area surrounding Rome: 'healthy', 'unhealthy', and 'very unhealthy'. Like Lancisi, he clearly regarded the empirical construction of the general environmental context as the key determining factor in this differentiation. This understanding was complemented in the text by detailed judgements on the degree of salubrity of different parts of the city itself, creating a perplexingly variegated jigsaw.[15] Such an uneven distribution necessitated explanations of why two places close together might fall into different categories. Indeed, Michel observed that 'mal'aria' was unevenly localised, to the extent that it might strike, not just in a particular street, but even a particular house within a street that was otherwise free from the problem.[16] This was a tangible and perhaps predictable result of what Michel proposed as the dominant feature of Rome's climate, its inconstancy (an idea dependent on the view that sudden changes of temperature, wind direction and humidity were always harmful because of the way they altered the body's condition), which in turn rendered medical advice highly unreliable.[17]

211

The creation of more precise medical records had the effect of demonstrating that specificity of location on its own was inadequate as an explanation for the incidence of 'mal'aria' as for many other conditions and diseases. Moreover, in the case of Rome, the apparently plausible association between insalubrity and disease was challenged by the notorious case of the Jewish Ghetto (on the north bank of the Tiber above the Isola Tiberina). On the one hand, this was agreed to be the dirtiest part of central Rome; on the other hand, it was acknowledged that it was not afflicted with 'bad air'.[18] The paradox of the Ghetto's unexpected salubrity was explained in the same manner adduced by Lancisi in the link he made between the course of winds being altered by the presence of woodland. In the case of the Ghetto, it was argued that it was its very congestion which obstructed the influx of tainted air. This example challenged the relevance of the common sense aesthetic criterion for associating the presence of disease with dirt, and further exposed the shortcomings of medical understanding of 'mal'aria'.

Nonetheless, without more convincing forms of explanation for the incidence of disease, the disturbing impression of ubiquitous filth continued to persuade observers of the city's unhealthiness. James Johnson claimed that Rome was the filthiest city in Europe, second only to Lisbon.[19] This caused him to misread the plaques regarding 'Immondezaio' that were found on some buildings in central Rome. He thought that they instructed Romans to 'throw dirt into the street', whereas Romans needed no such encouragement. In fact, these plaques reminded passers-by that legislation forbade the depositing of rubbish at these places. He also suggested that the tendency to nervous afflictions found amongst Romans and long-term residents was caused by the perversion of the olfactory nerves wrought by the stink of the Roman streets.[20] This gives an added dimension to the perception of a tension between past grandeur and present decrepitude which informs all Roman travel narratives. Modern detritus did not just impede apprehension of Antique Rome, it was physically offensive and believed to be potentially infectious. Like the pitiful condition of Roman peasants, such manifest neglect was also a stimulus to critiques of Rome's administration and its parlous state of civic decrepitude.

Comparative studies of diseases in different places also weakened the idea that they were as particular as their locations. For example, James Clark pointed out that the malarial fevers experienced in Rome were precisely the same as those found in the Lincolnshire fens, or Holland.[21] The idea that there was a specific condition known as

'Roman fever' ceased to be medically respectable by the mid nineteenth century. However, even at the very end of the nineteenth century, the term could be used as the title of a lengthy study of malarial fevers in Rome, although the author states at the outset that the weight of available evidence militated against accepting that such a particular condition existed (see W. North, *Roman Fever. The Results of an enquiry during three years residence on the spot into the origin, history, distribution and nature of the malarial fevers of the Roman Campagne, with especial reference to their supposed connection with Pathogenic organisms* (London: 1896). North includes a useful summary of nineteenth-century thinking as well as numerous maps which address the question of malarial distribution.) This recognition was combined with acknowledgement that, regarding the therapeutic effects of climate, different sites were only beneficial for particular conditions, to the extent that the best advice might be to stay at home.

Furthermore, in the case of Rome, focusing on the precise locations where 'mal'aria' struck brought to the fore the fact that bad air and its pathological effects were on the move.[22] Changed circumstances, especially depopulation, could expose new areas to invasion (the repopulation which might reclaim areas needed official action which was lacking until Rome became the nation's capital after 1870). In line with the continued influential role of Hippocratic principles, concern over exposure to winds identified the removal of ancient woods, which had provided a protective barrier, as having caused the changed character of, for example, the Pincio hill, which had succumbed to malarial presence, having once been thought of as an unusually salubrious area. This was partly why the French Academy was relocated to the Villa Medici at the time of its re-establishment after the Revolution.[23] Travel writers such as Hazlitt strongly recommended visitors to seek their lodgings in the hotels found in this area.[24]

Complementary to 'recherches médico-topographiques' was the evolving literature on climatology.[25] This was primarily oriented towards recommending therapeutic places rather than identifying causes of disease in unhealthy places. Progressively, different places were identified as beneficial for the treatment of certain conditions. However, nationalism and local partisan feeling, fuelled by the economic benefits of popularity amongst health tourists, played a significant role. In the case of Rome, however, the recognition that its climate was only beneficial for certain conditions, and then only at certain times of the year (for example, that consumptives should only make Rome their residence in winter), was slow to become accepted.[26]

Visitors to Rome were drawn by the general myth of the Warm South, what T. H. Burgess skeptically referred to as the 'talismanic efficacy of foreign climes';[27] Emile Decaisne more enthusiastically termed Italy 'the promised land of invalids', where they would be delivered from their afflictions.[28] This informed the deep-seated belief that the city was both a source of health and also cultural and artistic stimulation. But as the recognition gained ground that Rome could only be viewed as a therapeutic site at certain times of the year, and in relation to different conditions, so did the perception that the seasonal and topographical variations of climate meant that even healthy travellers should avoid particular places at specific times. Recommendations on visiting Rome reflect these ambiguities. One of the best known of these problematic sites was the Colosseum at midnight, preferably illuminated by moonlight. Since the later eighteenth century, a moonlit visit to it had become one of the obligatory ports of call for tourists to Rome. But by the later nineteenth century, it had become what Henry James, in *Daisy Miller*, termed a 'nest of malaria'. Hence, nocturnal meditations there were, as James put it, 'recommended by the poets, but deprecated by the doctors'.[29]

One aspect of medical uncertainties about Rome, was the question of whether the pursuit of culture was likely to be more injurious than therapeutic. While the inspirational effects of Roman landscape, light, and the atmosphere which created such effects were recognised not only to lift the spirit, but also to have a restorative effect on ailing constitutions, pursuing cultural itineraries was, nonetheless, not without its problems and dangers. On the one hand, Jean-François Dancel, in his study of travel and illness, viewed Rome's art treasures as a beneficial array of 'distractions' which could enhance the restorative effects of travel by providing a stimulating psychological boost.[30] On the other hand, James Clark spelt out the dangerous aspects of cultural tourism, particularly the extreme constrast of temperature and humidity experienced in moving from sundrenched ruins to dark, dank churches, whose chilled marble floors were especially dangerous for lightly shod women.[31] Indeed, T.H. Burgess extended this observation to the extent that he argued that, when talking of 'the climate of Italy', a distinction should be made between external conditions, and those found within churches and galleries.[32]

The pursuit of culture in Rome was all the more dangerous in so far as it was irresistible. Writing home from home in 1843, the painter Isidore Pils acknowledged the dangerous contradiction he was living: 'Je suis las de mon séjour en Italie; il me semble que le climat me tue; et cependant il est si beau!'[33] For one thing, in medical

214

terms, James Johnson suggested that the 'excitement of novelty and the exhilaration of travelling' disguised the initial effects of disease, thus delaying remedial action.[34] The city's riches induced overexertion and excitement which frequently resulted in a state of serious debilitation. This was itself sometimes classified as a pathological condition, what Burgess called 'the inveterate sight-seeing mania'.[35] For artists and architects, this could also lead to – or perhaps be confused with – a psychological crisis, in so far as the long-awaited rush of inspiration and the sense of a state of creative regeneration associated with the encounter with Rome might fail to materialise. In this respect, the stakes were raised regarding the heightened sense of expectancy with which new arrivals encountered the city, as there seems almost to have been an initiatory rite of passage which consisted of a high speed tour of the major sites before any kind of acclimatisation – or merely recovery from the rigours of the journey – had been possible. Excess of enthusiasm crossed over into disquietingly pathological reactions. There is a psychological dimension here, generated by the weight of expectation attached to the encounter with Rome, reinforced, and perhaps precipitated by, extreme physical states associated with the encounter.

The other type of cultural professionals whose activities were likely to expose them to risk were archaeologists, because excavations removed the barrier that had existed between the modern atmosphere and potentially noxious archaic miasmas, trapped beneath layers of stone and rubble.[36] Indeed, one explanation for the surprising salubrity of parts of central Rome was precisely the insulation provided by several layers of masonry accumulated over centuries of demolition and the collapse of monuments.[37]

The threat of 'mal'aria' interfered with other forms of artistic practice in the city. The Roman activities of the French artist François Marius Granet in the early nineteenth century provide a good example of this. Granet specialised in images of Italy, in particular his paintings and drawings of religious communities and scenes from past artists' lives. Both were based on extensive firsthand study of architecture and topography in Rome and elsewhere in Italy. Granet's engagement with Rome in the early nineteenth century exemplifies a reckless determination to pursue Romantic picturesqueness regardless of the consequences. In his case, he was specifically warned by his local guide that working in cold and damp crypts and the like was almost certain to damage his health. In his memoirs, he ruefully recollected the ambient dangers which artists who worked on Roman sites risked. When he set out to work in the vaults of San Martino ai Monti, formerly part of the Baths of Titus, he was alerted by monks there to its 'deadly' atmosphere. Granet's guide similarly urged him to make haste because of the bad air.[38] As he ruefully records, he was mistaken to spurn local advice and did, indeed, succumb to a prolonged bout of fever. His self-portrait while in the grip of fever appears at first sight to be an interesting example of the Romantic convention whereby extreme physical states were cultivated in order to gain access to new kinds of inspiration (Fig. 1). Granet, however, avoids self-heroization. Indeed, it might rather be seen as a kind of forensic self-reproach,

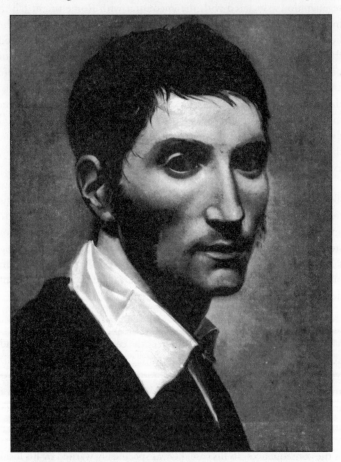

Figure 1
François-Marius Granet: *Selfportrait when ill,* c. 1811, oil on canvas,
40 x 31.4 cm. (Musée Granet, Palais de Malte, Aix-en-Provence).
Photo: Bertrand Terlay

216

documenting the wasted state that his illness had reduced him to, leaving him housebound and obliged to use himself as a model.[39]

The other quintessentially Roman resource much appropriated by visiting artists were the Romans, who were celebrated as evidence that earlier artists had merely copied the beauties they saw before them. This vision of Rome's populace relied on the ascription of long-term cultural aesthetic continuities that shaped the physiognomy of the special local identity – parallel to the belief in an ambient cultural catalyst in the form of 'something in the air' which was assumed to be the root cause of visiting artists' inspiration. In the images of Italian peasants in which he specialised, the Swiss artist Léopold Robert conjures up images of Raphaelesque nature as if they were spontaneously generated, and were an unchanged aspect of the inherently artistic Warm South. He fuses precise depiction of local costume with patterns of idealised form defined by early Renaissance art.

By the mid nineteenth century, academic naturalism in French artistic conventions gave way to a poetic realism that was willing to embrace diseased Roman peasants as pathetic but picturesque victims of their environment. This shift in perception is captured in Ernest Hébert's *La Mal'aria* (1850-1; Musée d'Orsay, Paris) (Fig. 2).[40] Hébert's painting applied in an ethnographic mode the possibility of representing disease and the diseased that had been spectacularly introduced in high art by Gros and Géricault, but which can be traced back to images dealing with the effects of plague such as David's *St Roch interceding with the Virgin for the healing of the plague-stricken* (1780) (Marseille, Musée des beaux-arts) and beyond. These were variations on the theme of the expressive body in a condition of noble suffering. Géricault added a psychological dimension to the representation of corporeal decrepitude, in tune with the idea, articulated in Cabanis's *Rapports du physique et du moral de l'homme* (1804), that the physical and the moral were coextensive. Hébert represents Roman peasants as inescapably rooted in their environment, and as distinctive expressions of it. In a sense, the painting made the indecorous phenomenon of disease visually acceptable by combining it with the old idea of the beautiful, quintessentially picturesque Italian peasant.[41] Similarly, Pierre François Eugène Giraud's *Le fiévreux dans la campagne romaine* (Fig. 3) transforms a study of a single figure chosen for its exemplification of a particular expressive register and anatomical configuration into something topographically and pathologically specific.[42] Such unfortunates were an equivalent to the 'deserving poor' in so far as they were understood to be emotive evidence of long-term

217

agricultural neglect and demographic degeneration. Their plight, and their wasted physique, were understood to be symptomatic of the shortcomings of local government – the expressive body was recognised to be shaped by contingent political conditions. Thus, the pathological and the political were directly linked. Protests by liberal French commentators in the early nineteenth century accused Rome's administration – whether the Austrians or the papacy – of simultaneously exploiting and ignoring the people of Rome, and insistently focused on evidence of contemporary neglect, rather than celebrating the splendour of artistic survivals from Antiquity.[43]

On a political and scientific level, the spectacle of disease was open to a general critique based on universal principles. But firsthand experience of the locale and its climate also tended to encourage the idea that, because 'mal'aria' was a localised, topographically specific problem, native knowledge accumulated over generations might provide the right advice as to how to avoid it. On the one hand, local knowledge, customs and sayings were noted and given credence – or at least recycled for consideration. For example, 'None but Englishmen and dogs walk on the sunny side of the street, Christians walk in the shade';[44] on location of residence: 'where the sun does not

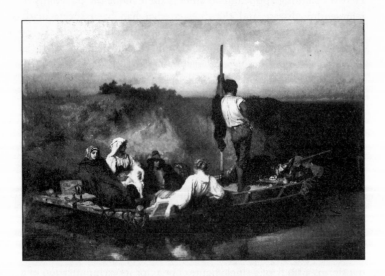

Figure 2
Ernest Hébert: *La Mal'aria*, 1850-1, oil on canvas,
135 x 193 cm. (Musée d'Orsay, Paris).

enter, there the physician invariably must'.[45] Berlioz reported that Romans disappeared from their promenade on the Pincio 'like a cloud of gnats' at 7.00 p.m. in the evening.[46] J.B. Michel notes the existence of a pseudo-scientific local vocabulary for different kinds of air: 'bad', 'heavy', 'fine', and 'subtle'.[47] In his advice to foreign visitors to Italy, Giacomo Barzellotti encouraged emulation of local customs as a means to minimize health risks.[48]

However, the impact of modern scientific ideas led to a more critical view of this source of knowledge. The persistence of popular beliefs about, for example, the contagious nature of consumption, which in institutional medical terms led to separate wards being set aside for its victims, was condemned as cruel and out of date by commentators who regarded Northern European medical practices as more enlightened and modern.[49] Foreign opinion on doctors in Rome also reflects this ambivalence. Baedeker advises consulting English and German doctors, nonetheless with the proviso that local maladies might respond better to 'native' skill.[50] Similarly, the entry on health in Murray's guide to Rome was written by a 'local authority', but one who had trained abroad.[51]

Such skepticism fitted in with the expectation that local advice

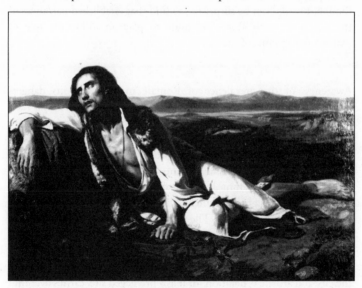

Figure 3
Pierre-François-Eugène Giraud: *Le fievreux dans la campagne romaine,*
1845, oil on canvas, 130 x 161 cm.
(Musée des beaux-arts, Clermont Ferrand).

219

might be disingenuously designed to reassure foreign visitors, and in the case of invalids travelling in pursuit of health, encourage trade. Examples of this can certainly be found in medical writing as far back as the mid eighteenth-century text by Giovanni Girolamo Lapi, *Ragionamento contro la volgare opinione di non poter venire a Roma nell'estate (Argument against the common opinion that one should not come to Rome in the Summer)* (Rome: 1749).[52] More generally, as has already been noted, climatology was inherently partisan, resulting in the most extreme form of skeptical recommendation that it was safer to stay at home. In so far as cultural and also therapeutic travellers constituted one of Rome's crucial economic resources, one can see that it was in the interests of Roman inhabitants and authorities to promote understanding of the causes of 'mal'aria', and to play down the notion that it was ineradicably rooted in the Roman environment. But much of this 'public relations' work was done in advance by the persuasive generic myth of the Warm South and its regenerative properties. In the case of Rome, one reason that this myth was able to retain its potency was because it was not until the 1880s that the causes of malaria in its modern sense were identified. The impact of this new knowledge on subsequent writing on Rome is something I have yet to explore – though it would not be surprising to find that established narratives of the encounter with Rome continue to play an influential role in shaping perceptions of the city.

Awareness of the prevalence of Roman 'mal'aria' and its dangers impinged on cultural tourism and art practice in several ways. As a threat, in tension with the prospect of inspiration and regeneration, and as a complement to the experience of destabilising excesses of enthusiasm. And, when its effects were observed in the wretched condition of Roman peasants, who were unable to escape their environmental and ethnically determined destiny, as a disturbing curiosity which might nevertheless become artistic raw material and thus, in a sense, be defused. The problem with the belief that Rome's unique culturally catalytic character was dependent on climate was that this also brought with it the corollary that Rome could not escape its pathological identity. This overlap between medical comprehension of the city and artistic veneration for it as a privileged site, carries over into the language of scientific analysis used to account for its infectious insalubrity. It was generally agreed that the causes of 'mal'aria' eluded all available instruments and empirical modes of enquiry. Hence Macculloch's rueful remarks, which I quoted at the beginning of the paper, in which what normally remained a pathological subtext, or an ominous aside, is made explicit. Macculloch seems to resent the need to rely on poetic language to pay a despairing, exasperated tribute to his elusive quarry. Other writers on the subject use similar terms of reference less ironically, indeed almost as if to play up the courageousness of their enquiries into the mysterious and at times dangerous workings of nature.

One way to make sense of the intersection of these ideas on Roman climate and its insidious effects would be to set out to trace the impact of scientific ideas on other types of discourse. However, it is also apparent that we need to recognise the considerable degree to which medical texts themselves rely on what we may call a poetics of pathology. They build up a picture of the nature of disease using not just tables of statistics and maps – although these may be their preferred, and most reassuring, mode of expression – but also drawing on a much wider linguistic repertoire. Indeed, paradoxically, the authority of their conclusions was enhanced, not diluted, by being able to quote poetry, and by adopting an explicitly literary idiom.

The vividness and detail of John Pemble's picture of later nineteenth-century travel, *The Mediterranean Passion*, encourages one to associate the heyday of travel for health with the later Victorian and Edwardian period.[53] The example of Rome, however, makes abundantly clear that, firstly, different forms of travel for health or to investigate disease were common throughout the eighteenth and early nineteenth century and earlier, and, secondly, that awareness of such issues also informed much of the extremely diverse literature of travel. In the case of Rome, the uniquely contradictory components of its reputation for cultural and therapeutic effects as well as the city's more sombre history as a place of disease and death necessitated the deployment of an elaborate range of discursive strategies for making sense of the experience. The undimmed popularity of the city through the eighteenth and nineteenth centuries as a destination for travellers resulted in the relation between these two sides of the city remaining as enigmatically compelling as they were complex.

•

For advice, encouragement and salutary criticism in my preparation of this text, I would particularly like to thank Chloe Chard and Jonathan Andrews. More generally, my preparation of this text has benefitted from the pleasurable stimulus of discussions with George Revill on the theme of pathologies of travel, amongst many other things. Kathy Maclauchlan generously supplied me with several valuable references arising from her work on the French Academy in Rome in the nineteenth century. I gratefully acknowledge the role played by a grant from the British School in Rome in initiating the research on which this study is based.

Notes

1 As noted by Mary Dobson, 'Marsh Fever: the Geography of Malaria in England', *Journal of Historical Geography*, vi: 4 (1980), 357-90. For a modern account of the impact of malaria and the development of its understanding, see Leonard Jan Bruce-Chwatt, Julian de Zulueta, *The Rise and Fall of Malaria in Europe: a historico-epidemiological study* (New York: Oxford University Press, 1980).

2 John Macculloch, *On Malaria: an essay on the production and localities of the places by which it is produced: with an enunciation of the diseases caused by it, and the means of preventing or diminishing them, both at home, and in the naval and military service* (London: 1827), 6, 381. John Henner strikes a similar note in characterising the conflict between the cultural historical reputation and medical reality of the Mediterranean: 'To the Medical Topographer, belongs the less pleasing task of describing these far-famed scenes as they at present exist: – no longer the seat of science, the chosen residence of demi-gods, and the fruitful nursery of sages and heroes; but now, alas! too often the residence of squalid misery and sordid ignorance; immersed in the noisome vapour of untrodden marshes, and fanned by no zephyrs but those which scatter disease and health from their wings' (*Sketches of Medical Topography of the Mediterranean: comprising an account of Gibraltar, the Ionian Islands, and Malta; to which is prefaced a sketch of a plan for memoirs on medical topography* (London: 1830), 1).

3 To this extent, this study complements the excellent article by Christopher Hoolihan, 'Health and Travel in Nineteenth-Century Rome', *Journal of the History of Medicine and Allied Sciences* (1989), 462-85, which primarily focuses on English responses, and provides a fuller account of prevailing medical opinions and prescriptions.

4 Auguste Creuzé de Lesser, *Voyage en Italie et en Sicile fait en 1801 et 1802* (Paris: 1806), 325.

5 For fuller discussion of Roman air and its 'antique perfume', see Richard Wrigley, 'Infectious Enthusiasms: Influence, Contagion and the Experience of Rome', in *Transports: Travel, Pleasure and Imaginative Geography 1600-1830*, Chloe Chard and Helen Langdon (eds) (New Haven and London: Yale University Press, 1996), 75-115.

6   Henry Matthews, *The Diary of an Invalid, being the Journal of a Tour in Pursuit of Health, in Portugal, Italy, Switzerland, and France in the Years 1817, 1818, and 1819* (London: 1820), 389.

7   See James C. Riley, *The Eighteenth-Century Campaign to Avoid Disease* (Basingstoke and London: 1987), 50-5, and Alain Corbin, *Le Miasme et la jonquille: l'odorat et l'imaginaire social, XVIIIe-XIXe siècles* (Paris: 1982), 16.

8   See James Johnson, *Change of Air, or the Pursuit of Health; an autumnal excursion through France, Switzerland, and Italy, in the year 1829 with observations and reflections on the moral, physical, and medicinal influence of travelling-exercise, change of scene, foreign skies, and voluntary expatriation* (London: 1831), 29-30; P. Foissac, 'Le miasme paludéen … échappent à tous les instruments' (*De la Météorologie dans ses rapports avec la science de l'homme et principalement avec la médecine et l'hygiène publique* (2 vols; Paris: 1854), ii, 509. It is interesting to note Mary Dobson's remarks on the work of her 'predecessors' in the seventeenth and eighteenth centuries: 'This book sets out to produce the type of regional and medical topography and chronology envisaged, but never produced on a large scale in England during the seventeenth and eighteenth centuries. Its findings ironically serve to reinforce the convictions, the certainties and the confusions of the early modern medical environmentalists' (*Contours of Death and Disease in Early Modern England* (Cambridge: Cambridge University Press, 1997), 41-2.

9   See Volney, 'Questions de statistique à l'usage des voyageurs' (1795) in *Oeuvres complètes* (Paris: 1846), 748-52, and James C. Riley, *The Eighteenth-Century Campaign to Avoid Disease*, chapter 2, 'Medical Geography and Medical Climatology', 31-52.

0   *Opuscula varia* (Rome: 1603), [55] unpaginated.

1   See Giorgio Cosmacini, *Soigner et réformer. Médecine et santé en Italie de la grande peste à la première guerre mondiale*, trans. Françoise Felce (Paris: 1992), 221-5.

2   *De noxiis paludum effluviis, eorumque remediis*, in *Opera* (3 vols; Geneva: 1718), i, 124-5.

3   For example, Frédéric Sullin de Chateauvieux, argued that Rome was 'about to fall prey to an invisible enemy [i.e. malaria], which a vigilant and wise administration would have enabled it to resist' (*Lettres écrites d'Italie en 1812 et 1813 à Mr Charles Pictet, l'un des rédacteurs de la Bibliothèque britannique* (Paris: 1816), quoted in the review in *Edinburgh Review* (March 1817), 58); A. Vieusseux, *Italy and the Italians in the Nineteenth Century* (2 vols; London: 1824), ii, 165.

4   Only the first volume of the two announced seems to have been

published.

15 *Recherches médico-topographiques*, i, 111-55.

16 Mary Dobson has pointed out to me that this kind of unpredictable distribution conforms to the habits of mosquitoes.

17 *Recherches médico-topographiques*, i, 30.

18 See Johnson, *Change of Air*, 77, 122; Michel, *Recherches médico-topographiques*, i, 140; Macculloch, *On Malaria*, 292-3. W. North, *Roman Fever. The Results of an enquiry during three years residence on the spot into the origin, history, distribution and nature of the malarial fevers of the Roman Campagne, with especial reference to their supposed connection with Pathogenic organisms* (London: 1896), 24; Dr Philip, *The Ghetto in Rome* (Florence: 1875).

19 Johnson, *Change of Air*, 178.

20 *Ibid.*, 274.

21 James Clark, *The Sanative Influence of Climate*, 3rd edition (London: 1841), 225.

22 J. Forsyth: 'This mal'aria is an evil more active than the Romans, and continues to increase' (*Remarks on Antiquities, Arts, and Letters, during an Excursion in Italy in the years 1802 and 1803* (London: 1813), 266), cit *Oxford English Dictionary*; Johnson, *Change of Air*, 122-4; Macculloch, *On Malaria*, 253-5; Frédéric Sullin de Chateauvieux noted that the areas now infected included the Quirinal, the Perician, the Palatine, the area surrounding the Villa Borghese, the Monte Mario, and the surroundings of the Villa Pamfili (*Lettres écrites d'Italie en 1812 et 1813*, quoted in *Edinburgh Review* (March 1817), 56-8).

23 J. B. Michel described the complex microclimate of the Academy created by its being subject to different winds, and spaces variably responsive to the external climate (*Recherches médico-topographiques*, i, 125).

24 Hazlitt, *Notes of a Journey through Italy and France* (New York: Chelsea House, 1983 [London: 1826]), 231; the abbé Richard pointed out that a further reason for the Pincio's favourable atmosphere was the absence of smoke from street kitchens which marred the rest of Rome (*Description historique et critique de l'Italie, ou Nouveaux Mémoires sur l'état actuel de son gouvernement, des sciences, des arts, du commerce, de la population et de l'histoire naturelle* (6 vols; Dijon and Paris: 1766), vi, 139-40; *A Handbook of Rome and its Environs; forming part II of the Handbook for travellers in Central Italy* (London: 1858), 285. See also Macculloch, *On Malaria*, 253-7.

25 E. Carrière reviews the literature: *Fondements et organisation de la climatologie médicale* (Paris: 1869). See also P. Foissac, *De la*

Météorologie dans ses rapports avec la science de l'homme et principalement avec la médécine et l'hygiène publique (2 vols; Paris: 1854), and *De l'influence des climats sur l'homme et des agents physiques sur le moral* (Paris: 1867). See also John Pemble, *The Mediterranean Passion. Victorians and Edwardians in the South* (Oxford: Clarendon Press, 1987).

26 See David Young, *Rome in Winter, the Tuscan Hills in Summer* (London: 1880); Toscani, *La Saison d'hiver à Rome* (Rome: 1881).

27 T.H. Burgess, *Climate of Italy in Relation to Pulmonary Consumption: with remarks on the influence of foreign climates upon individuals* (London: 1852), 1.

28 *Guide médical et hygiénique du voyageur* (Paris: 1864), 195.

29 Henry James, *Daisy Miller* (Harmondsworth: 1978 [1878]), 81.

30 *De l'Influence des voyages sur l'homme et sur les maladies* (Paris: 1846), 63; Decaisne, *Guide médical*, 198.

31 *Medical Notes on Climate, Disease, Hospitals and Medical Schools in France, Italy, Switzerland; comprising an inquiry into the effects of a residence in the South of Europe in cases of pulmonary consumption, and illustrating the present state of medicine in these countries* (London: 1820), 106.

32 *Climate of Italy*, 106; he noted that St Peter's was an exception to these problems with cold, damp churches; its huge volume of air seemed to remain mild in winter, and cool in summer (172).

33 Quoted in L. Becq de Fouquères, *Isidore-Alexandre Auguste Pils: sa vie et ses œuvres* (Paris: 1876), 20. I am extremely grateful to Kathy Mclauchlan for drawing this reference to my attention.

34 *Change of Air*, 127.

35 *Climate of Italy*, 106. The most notorious cognate modern form of this recognition has been dubbed the 'Stendhal syndrome'; see G. Magherini, *Le Syndrome de Stendhal. Du voyage dans les villes d'art* (Paris: 1989).

36 See Angelo Celli, *The History of Malaria in the Roman Campagna from Ancient Times*, Anna Celli-Fraentzel (ed.) (London: 1931), 121 (on the illness of workers at the archaeological excavations at Ostia in 1857), and 136 (citing J.G. Keysler, *Travels through Germany, Bohemia, Hungary, Switzerland, Italy and Lorrain*, trans. from 2nd end. of German original, (4 vols; London, 1756), ii, 25-7, 30, 337).

37 See Johnson, *Change of Air*, 119. Edward Diccy extended this idea to reclaiming the *campagna*, suggesting that one solution would be to pave it over, so as to seal off the rising miasmas (*Rome in 1860* (Cambridge and London; 1861), 46-7). This reference was kindly pointed out by Kathy Maclauchlan. On the role of paving as a barrier

to the exhalation of 'mal'aria', see Pietro Balestra, *L'Hygiène dans la ville de Rome et dans la campagne romaine* (Paris: 1876), 205-7.

38 *François Marius Granet. Watercolours from the Musée Granet at Aix-en-Provence*, with the 'Memoirs of the Painter Granet', translated and annotated by Joseph Focarino (New York: Frick Collection, 1988), 21-2.

39 This selfportrait takes on a further degree of pathos if we recall Ingres' portrait of Granet (Musée Granet, Aix-en-Provence), a veritable icon of the self-possessed Romantic artist, standing imperiously against a Roman backdrop made up of a lowering sky above the campanile of Trinita dei Monti, adjacent to the French Academy. On the selfportrait, see Bernard Terlay, 'Les Portraits de Granet', *Impressions du Musée Granet, Association des Amis du Musée Granet, Aix-en-Provence*, 7, 1992, 6-14.

40 Hébert conceived the picture in Rome, but executed it in Paris. See René P. d'Unkermann, *Ernest Hébert 1817-1908* (Paris: Editions de la Réunion des Musées Nationaux, 1982), 62-6. Unkermann quotes Théophile Gautier's approving judgement of the picture in terms of its successful evocation of the diseased Roman locale: 'Si *La Mal'aria* est une belle œuvre, c'est que la fièvre émane de la toile et qu'on éprouve le poids du ciel, de l'eau, de l'air, on se sent oppressé par l'atmosphère pestilentielle; l'artiste a littéralement peint le mauvais air' (*Des Beaux-arts en Europe* (Paris: 1855), 63). The picture was bought by the state and exhibited in the Musée du Luxembourg; see *Le Musée du Luxembourg en 1874: peintures* (Paris: Editions de la Réunion des Musées Nationaux, 1974), 98-9.

41 On myths of Italy, see Michel Crouzet, *Stendhal et l'italianité. Essai d'une mythologie romantique* (Paris: Corti, 1982); James G. Shields, 'Stendhal et Cabanis: le mythe italien à travers le prisme de physiologie', in *Stendhal, Paris et le mirage italien: Colloque pour le cent-cinquantième anniversaire de la mort de Stendhal* (Paris: 1992), 123-40, and Jacques Misan, *L'Italie des doctrinaires (1817-1830). Une image en élaboration* (Florence: Bibliothèque dell'Archivium Romanicum, 1978). Carlo Fea argued that the disagreeable climactic conditions were, in fact, suited to the encouragement of the fine arts; see *Discorso intorno le belle arti a Rome* (Rome: 1797), 21-2, 27-8. Catherine Guégan kindly drew this reference to my attention. See also G. Taussig, *The Roman Climate, its influence on health and disease, serving as an hygienical guide* (Rome: 1870): 'Thus the culture of the fine arts is carried on in every part of Rome and elevates and enobles the feelings of even the lower classes' (42).

42 See *Les Années romantiques 1815-1850* (Paris: Editions de la Réunion

des Musées Nationaux, 1995), 391.

43   On the question of why Roman splendour had given way to modern decrepitude, see Wrigley, 'Infections Enthusiasms'. The role of disease in determining degrees of cultural fertility in Ancient Rome, and also Greece, is considered in Leonard Jan Bruce-Chwatt and Julian de Zulueta, *The Rise and Fall of Malaria in Europe. A historico-epidemiological study* (New York: Oxford University Press, 1980), 89-105. See also W.H.S. Jones, *Malaria: a neglected factor in the history of Greece and Rome* (Cambridge: Bowes and Bowes, 1907), and *Malaria and Greek History: disease's role in cultural decline* (Manchester: Manchester University Press, 1909). 'On se promène en ce pays comme en un vaste Salon d'exposition publique où sont rassemblés les chefs-d'œuvre des grands maîtres du temps de Léon X, et les monuments de l'antiquité: pour le peuple, on n'y songe seulement pas. Sous l'épée française, ou sous le baton autrichien, qu'importe cet esclave malheureux et pourtant si plein de génie? Qu'est-ce que cela fait à l'artiste, au poète, au reveur?' (*Le Globe* (2 Nov. 1824), 97, cit. Jacques Misan, *L'Italie des doctrinaires (1817-1830)*, 29. Not surprisingly, French commentators claimed much progress was made to counteract this historic neglect during their occcupation of the city; see Comte de Tournon, *Études statistiques sur Rome et la partie occidentale des états romains*, 2nd edn (2 vols; Paris, 1855).

44   Karl Baedeker, *Italy. Handbook for Travellers, first part, Northern Italy* (Leipzig and London: 1877), xxiii.

45   *A Handbook of Rome and its Environs; forming part II of the Handbook for Travellers in Central Italy*, 5th edition (London: John Murray, 1858), 283.

46   Hector Berlioz, *The Memoirs of Hector Berlioz, Member of the French Institute, including his travels in Italy, Germany, Russia and England 1803-1865*, trans. David Cairns (ed.), (Frogmore: Panther, 1970), 176.

47   *Recherches médico-topographiques*, i, 56. A similar range of vocabulary was noted by the comte de Tournon: 'aria pessima, aria cattiva, aria sospetta, aria sufficiente, aria buona, aria fina, ou ottima' (*Études statistiques sur Rome*, i, 238-9).

48   Giacomo Barzellotti, *Avvisi agli stranieri che amano di viaggiare in Italia o dimorarvi per conservare o recuperare la salute* (Florence: 1838).

49   Clark, *Medical Notes*, 94.

50   *Italy. Handbook for Travellers*, xxiii. See also Hoolihan, 'Travel and Health', 484.

51   *A Handbook of Rome and its Environs*, 283.

the Italian and edited with an additional chapter on 'Rome as a
Health Resort' by John J. Eyre (London: 1897), translator's preface.
53 John Pemble, *The Mediterranean Passion: Victorians and Edwardians
in the South* (Oxford: Oxford University Press, 1987).

7

The Railway Journey
and the Neuroses of Modernity

Ralph Harrington

For the Victorians, the railway was a source of a highly significant collective experience of technology, and of a powerful, liberating and disturbing vision of what technology offered. Railways could be seen as a symbol of progress, promising economic and social betterment, democracy, energy, freedom from old restrictions, all the benefits and opportunities of the constantly circulating liberty of modern mechanized civilization. Yet they were also associated with pollution, destruction, disaster and danger, threatening the destabilization and corruption of the social order, the vulgarization of culture, the despoliation of rural beauty, the violence, destruction and terror of the accident.[1]

As both a collective and an individual experience, the journey was at the heart of evolving perceptions of the railway, and it assumed a central role in the perception of the railway as the source of a degenerative assault on the human mind and body. The bureaucratic demands of the crowded booking hall, the claustrophobia of the compartment, the jolts and vibrations of train travel, the blurred view from the carriage window, constituted aspects of the mechanization of travel associated with the railway, a process often experienced as an assault on the human constitution. It was through the journey that the railway as a disruptive, alarming, threatening agency was most widely and directly experienced by the Victorians. Few people suffered the horrors of direct involvement in railway accidents, or were the victims of criminal assault on a train, or even witnessed such events, but every traveller could draw on the collective experience of the railway journey. Every railway passenger had heard and read about accidents and assaults on trains, and had experienced unexplained halts and delays, the discomfort of poorly-sprung carriages, the darkness and foul air of tunnels, the noise and confusion of stations. Every railway passenger had internalized the mental structures of anxiety which were the collective heritage of Victorian travellers, and which were augmented and renewed with every year's new tally of collisions, derailments and other mishaps. The railway journey was not merely an event or a process; it was a shared cultural location through which the ill-defined but potent anxieties associated with the advent of mechanized mass transportation were focussed, collected and transmitted. It constituted the paradigmatic experience of the railway age, serving as a link between the public, externalized, shared fears and anxieties provoked by the railway and the private, internal trauma of the individual railway traveller, confronted with the dangers, discomforts, and industrialized stresses of train travel.

The railway journey was first and foremost a collective, social experience. Railways were the first mass transit system. By means of the train, more people than ever before could travel, and in greater numbers. The crowds of people at railway stations, the passengers who filled the trains, constituted an entire society on the move: one observer commented in 1855 on 'the railway engine dragging in its train, what seems at times like a street in motion, with its numerous apartments and various classes of a living population'.[2] As H. G. Wells observed in 1902:

> When the historian of the future speaks of the past century as a Democratic century, he will have in mind, more than anything else, the unprecedented fact that we seem to do everything in heaps – we read in epidemics; clothed ourselves, all over the world, in identical fashions; built and furnished our houses in stereo designs; and travelled – that naturally most individual proceeding – in bales.[3]

Railway trains, like the society they served, were divided into a hierarchy of classes. However, the significance of this system of class distinction was strictly limited. It did not alter the fact that the railways were open to all who could afford to ride, and that all passengers of whatever class travelled at the same speed and reached their destinations at the same time. Furthermore, despite the efforts of railway companies to provide entirely separate facilities for the different passenger classes, it was in practice impossible to keep them apart entirely and people of all sorts and conditions inevitably met and mixed, particularly at stations. Finally, for many critics of the railway the system of passenger classes was an irrelevance; the fact that representatives of almost all levels of society were able to travel as never before was a negative factor in itself. With the coming of the railway, the mob had become mobile.

It was universally accepted that the railways were having a 'democratizing', 'levelling' effect on society. Critics and supporters of the railways alike would have agreed with the economist and journalist James Jeans's statement of 1887 that 'Railways are the great levellers of the world'.[4] 'Theories of democracy were useless prior to railways', was the view of the railway writer E. Foxwell in 1884:

> For fifty years ... people of every sort and variety have come across each other, and have been intimately mixed up in the affairs of life. This constant rubbing against one another has taught them to be more kindly disposed to all sorts and conditions ... and while it has in consequence created a wish to level everyone up to those best possibilities of which his human composition renders him capable, the incessant contact of ideas has bred feasible plans for the wiser treatment of that stuff of which high and low are only variations. This is Democracy, and this is the work of railways.[5]

Foxwell celebrated the phenomenon of wider social interaction, greater tolerance, the breaking down of class barriers, the liberation of people from the bonds of custom and deference; others saw the very foundations of civilization being eroded by the influence of the railway. Members of the aristocracy felt this danger particularly keenly. In 1842 an anonymous pamphleteer observed that 'Railways are decidedly unpopular with the aristocracy', and suggested that one reason for this lay in the fact that 'the mode of carriage is not sufficiently exclusive and that the same speed conveys the poorest and greatest man to his destination'.[6] Indeed, upper-class travellers, accustomed to the freedom and status of travel in their own, private horse-drawn vehicles, did have reason to feel particular discomfort and resentment at the restrictions imposed by rail travel.[7] The new form of transport was open to all, and the discerning traveller could no longer rely on the possession and use of a status-confirming means of transport to exclude the lower orders. In Benjamin Disraeli's novel *Sybil* (1845), Lord De Mowbray declares that the railway has 'a dangerous tendency to equality' and is one of the foremost representatives of 'the levelling spirit of the age' against which the nobility must 'make a stand'. Lady Marney, agreeing with him, recounts the experience of her friend Lady Vanilla, who found herself sharing her compartment with two arrested pickpockets, chained together: '"A countess and a felon! So much for public conveyances," said Lord Mowbray.'[8]

Such concerns related to a complex of fears about technological modernity itself, and its association with an urbanized, socially and culturally degenerate mass civilization. The poet John Davidson articulated this concern through his elitist character Sir John Simplex, in 'The Testament of Sir John Simplex concerning Automobilism' (1907). Simplex complains that railway travel 'Unites one with a vengeance to the Mob':

> Bankers and brokers, merchants, mendicants,
> Booked in the same train, like a swarm of ants ...
> In the guard's van my sacred luggage knocks
> Against the tourist's traps, the bagman's box;
> And people with inferior aims to mine
> Partake the rapid transit of the line.[9]

This fear of the enforced social mixing extended throughout the upper and middle classes. For the middle classes, identified with the bourgeois values of order, decency, and self-restraint, the urban masses were increasingly perceived as disorderly, indecent, unrestrained, and much of Victorian middle-class culture can be understood in terms of structures of exclusion designed to keep the perceived threat of the masses at bay. The phenomena which constituted middle-class civilization and expressed the ideology of progress which was central to middle-class identity embodied the ideal of free movement, of unimpeded physical, commercial, cultural and intellectual circulation. Yet the very openness of such systems of circulation and exchange made them vulnerable to infiltration from the unimproved, regressive elements of mass society, variously conceived as a cultural, social, or biological threat.[10] The railway, the most striking and public exemplar of the concept of free movement and circulation, was at the heart of this paradox.

Against this background, the railway can be viewed not only as a system of circulation and exchange, but as an arena of contested social spaces: the station, the platform, the railway carriage. The railway compartment in particular played a significant role in this discourse. In 1887 the medical periodical *The Lancet* drew on the anxiety and unease associated with the compartment when it commented:

> The forcible intrusion of persons often in the dirtiest condition among the occupants of first and second class carriages, who have purchased the comparative comfort in which they choose to travel, is a matter of serious public inconvenience. The company of these intruders is not only objectionable on aesthetic grounds, but it is equally undesirable on sanitary principles ... the possible transference of infection and other *contagium vivum* of parasitic

nature is no mere shadow of imagination when one's travelling companions have come from the slums of the great city.[11]

While ostensibly concerned solely with issues of public health, this passage is fraught with many other layers of meaning. The status of first- and second-class passengers, and the right of those who have more money to occupy a great share of space and secure more comfortable facilities, is represented as a matter of public good rather than private privilege. The 'intruders' complained of are represented as a threat to health, not merely as unsightly and unpleasant objects; but the validity of objections to them 'on aesthetic grounds' is implicitly admitted. In short, it is assumed that intruders from outside the sequestered comfort of the first- or second-class compartment will use violence ('forcible intrusion') to gain admittance, will be insanitary and dirty, of offensive appearance and behaviour, and quite possibly highly infectious. The reference to '*contagium vivum* of parasitic nature', it is clear, does not refer only to the diseases these intruders may be carrying; it refers to the intruders themselves.

John Davidson spoke for many when he portrayed the train as the symbol of a society which embodied the triumph of the crowd; the representatives of the railway-travelling middle classes who articulated these concerns were haunted by the spectre of the mob. The potential for disorder and violence inherent in all large bodies of people made the station in particular a place of uneasy and fragile balance between order and chaos, in which a veneer of regulation and control overlaid a disturbing potential for turbulence and disorder. Wilkie Collins provided a brief but vivid sketch of York station in his 1862 novel *No Name*: 'Three different lines of railway assemble three passenger mobs, from morning to night, under one roof; and leave them to raise a travellers' riot'.[12] Collins's account is humorous, but nevertheless conveys the threat of violence and disorder which he perceived in the crowd. The terms he uses – 'mobs', 'riot' – are not neutral or dispassionate. They draw on perceptions of the crowd as frightening, unmanageable, threatening, and reflect an image of the station as an arena of inadequately contained disorder and turmoil.

The railway station provided a concentration of many of the aspects of modern life which were widely believed to be injurious to health: anxiety, pressure, worry, noise, bustle, crowds, constant movement. A physician writing in the *Association Medical Journal* (the forerunner of the *British Medical Journal*) in 1856 recounted how a friend who was a regular commuter on one of the lines into

London 'fell down dead on the platform of a railway station; his life being the forfeit paid for the exertion which he had made to reach the starting train'; although he was careful to point out that the individual in question suffered from 'an affection of the heart'.[13] A physician writing in *The Lancet* in 1862 commented that years of observing travellers from his home near a large station had convinced him that 'the frequent excitement, and constant hurry and anxiety which he witnessed on the part of passengers arriving' were 'a mischievous circumstance. In certain unhealthy conditions of the heart it has many times proved fatal.'[14] Medical commentators agreed that people with already weakened constitutions were especially vulnerable to the effects of hurry and anxiety, but that all travellers were at risk in the mentally and bodily exhausting environment of the railway[15] and that the station was a particularly dangerous location. It was at the station that the railway system connected with the rest of the social and economic infrastructure of society; it was from the station that the invisible but inexorable demands of the railway extended across society; and it was upon entering the station that the traveller felt the imposition of railway time and railway regulation. The railway station stands as a symbol of the often traumatic Victorian encounter between technological modernity and the human constitution.

Not least among the threatening forces associated with the Victorian railway was crime. Trains provided new opportunities for the rapid and unimpeded movement on the part of criminals, as well as a new arena for their activities in the confines of the carriage, among the contents of luggage vans and goods wagons, and at the station which, with its transient population, its mixing of all sorts and conditions of people, its constant bustle and confusion, was a magnet for thieves, pickpockets, prostitutes, misfits, idlers and ne'er-do-wells. Authors were quick to exploit the potential of railway crime, and railways made frequent appearances in Victorian crime stories; train chases in particular, in which the escaping criminal was pursued across the network, became a common feature of sensational literature in the latter half of the nineteenth century.[16]

The dangers of one particular aspect of railway travel, the compartment, were thrown into a lurid light by a number of highly-publicized assaults and murders which took place on trains in the 1860s. The murder of Chief Justice Poinsot on a train between Mulhouse and Paris in December 1860 caused concern throughout Europe,[17] and a number of similar occurrences in Germany were also widely reported.[18] The resulting climate of anxiety provoked a British journal to comment in 1863 that 'murder, or violence worse than murder, may go on to the accompaniment of a train flying along at sixty miles an hour. When it stops in due course, and not until then, the ticket collector coming up may find a second-class carriage converted into a "shambles". We are not romancing.'[19]

In July 1864 the public's fears received ghastly confirmation with the murder of Thomas Briggs, brutally assaulted in broad daylight on a stopping train in the London suburbs.[20] The facts of the case were shocking: aboard a busy train, in the brief interval between two closely-spaced stations, Briggs was stabbed, robbed, and thrown out onto the tracks to die. The crime was not discovered until a passenger got into the first-class compartment formerly occupied by the victim and noticed blood on the seats and floor. 'It is the glory of an age of scientific progress to have invented a perfectly new and unique description of social torture', observed the *Saturday Review* in the wake of this crime:

> The English railway-carriage – more especially, the English first-class railway-carriage – may be defined as an apparatus of unexampled efficiency for isolating a human being from the companionship and protection of his fellow-creatures, and exposing him a helpless prey to murderous outrage.[21]

The Briggs case led to what the *Saturday Review* called a 'frenzy of the public mind about the dangers of railway travelling'.[22] In fact, murders were almost unknown on British railways: the next case of a railway passenger being murdered on a moving train did not occur until 1881, and there were only five such murders between 1864 and 1914;[23] but the anxiety created by the idea of such crimes was out of all proportion to the reality. More than thirty years after the Briggs murder, the furore provoked by the publication in 1897 of John Oxenham's short crime story *A Mystery of the Underground* illustrates the power such anxiety continued to wield in the public mind. The story was published as a serial in the popular magazine *To-Day*, beginning on 27 February 1897; it described, through apparently authentic extracts from London newspapers, how the London underground railway system was being terrorised by a serial killer who struck at the same time every Tuesday, week after week, shooting innocent passengers dead in their seats. The magazine's circulation surged, and alarm spread among underground travellers; railway officials claimed that passenger numbers actually dropped on Tuesday evenings, and representatives of the companies which ran the underground system wrote a formal letter of protest to the magazine, leading the magazine's editor to consider dropping the story.[24]

One of the most important factors in the scale and longevity of the impact of the Briggs case was the peculiarly middle-class sense of security which was outraged by the crime. Writing one year after the murder, Matthew Arnold articulated this class dimension when he remarked on the profound effect which the crime had had on his fellow travellers on the Woodford branch of the Great Eastern Railway:

> Every one knows that the murderer, Müller, perpetrated his detestable act on the North London Railway, close by. The English middle class, of which I am myself a feeble unit, travel on the Woodford branch in large numbers. Well, the demoralisation of our class ... caused by the Bow tragedy, was something bewildering.[25]

There is more to this 'demoralisation' than the sense of vulnerability to crime which is one of the constant themes of middle-class Victorian life. The railway had a very particular significance to the middle classes, as one of the commercial and technological achievements which made possible the comfort and security of their lives. It was woven into the texture of middle class civilization, carrying families to holidays, men (and, increasingly, women) to and from work, conveying newspapers, luxuries and essentials, innumerable home comforts. The railway-travelling middle classes felt profoundly the assault on Mr Briggs as an assault on their whole class. The nexus of the anxiety provoked by the murder was located in its transgression of the structures of security, privacy and protection which had developed around the middle-class railway passenger since the 1830s, and which were physically embodied in the phenomenon of the upholstered, enclosed compartment. The Briggs case dramatized the highly ambiguous form of security offered by the compartment, beset as it was by the paradox that for the passenger it was as much prison as it was protection. The helpless traveller could find him- or herself confined with someone 'from an infectious sick bed, or ... unconsciously himself the seat of an incubating fever',[26] or with a violent criminal, a lunatic, a garrotter, or a rapist. The dream repeatedly experienced by one of Freud's patients, in which 'a lunatic was being conveyed in a compartment on an Italian line, but through carelessness a traveller was allowed in with him', and which ended with the lunatic killing the other traveller, echoed a widespread fear.[27]

The anxiety associated with enclosure in the compartment was intensified when combined with the fears provoked by the tunnel.

Tunnels were, under any circumstances, frightening for the nervous railway traveller; the danger that they might give the assailant with whom one was closeted in one's compartment the opportunity to strike gave them particular horror. 'Male passengers have sometimes been assaulted and robbed, and females insulted, in passing through tunnels', warned *The Railway Traveller's Handy Book*, a manual of advice and information for railway travellers, in 1862; 'In going through a tunnel, therefore, it is always as well to have the hands and arms ready disposed for defence, so that in the event of an attack, the assailant may be instantly beaten back or restrained.'[28] Considerable effort was expended on devising mechanical means whereby the occupants of a compartment could communicate with the outside world. *The Handy Book*'s suggestion was 'to tie a coloured handkerchief on to the end of a stick, and hold it out as far beyond the carriage as possible'[29] •– although what use this would be in a tunnel, and how one could do it while holding the hands and arms ready disposed for defence, was not explained. There was very little support, however, for the idea of moving away from the compartment altogether towards the American model of open carriages; the shared space of the open car might suit the 'democratic' American temperament, but was felt to offend against the important European right to privacy and quiet. Despite the perceived dangers of 'railway imprisonment', the British middle classes, like their French and German counterparts, were reluctant to abandon their structures of enclosure and exclusion.

Such structures were important, given the transformation in social relations brought about by railway travel. In particular, the railways brought new opportunities for women travellers. As early as 1844, the *Quarterly Review* observed approvingly that railways had brought about 'the emancipation of the fair sex, and particularly of the middle and higher classes, from the prohibition from travelling in public carriages, which with the majority was a prohibition from travelling at all.'[30] The emergence of opportunities for relatively free travel for women led to a reshaping of social relations and public spaces, and the development of new areas of cultural and sexual negotiation and friction. In the case of the railway, the character of the public spaces occupied by travellers, and in particular the compartment, became the focus for new anxieties. The British railway compartment, as we have seen, was a very particular kind of space; whereas the openness of the American railroad car provided the security of visibility,[31] the compartment enclosed its occupants in a self-contained environment, shielded from public scrutiny. It also provided a secluded arena for sexual assault. Cases of sexual assault in railway carriages continued in a steady flow throughout the nineteenth century; they were never common, but as with other aspects of railway anxiety it is the public perception of the danger that is more significant than the reality.

Such cases as did occur were widely reported, in full and often salacious detail, encouraging the development of a climate of alarm over the safety of the railway compartment; in the words of the *Saturday Review*, 'Everybody feels that no man's life and no woman's honour is safe inside a railway carriage'.[32] As well as providing a secluded arena for male sexual fantasy, and sometimes for actual sexual assault, the compartment confronted men and women with each other, in a luxurious, rhythmically moving environment. E. M. Forster encapsulated the sensuality and the erotic promise of the railway compartment in *Howard's End*: '"Male and female created He them"; the journey to Shrewsbury confirmed this questionable statement, and the long glass saloon, that moved so easily and felt so comfortable, became a forcing-house for the idea of sex.'[33]

Many contemporaries were convinced that railway travel created conditions in which female passengers of an 'imaginative' or 'hysterical' tendency might be led to invent, either consciously or unconsciously, stories of assault, leading to the unjust impugning of innocent men, and even to blackmail. The *Saturday Review* commented on a recent case which had brought out 'this special evil which railway travelling has aggravated' in 1864:

> There is a danger to which the unprotected male passenger is liable which does not affect his life, but which compromises interests that are even dearer than life. We mean the liability which every man incurs of being charged with indecent assault ... Poor Mr. Briggs found in a first-class carriage, and in a train stopping every five minutes, no security for his life. A respectable young man, Rutherford, found the crowded benches of a third-class van on the North Kent line no security against a charge preferred by a 'modest and respectable young woman,' as we are assured, who was stimulated into semi-insanity by the terrors of a tunnel and the newspaper reports of assaults which have been made, under similar circumstances, on female chastity.[34]

The experience of Sir William Hardman two years later would seem to indicate that it was not only women who were susceptible to over-stimulation in the prevailing climate of alarm. Hardman was greatly disturbed by the behaviour of a woman who got into his

238

compartment and changed her seat a number of times: 'three seats in as many minutes! I began to speculate as to where she would sit next – perhaps on my knee, and then would charge me with sexual assault.' She got out at the next station, but Hardman's ordeal was not over, for she re-boarded the train, this time getting into the next compartment:

> Perhaps she was relating to her new companion how she had just been grossly insulted by a lewd gent in the place she had just left ... These unfounded charges of indecent assault have been very common of late, and I have determined to object in future to the entry of any unprotected female into a carriage where I may be alone.[35]

In 1866 *Punch* supported the provision of 'distinct carriages for unattended females', but their concern was not primarily with the safety of women travellers but rather with 'the dangers of extortion to which male passengers are exposed.'[36] The risks run by women railway travellers in the nineteenth century were real enough; yet the issue which concerned much of the periodical press and many individual male travellers was the danger presented by women making false accusations of assault against innocent, respectable men. Perhaps this was in part a reaction to the successful claiming by women of the new freedom to travel which the railway brought, and their consequent presence in the public spaces of the railway. It can thus be seen in the context of the railway's role as an agent of social mixing, and as a disrupter of established codes of conduct. As the American scholar Patricia Cline Cohen has observed of the railway, the 'possibility of movement, both rapid and far from home, untied people from obligations, restrictions and expectations.'[37] The etiquette of travel remained uncertain and fluid in Victorian Britain, the established structures of social differentiation and division inadequate to the new circumstances of mass industrialized transportation.

The railway brought new opportunities and freedoms, but it also imposed regulation and rigidity. 'To make a journey': the phrase suggests that the traveller possesses a degree of creative autonomy, and can shape the journey according to his or her particular requirements. One of the chief complaints against the train from its earliest days was that the railway traveller was denied the freedom to 'make' a journey, and was transformed from an autonomous and creative agent into a passive commodity being transported within a rigid system of routes and stations. Railway journeys were laid out in advance, times of departure and arrival pre-ordained, routes pre-

239

planned, with travellers collectively serving as the raw material for what was in effect an industrial system, the end-product of which was mass transportation.[38]

In 1883 James Nasmyth, chairman of the Metropolitan Railway, presided at a meeting of the railway's shareholders at which he performed an interesting demonstration:

> At a recent meeting of the Metropolitan Railway Company I exhibited one million of letters, in order to show the number of passengers (thirty-seven millions) that had been conveyed during the previous twelve months. This number was so vast that my method only helped the meeting to understand what had been done in the way of conveyance. Mr. Macdonald, of The Times, supplied me with one million type impressions, contained in sixty average columns of The Times newspaper.[39]

Nasmyth's attempt to illustrate in concrete terms the abstract statistical concept of the 37 million journeys made on the Metropolitan Railway during the year 1882-3 clearly conveys both the unprecedented scale of railway activities and the difficulties sometimes experienced by contemporaries in grasping such a large and complex reality; but it also gives expression to the transformation of railway passengers into numbers to be counted, flows to be controlled, commodities to be transported. The individuality of the railway traveller became subsumed into the flow of 'passenger traffic'; people became atoms, pulsing, coalescing and dispersing across the railway network. Nasmyth's demonstration embodied in graphic form the new conceptualization of the crowd in the age of mass transit, in which millions of individuals were transformed into stereotyped representations. It is within this context that Ruskin's famous complaint of 1856, that he did not consider going by railway as travelling at all but merely as '"being sent" to a place, and very little different from becoming a parcel',[40] should be understood.

One of the most important aspects of the industrialization of travel brought about by the railway was the high degree of regulation and control experienced by the passenger. At every stage of the journey, the traveller was confronted by the regulated, systematic, mechanical nature of the railway, in the apparatus of tickets, luggage labels, timetables, clocks, bells, uniformed officials, in the numbering of carriages, compartments, seats, tickets and platforms. To a degree unprecedented in civilian life, railway passengers were subjected to bureaucratic procedures, counted, regulated, ticketed and controlled. This phenomenon was dictated by the nature of the railway, which did not permit free and unregulated access by people driving their own vehicles and following their own itineraries as on any other highway, but had to be a closed system to which all access was controlled, and within which all movement was regulated. As a writer observed in 1846, 'The wheels, rails, and carriages are only parts of one great machine, on the proper adjustment of which, one to the other, entirely depends the perfect action of the whole.'[41] The passengers were as much a component of the great railway machine as the tracks and trains, and just as all the movements of the mechanical components had to be controlled if the machine was to operate effectively, so the behaviour of the human traveller had to be regulated with mechanical efficiency.

The Railway Traveller's Handy Book conveys both the extent of that regulation and the powerful effect it had on the minds of contemporary railway passengers, in its advice to the traveller who wishes to avoid unnecessary stress and confusion:

> About five minutes before a train starts a bell is rung as a signal to passengers to prepare for starting. Persons unaccustomed to travel by railway connect the ringing of the bell with the instant departure of the train, and it is most amusing to watch the novices running helter-skelter along the platform, tumbling over everything and everybody in their eagerness to catch the train which they believe is about to go without them. At the same time the seasoned traveller, who understands the intention of the bell, stands by the carriage door coolly surveying the panic-stricken multitude ...[42]

A contributor to the *Association Medical Journal* in 1854 similarly suggests the extent to which passengers felt pressurised by the railway's regulated, timetabled operations. The chief medical evils of railway travel, he writes, result from 'the excitement, anxiety, and nervous shock consequent on the frequent efforts to catch the last express; to be in time for the fearfully punctual train ... Cases of sudden death, produced by the hurry and eagerness often required to reach the train on time, are on record.'[43]

The implication is that the railway pressurizes, exhausts, dehumanises, with what the *Handy Book* calls its 'straight-laced punctuality'[44] and its rigid concern with rules and regulations. 'The station, with its timetables, tickets, uniformed staff, and ubiquitous clocks, is an inherent supporter and encourager of discipline and order.'[45] comment Jeffrey Richards and John MacKenzie in their *Social History of the Railway Station*, while the railway historian Jack Simmons observes that the railways 'enforced a new observance of

241

punctuality. Through them the clock came to guide – even to rule – lives as it never had before.'[46] No more potent symbol could be found for the enforcing, regulating aspect of the railway than the prominence of the clock in station architecture,[47] and the establishment in Britain, the United States and wherever else the trains ran of 'railway time' as a unified national standard.

The transformation from autonomous individual into passive subject of an industrial process was experienced by all classes of traveller, and was as clear for the first- or second-class passenger, travelling in upholstered and well-appointed comfort in enclosed carriages as it was for the third-class passenger in more spartan (but less constricted) accommodation. The provision of seat cushions, padded doors, lace and gilt trimmings, mirrors, framed pictures and all the accoutrements of a comfortable drawing room could only disguise, not obliterate, the mechanical, industrial nature of the process.[48] In the early days of the railway, attempts had been made to combine the freedom of travel in a private road vehicle with the speed and facility of rail travel by permitting aristocratic and wealthy travellers to make their railway journeys in their own vehicles. The road carriage, sometimes with its wheels removed, would be secured to a flat wagon attached to the train;[49] the horses would be conveyed in a van in the same train, and on arrival horses and carriage would be reunited and the journey would be continued by road, without the necessity for the passengers ever to leave their own vehicle. This was a short-lived experiment, however; apart from the resulting delay and complication during the marshalling of trains at stations, it was also inherently unsafe.[50] By the end of the 1840s the practice had been abandoned on British railways, and all passengers travelled in self-contained railway vehicles of some description. The practice of conveying passengers in their own road vehicles mounted on railway wagons can be seen as a transitional stage both in the technological development of the railway carriage and in the adjustment of peoples' attitudes to the demands of the new mode of transport.

The abandonment of the practice did not mark the end of this transitional mode, however; until the 1850s even purpose-built railway carriages long remained little more than road carriage bodies mounted on railway underframes. Even with the appearance by the 1890s of bogie carriages, corridor connections, heating, and on-board lavatories,[51] the British railway carriage remained indebted to its horse-drawn forebears in the crucial matter of the provision of compartments. The compartment, intended to minimise the shock and discomfort of rail transportation for the bourgeois or aristocratic traveller by reproducing the privacy, status and comfort of horse-drawn travel, tended in fact to have exactly the opposite effect. Rather than bestowing upon the new means of travel the spirit and character of the old, the compartment emphasized the gulf between the two. Many travellers may have found it reassuring; but for others it simply made the restricted, enclosed, mechanical nature of rail travel all the more apparent. To take just one example, while journeying by road offered the pleasures of an ever-changing scene and the chance of conversation with people met upon the road, the railway compartment merely trapped the traveller in boredom and monotony, with nothing to look at but the faces of those sitting opposite. In 1838 a letter appeared in the *Railway Times,* signed 'An Enemy to Imprisonment for Debt and in Travelling' which suggested that the seating in some compartments be placed back to back, enabling the passenger to 'see all the country within view of both sides of the road; and, surely, this would be pleasanter than a three or four hours' study of physiognomy at a stretch, for want of any other occupation.'[52]

Railway travel transformed the traveller's experience of the passing scene. The view from the window became commodified, like a picture on a wall; a commodification of experience, a place or event transformed into product to be used or ignored as the consumer desires. Ralph Waldo Emerson commented on the same phenomenon in 1843, observing that the towns through which his train passed on its journey from Philadelphia to New York 'make no distinct impression. They are like pictures on a wall. The more, that you can read all the way in the car a French novel.'[53] In an article published in the *Magazine of Art* in 1880, the essayist Edward Bradbury drew the attention of railway travellers to 'the "hurrygraphs" of scenery that come and go like the sliding scales of a magic lantern':

> The average traveller allows these choice vignettes to pass unheeded. He – 'good, easy man!' – seats himself in his favourite corner of the carriage, pulls his rug over his knees, his Times out of his pocket, his pipe out of its case, and settles down into the foreign telegrams and the share market, or falls into a tobacco trance. The windows – framing picture after picture – are only referred to for purposes of ventilation ...[54]

These perceptions of the external scene as forming 'pictures on a wall' or a series of magic lantern slides reflect two important aspects of the railway journey which were widely noted by contemporaries. The first relates to the nature of the view obtained from a moving railway train. As Bradbury's intriguing term 'hurrygraphs' indicates, it is the effect of the speed of the train which gives the passing scene as viewed from the railway carriage its particular character. Because nearer objects pass too quickly to be perceived as anything other than flashes of colour, the traveller's gaze is drawn to more distant objects, which move more slowly. Jules Verne commented on this phenomenon in 1869, when the narrator of his *Twenty Thousand Leagues Under the Seas* observed that from the window of the speeding submarine Nautilus he 'saw of the Mediterranean's depths merely what the traveller on an express glimpses of countryside passing before his eyes: far-off horizons, and not the close-ups which pass by in a flash.'[55] The effect of this phenomenon was to confuse the traveller's senses of distance and movement, and flatten out the prospect visible from the window. The second point relates to the relationship between the viewer and the view. The passenger, dissociated from the passing prospect by this disturbed perception and physically separated by the walls and windows of the carriage itself, becomes not an active participant in the surrounding landscape, but a passive consumer of it, and very often – as Emerson suggests – ends up ignoring it, just as an uninteresting picture on the wall is ignored. This phenomenon came to be almost an expected part of railway travel, particularly with the advent of railway tourism from the 1850s. As James Buzard notes in his recent history of tourism:

> The detached perspective and imprecise panoramic vision ascribed to passengers of the new means of transport became vital ingredients of the 'tourist's frame of mind'. So too did passengers' boredom, augmented by the blurred landscape and assuaged less by looking out of the window than by ignoring that passing panorama in favour of some diverting reading matter.[56]

As an instance of the industrial commodification of experience, the view from the railway carriage window is in the same category of nineteenth-century socio-cultural phenomena as the department store window display, photography, and, at the end of the century, cinema. The cultural critic Raymond Williams, in his discussion of the relationship between the observer and the city in nineteenth- and twentieth-century literature, identifies the 'fragmentary experience' of perceiving a constantly moving, constantly varied scene as one of the key forms of modern imagery. He goes on to claim that 'the perceptual experience itself does not necessarily imply any particular mood, let alone an ideology',[57] and in the case of a figure moving through the modern city – in Virginia Woolf's *Orlando* or James Joyce's *Ulysses*, to cite Williams's examples – this is to an extent true; a variety of moods and meanings can be read into the experience of urban movement. Similarly, the experience of railway travel can be used to convey exhilaration or despair, according to the author's purposes. Robert Louis Stevenson's poem 'From a Railway Carriage' conveys the former: 'Faster than fairies, faster than witches, / Bridges and houses, hedges and ditches';[58] while Dombey's journey to Birmingham in Dickens's *Dombey and Son* expresses the latter,[59] although making a similar use of the rhythms and fragmented glimpses of railway travel. But in the case of the railway, which Williams does not address, the isolation of the traveller from the scene outside the carriage introduces an extra level of meaning: much more than the journey through a city street, an environment with which the observer can freely interact, the railway journey is characterized by alienation and passivity.

In this sense the sensory experience of the railway journey is a direct forerunner of the sensory experience of cinema; the railway journey literally 'trained' audiences in the cinematic gaze. It is significant that railways played a prominent role in early cinematic productions. The arrival of a train at a station, trains passing at speed, the view from inside a train, produced visual effects which fascinated pioneering cinematographers, as such 1890s film titles as 'Arrival of a Train at La Ciotat' (1895) and 'Arrival of the London Express at Brighton' (1896) suggest. A series called 'Phantom Rides' offered views from the cabs of moving trains: 'Railway Ride over the Tay Bridge' (1897), 'Down Exeter Incline' (1896) and 'View from an Engine Front' (1900) are notable surviving examples of what was a very popular genre with filmmakers and their audiences.[60] The close relationship between the passing view from a train and the experience of cinema is perhaps demonstrated most directly in films which feature scenes set within moving railway carriages, in which the world going by outside the window is simulated by a moving film within the film. The connections between railway travel and cinema are a particularly striking illustration of the way in which, with the coming of the railways, the journey itself becomes both process and commodity; in the words of the cultural historian Anne Friedberg, 'Transportation ... alters the commodity, but it also becomes a commodity itself – the train ticket.'[61] This phenomenon is a prerequisite for the rise of tourism. With the railways, for the first time in human history the journey enters the arena of the market place and becomes itself a product for which desires must be created and satisfied. The phenomena of mass tourism, holidays and excursions, marketed by advertising and publicity, were creations of the railway age and expressed powerfully the commodification of the railway traveller and the railway journey.

The perceived degenerative threat of the railway journey was not limited to its cultural, social, moral and aesthetic influence on the external world; it was also widely believed to consist in more insidious influences, and particularly in the ways in which the deleterious environmental and sensory influences associated with railway travel acted upon the human mind and body from within. Just as the railway undermined the social and cultural differentiations and hierarchies upon which the stability of Victorian and Edwardian society rested, so, it was supposed, it attacked the delicate balance of biological energies and functions which sustained the workings of the human body. It was widely accepted that the greater freedom of travel created by the coming of the railways had brought great benefits to health, particularly for the urban labouring population, who were able to escape the crowding and foul air of the cities and travel to the seaside and the country with more freedom and in greater numbers than ever before. Some went further, asserting that railways were beneficial to public health not only because they brought people to healthful locations, but through the influences which worked upon them during the journey itself. Under the heading 'Health Seekers', the *Railway Traveller's Handy Book* declared that 'being whirled through space at the rate of thirty or forty miles an hour is most pleasurable in its effects. To the over-wrought brain, or the over-strained mental faculties, to the toiler who has sunk into a state of exhaustion, this rapid locomotion acts as an agreeable fillip.'[62] E. Foxwell agreed, writing in 1884 that 'Many a modern brain, aching from inward collision, receives an unrivalled tonic from the pleasant broadside of life that plays upon our rapid course with such a kind profusion' as the train 'Whirl[s] with a magnificent ease through a panorama of life so generously presented'.[63]

Such opinions tended to be in the minority, however. The general view was that travelling was a tiring activity whatever the means employed, and that railway travel produced particular discomfort. By the mid-nineteenth century it was widely believed that there was a particular, novel form of railway travel exhaustion, different in nature from the tiredness associated with other forms of travel. Sheridan Le Fanu describes it in *Uncle Silas* (1864): 'Fatigued with the peculiar fatigue of railway travelling, dusty, a little chilly, with eyes aching and wearied'.[64] Travellers throughout the Victorian age complained constantly about the poor riding qualities, noisiness, uncomfortable seating, inadequate lighting, and ineffective heating and ventilation of railway carriages. 'Railways are excellent things, and I wonder how the world got on without them', declared a character in Mortimer Collins's novel of 1870, *The Vivian Romance*:

> but twenty or thirty miles on the best line in England thrills every nerve in my body, and makes my brain throb, and causes me to feel so grim, that I abhor myself. Then the hideous smell of the engine, the dust and ashes that attack your eyes and nostrils, the fustiness of the carriages, the maniacal scream of the steam-whistle, the grinding and groaning noises of the whole machine – are not these abominations?[65]

The environment of the railway carriage, as we have seen, offered the ambiguous security of enclosure and protection. The carriage was enclosed, shielded from the elements, padded and furnished inside, but the industrial nature of the railway travel process was vividly conveyed to the passenger by the noise, smoke and steam of the locomotive, the sound of the whistle, the jolts and vibrations which were conveyed through the structure of the carriage. Travel in road vehicles shared some of these qualities: the ride was frequently uncomfortable, and the interior was often too hot or cold; but the noisy, smelly presence of the steam locomotive, the rapidity of railway travel, and the fact that the passenger could not break his or her journey, step out of the carriage for a while, or in other ways interact with the landscape through which the train passed, made the conditions of the train journey novel and disturbing. 'Railway fatigue' was not only new and distinctive; it was also worrying, seeming to hint at some deep insidious damage being done by the railway to the human constitution. The vibration and shaking to which railway travellers were subjected formed an early focus of concern for those seeking to investigate the consequences of railway travel for human health. The French doctor E. A. Duchesne, who published his *Des chemins de fer et leur influence sur la santé des mécaniciens et des chauffeurs* in 1857,[66] suggested that a *maladie des mécaniciens* could be identified among railway workers, particularly those who worked on locomotive footplates, exposed to extremes of heat and cold. He described this 'engineer's malady' as including pseudo-rheumatic pains and 'generalized, continuous and persistent pains, accompanied by a feeling of weakness and numbness',[67] caused by the peculiar vibrations and jolts experienced on the engines.

These aspects of travelling on the footplate were confirmed and commented on by journalists and others who had occasion to make a journey by railway in the company of the locomotive crew. Thus Frederick Williams, describing a ride he had taken on the footplate of the London to Dover night mail train, remarked that his thoughts were 'shaken into hopeless jumble by the incessant vibrato which my anatomy was undergoing', and complained that he suffered from 'extremes of temperature, a bleak wind ... freezing me to my waist, while the heat from the furnace bakes my legs.'[68] The effects of vibration were not limited to locomotive crews; the same influences acted upon passengers in the train. The mid-nineteenth-century railway carriage shook, rattled and jolted to an alarming degree, a fact commented upon by many travellers. Dante Gabriel Rossetti recounted in verse 'the sore torment of the route;— / Toothache, and headache, and the ache of wind' which he had suffered on his railway trip from London to Brussels in 1849; 'This cursed pitching is too bad,' he complained, 'my teeth / jingle together in it'.[69] When the medical journal *The Lancet* came to examine the effects on health of railway travelling in 1862, much attention was paid to the jolts and vibrations experienced in the course of a journey. 'The frequency, rapidity and peculiar abruptness of the motion of the railway carriage keep ... a constant strain on the muscles;' observed *The Lancet*, 'and to this must be ascribed a part of that sense of bodily fatigue, almost amounting to soreness, which is felt after a long journey.'[70]

The nature and consequences of the 'incessant vibrato' associated with the railway journey were questions which would assume great importance in subsequent medical investigations of railway travel. It was not that the ride on a train was bumpy in the sameway as the ride in a stage-coach or on a horse-drawn wagon; on the contrary, it was far smoother, giving rise to the idea that rail travel was akin to 'flying', unaffected by the ruts, potholes and rough surfaces of the common roads. The point was that railway travel subjected the traveller to a new kind of vibration consisting of a rapid and continuous succession of minor jolts and jars. Duchesne was clear that the symptoms of his *maladie des mécaniciens* were largely due to this vibration: 'Without exception, all the firemen and drivers complain about the vibration of the machine, the regular but perpetual movements that it transmits to the entire body and the lower extremities in particular'.[71] This vibration was so fatiguing, Duchesne went on to relate, that drivers contrived what means they could to cushion themselves against it, ranging from the placing of a doormat under the feet to the installation of 'an elastic stool on which they can sit down from time to time.'[72] The seats and upholstery in first and second class carriages were partly a response to this vibration, intended to protect the passenger mechanically, through the provision of springs and cushions, and to distance him or her psychologically from the industrial nature of the process by making the railway compartment as far as possible an extension of the domestic environment. *The Lancet* stressed that this constant 'vibration and oscillation' affected not only the muscles but also the brain, the spinal cord and the nervous system as a whole, and the results of such 'commotion of the brain or spinal system of nerves' could be of the utmost seriousness: 'Cerebral or spinal concussions, in their higher degree, annihilate the functions of those organs. In the milder forms they lead up to a disease which, remaining for a long time latent, may still end in paralysis.'[73] *The Lancet* was not alone in perceiving in the vibrations felt by railway passengers an insidious degenerative threat of nervous and cerebro-spinal disease. It was generally accepted that exposure over a prolonged period to constant shaking and jolting could have potentially serious effects on the nervous system.

The more regular and intensive an individual's experiences of railway travel, the more liable he or she was to suffer ill effects. Commuters were seen as a particularly vulnerable group. Railway commuting had begun in earnest in the 1850s, soon becoming an established feature of working life for many people, but the possible health effects of daily, sometimes lengthy, railway journeys undertaken in addition to the normal pressures of work remained a cause for concern. *The Lancet*'s comments on this issue struck a chord of recognition beyond the confines of the medical profession. *The Spectator* saw season-ticket holders as more vulnerable than other travellers to the 'injurious and peculiar evils arising from railway travelling': '[these] travellers are a distinct class; many of them are constantly in motion; it is to these that accrue the evil effects.'[74] *The Cornhill Magazine* similarly warned that for rail commuters 'the muscular and nervous strain, daily repeated twice, will generally exert a baneful influence; and if there be already organic disease, that influence may be very serious.'[75] *The Lancet* cited 'the large number of instances in which season ticket holders have been compelled to desist from the practice of long daily journeys' because of the tiredness and strain which their journeys, on top of the usual fatigues of the urban working day, entailed. 'There is strong evidence, indeed,' *The Lancet* continued, 'in favour of the opinion that the privilege of country residence may be dearly bought at the cost of long daily journeys by rail.' In support of this claim, they reproduced the testimony of 'one of the leading physicians of the metropolis' on 'the rapid ageing of season-ticket holders':

> Travelling a few years since on the Brighton line very frequently, I became familiar with the faces of a number of the regular passengers on that line. Recently I had again occasion to travel several times on the same line ... I have never seen any set of men so rapidly aged as these seem to me to have been in the course of those few years.[76]

Another observer commented in 1868 that 'It has been over and over again observed that season-ticket holders, especially on the Brighton line, age very rapidly.'[77]

The claim of one medical authority in 1868 that the demands of railway travelling, particularly 'all this striving to do certain distances in certain given times' had 'engendered an irritability in our organs'[78] underlines the contemporary perception that the railway was attacking the very substance of the body itself, and that the whole cerebral, spinal and nervous structure of the body was implicated in railway fatigue. This view is emphasized by the attention paid by contemporaries to the exhaustion of the organs of sense which paralleled this muscular exhaustion; in the words of *The Lancet*:

> The influence of railway travelling upon the brain cannot, however, be measured solely by estimating the character and extent of the concussions to which it is subjected. The brain is not only affected by the mind, but also through the avenues of the eye and ear; and by the excitement of the respiratory and circulatory systems.[79]

It was widely believed that the rapidity of railway travel placed new demands on the eyes and brain, taxing them to a far greater degree than slow, pre-industrial road travel. *The Lancet* commented:

> The rapidity and variety of the impressions necessarily fatigue both the eye and the brain. The constantly varying distance at which the objects are placed involves an incessant shifting of the adaptive apparatus by which they are focused upon the retina; and the mental effort by which the brain takes cognizance of them is scarcely productive of cerebral wear because it is unconscious; for no fact in physiology is more clearly established than that excessive functional activity always implies destruction of material and organic change of substance.[80]

The key term here is 'excessive functional activity'. The visual stimuli associated with railway travel transformed the demands placed upon the eyes and brain, above all by greatly increasing the sheer quantity of stimulation with which they had to deal; and this increased level of activity, it was suggested, threatened to inflict physical damage on the organic substance of the body.

The pathological disruption produced by the effects of railway travel on the eyes must be placed in the context of the adjustment required of the nineteenth-century traveller by the particular conditions of railway travel. The demands placed on the visual apparatus of the passenger by the speed of movement on the rails represent an aspect of the pressures placed on the human mind and body to adapt to the demands of industrialized travel. *The Lancet's* strictures on the dangers of over-taxing the eyes can be read as a warning of the pathological consequences of employing the pre-industrial gaze in the industrialized context of the railway journey: strained muscles and nerves, exhausted eyes, aching brain. Travellers on the road had no difficulty observing the passing scene, deciding what they would look at and what they would ignore, examining particular aspects of the scene in as much detail as they wished. Ruskin advised travellers 'to be content with as little change as possible':

> If the attention is awake, and the feelings in proper train, a turn of a country road with a cottage beside it, which we have not seen before, is as much as we need for refreshment; if we hurry past it, and take two cottages at a time, it is already too much; hence to any person who has all his senses about him, a quiet walk along not more than ten or twelve miles of road a day, is the most amusing of all travelling; and all travelling becomes dull in exact proportion to its rapidity.[81]

Ruskin here makes three points about the interaction between the traveller and the landscape. First, it is as much a psychological matter of the state of mind of the observer as a physical one of the conditions of observation; the observer must have his or her 'feelings in proper train' – a feat impossible, Ruskin believed, for a harassed and hurried railway traveller. Second, the landscape must be allowed to unfold at its own pace; the traveller must accept what it offers and not 'hurry past it', seeking more stimulation for its own sake. Third, and related to the first two, rapidity itself is incompatible both with looking and with travelling.

Not everyone reacted to the new types of vision made possible by rail travel with hostility; some adjusted readily, and welcomed the new ways of seeing. Matthew E. Ward, an American traveller, wrote in 1853 that the English landscape was best appreciated 'when dashing on after a locomotive at forty miles an hour':

Nothing by the way requires study, or demands meditation, and though objects immediately at hand seem tearing wildly by, yet the distant fields and scattered trees, are not so bent on eluding observation, but dwell long enough in the eye to leave their undying impression. Every thing is so quiet, so fresh, so full of home, and destitute of prominent objects to detain the eye, or distract the attention from the charming whole, that I love to dream through these placid beauties whilst sailing in the air, quick, as if astride a tornado.[82]

The enjoyment of the landscape which Ward experiences is dependent upon his adjustment to a new type of vision; the very adjustment which Ruskin, conscious of the aesthetic and moral consequences of the industrialization of vision, resists. Ward does not attempt to watch everything, does not seek to dwell upon individual incidents and objects, but embraces the 'charming whole', the entire speeding vista with his vision and becomes, not the active, discriminating, psychologically engaged Ruskinian observer, but the passive consumer of a spectacle provided ready-animated and complete outside his carriage window.

In addition to the strain it inflicted on the eyes, the railway journey was believed to exert a baneful influence through the other senses as well. The hearing, argued *The Lancet*, was strained by 'The rattle and noise which accompany the progress of the train' which cause 'an incessant vibration on the tympanum'.[83] Poorly-heated and draughty carriages exposed the passenger to the effects of cold, which 'will surely and steadily chill the parts of the body exposed, and will as surely excite disease in those predisposed to it ... the speed of the railway intensifies the cold.'[84] In other cases, the lack of proper ventilation made for unhealthy heat and stuffiness. The journeys William Morris made between Calais and Ghent in 1874 were made unbearable, he complained, by the heat: 'I must say I had no idea what heat was before, it was like being in a Turkish bath.'[85] All these factors combined to produce a unique level of physical and mental fatigue in the railway passenger:

Assailed through the avenues of the eye and ear, and subject to concussions due to vertical movement and lateral oscillation communicated through the trunk, and actually transmitted through the bony walls of the head when it rests against the back of the carriage, the brain is apt to suffer certain physiological changes. Amongst the well-known effects are – occasional dizziness, headache, sickness, and mental fatigue.[86]

These symptoms represent an ameliorated form of Duchesne's *maladie des mécaniciens*. Railway passengers were protected from the extremes of heat and cold experienced on the footplate – although the inadequacies of heating and the persistence of draughts did cause them to develop colds, catarrhs, chills and similar ailments[87] – but they were exposed to the same vibrations, jolts and shakes. Like the drivers and firemen, they were part of the process of industrialized transportation, and were exposed to the wear and tear associated with that process.

The Victorian railway represented in a particularly dramatic and important form the ambivalence of the age towards technological modernity, and the pervasiveness and persistence of the anxieties it provoked demonstrate its central significance as a locus of that ambivalence. Other aspects of industrial civilization, from gas lights to steamships, were on occasion dangerous and destructive; but no other technological system required large numbers of ordinary people to surrender their security and safety to a vast, fast-moving machine driven by incomprehensibly powerful and barely controllable energies, nor did any do so as frequently, and on such a scale, as the railway. Against the convenience of the journey had to be weighed the isolation of the compartment, the discomfort and deleterious consequences for health of noise, draughts, vibration and jolts; travel was faster than ever before, but there was the constant sense of danger and the risk of catastrophic disaster; mobility was more widely available, but the bustle and confusion of the crowded railway station exhausted the nerves of travellers; the service provided by the railways was extensive and comprehensive, but passengers had to grapple with the complexity of timetables, connections and bureaucracy.

The pathologies of train travel were the consequences of the machine-dominated, urbanized, fast-moving civilization of industrial modernity; the civilization of which the railway, perhaps more than any other technological system, was the symbol and the embodiment. The railway, with its speed, power and danger, was a focus of nervous and psychological disorders; the neuroses associated with the shock of the railway's appearance in the landscape, the exhaustion and sensory disturbance of the journey, the catastrophe of the railway accident, were all aspects of the railway's potency as a focus and agent of the destructive, destabilizing, degenerative energies of technological modernity.

Notes

1 For more on the significance of the railway in the Victorian

imagination, see Wolfgang Schivelbusch, *The Railway Journey: the Industrialization of Time and Space in the Nineteenth Century* (Oxford: Blackwell, 1980); George F. Drinka, *The Birth of Neurosis: Myth, Malady and the Victorians* (New York: Simon & Schuster, 1984), ch. 5, 'The Railway God'; Ralph Harrington, 'The neuroses of the railway', *History Today*, vol. 44, no. 7 (July 1994), 15-21.

2   John Blakely, *The Theology of Inventions: or, Manifestations of Deity in the Works of Art* (Glasgow: William Collins, 1855), 134.

3   H. G. Wells, *Anticipations of the Reaction of Mechanical and Scientific Progress upon Human Life and Thought* (London: Chapman & Hall, 1902), 16 (footnote).

4   J. S. Jeans, *Railway Problems: an Inquiry into the Economic Conditions of Railway Working in Different Countries* (London: Longman, Green & Co., 1887), xvii.

5   E. Foxwell, *English Express Trains: Two Papers* (London: Edward Stanford, 1884), 37.

6   Anon., *Railways: their Uses and Management* (London: Pelham Richardson, 1842), 63.

7   For more on aristocratic reactions to railway travel, illustrated mainly with examples drawn from Germany, see Wolfgang Sachs, *For Love of the Automobile* (1984; Eng. trans. Berkeley & Los Angeles, Calif.: University of California Press, 1992), 92-7.

8   Benjamin Disraeli, *Sybil, or The Two Nations* (1845; Oxford: Oxford University Press, 1981), book II, chap. 11, 101-2.

9   *The Poems of John Davidson*, Andrew Turnbull (ed.), (2 vols., Edinburgh & London: Scottish Academic Press, 1973), vol. 2, 375.

10   For a suggestive discussion of this issue in the context of the movement for urban sanitary reform and improvement in the 1830s, see Mary Poovey, *Making a Social Body: British Cultural Formation, 1830-1864* (Chicago, Ill.: University of Chicago Press, 1995), 57-60.

11   *The Lancet*, 24 September 1887, 625.

12   Wilkie Collins, *No Name* (1862; Oxford: Oxford University Press, 1986), 187. The description is based on the York station of the 1840s, which was notoriously disorganized; *The Times* of 17 September 1847 called it 'ill-planned, worse managed, and far too small for the traffic.' It was rebuilt in the 1870s.

13   'Railway travelling and its effects on health', *Association Medical Journal*, vol. 4, no. Clx (n.s.), 26 January 1856, 72. This was a reprint of an article originally published in the *Quarterly Journal of Public Health* for December 1855.

14   *The Lancet*, 11 January 1862, 51.

15   See, for example, the monograph by Alfred Haviland, *Hurried to*

Death: Especially Addressed to Railway Travellers (London: Renshaw & Mitchell, 1868). I am grateful to Dr Nicholas Daly of Trinity College, Dublin, for bringing this publication to my attention.

16 For example: Mary Elizabeth Braddon, *Lady Audley's Secret* (1862), *Henry Dunbar: the Story of an Outcast* (1864); Arthur Conan Doyle, *The Final Problem* (1894); Richard Marsh, *The Beetle* (1897). Robert Louis Stevenson parodied the conventions of the sensational railway chase in *The Wrong Box* (1892).

17 See Schivelbusch, *Railway Journey*, 80-8. The Poinsot murder also provided part of the inspiration for Émile Zola's *La Bête humaine* (1890)

18 On the German cases see David Blackbourn & Geoff Eley, *The Peculiarities of German History* (Oxford: Oxford University Press, 1984), 214-5.

19 *The Globe*, 1863; quoted in Schivelbusch, *Railway Journey*, 79.

20 There is an account of the Briggs case in Jonathan Goodman (ed.), *The Railway Murders* (London: Allison & Busby, 1984), 11-44.

21 *Saturday Review*, 16 July 1864, 72.

22 *Ibid*, 23 July 1864, 106.

23 The cases concerned were the Briggs murder itself, and the murders of Frederick Isaac Gold in Balcombe Tunnel, Sussex, in 1881; of Maria Sophia Murray, near the same location, in 1905; of John Innes Nisbet, between Newcastle and Alnmouth, in 1910; and of Willie Starchfield, a child of five, near Broad Street Station, London, in 1914. All five cases received sensational press coverage. See Goodman, *Railway Murders*, for accounts of all these cases.

24 An account of these events can be found in the anthology *Murder on the Railways*, edited by Peter Haining (London: Orion Books, 1996), 337-9. The story itself is reprinted in the same collection, 340-68, as are three other stories dealing with similar railway murder cases: Baroness Orczy, *The Mysterious Death on the Underground Railway* (1901); Victor L. Whitchurch, *The Murder on the Okehampton Line* (*c.* 1903); and Thomas W. Hanshew, *The Riddle of the 5.28* (1910).

25 Matthew Arnold, *Essays in Criticism* (1865); from *The Complete Prose Works of Matthew Arnold* (11 vols., Ann Arbor, Mich.: University of Michigan Press, 1960-77), vol. 3, 288-9. Bow was the station at which the assault was discovered.

26 *The Lancet*, 25 October 1884, 745.

27 Sigmund Freud, *The Standard Edition of the Complete Psychological Works*, vol. 15: *Introductory Lectures on Psycho-Analysis (Parts I and II)* (London: Hogarth Press & Institute of Psycho-analysis, 1955), 197.

28 *The Railway Traveller's Handy Book of Hints, Suggestions, and Advice,*

Before the Journey, During the Journey, and After the Journey (London: Lockwood & Co., 1862), 93-4.

29   *Ibid*, 101.

30   *Quarterly Review*, vol. 74 (1844), 250.

31   For a discussion of American women travellers, see Patricia Cline Cohen, 'Safety and danger: women on American public transport, 1750-1850', in Susan Reverby & Dorothy Helly (eds.), *Gendered Domains: Public and Private Spheres in Historical Perspective* (Ithaca, N.Y.: Cornell University Press, 1992), and the same author's 'Women at large: travel in antebellum America', *History Today*, vol. 44, no. 12 (December 1994), 44-50. There is a lack of similar work on the experience of British women travellers.

32   *Saturday Review*, 23 July 1864, 106.

33   E. M. Forster, *Howard's End* (1910; Harmondsworth: Penguin, 1983), 209.

34   *Saturday Review*, 23 July 1864, 106. It is notable that the respectability of Mr Rutherford is taken for granted by the *Review*; the unnamed young woman's respectability is placed between questioning quotation marks.

35   Sir William Hardman, *The Hardman Papers*, S. M. Ellis (ed.), (London: Constable, 1930); quoted in Jack Simmons (ed.), *Railways: an Anthology* (London: Collins, 1991), 101-2.

36   *Punch*, vol. 51 (1866), 70.

37   Cohen, 'Women at large', 50.

38   For more on this point, see Schivelbusch, *Railway Journey*, 38-9.

39   James Nasmyth, *An Autobiography*, Samuel Smiles (ed.), (1883); quoted in Humphrey Jennings, *Pandaemonium: the Coming of the Machine as seen by Contemporary Observers*, Mary-Lou Jennings & Charles Madge (eds), (London: André Deutsch, 1975), 348.

40   John Ruskin, *Modern Painters* (1856), part IV, chap. XVII; in *The Works of John Ruskin*, E. T. Cook & A. Wedderburn (eds), (39 vols., London: George Allen, 1903-12), vol. V, 370.

41   C. H. Greenhow, *An Exposition of the Dangers and Deficiencies of the Present Mode of Railway Construction, with Suggestions for its Improvement* (London: John Weale, 1846), 4.

42   *Handy Book*, 70-1.

43   'Railway travelling and its effects on health', *Association Medical Journal*, vol. 4 (New Series), 1 December 1854, 1079.

44   *Handy Book*, 29.

45   Jeffrey Richards & John MacKenzie, *The Railway Station: a Social History* (Oxford: Oxford University Press, 1986), 14.

46   Jack Simmons, *The Victorian Railway* (London: Thames & Hudson,

1991), 347.

47   The first such clock in Britain was at Bricklayer's Arms in south-east London, opened in 1844. For examples, see Carroll L. V. Meeks, *The Railroad Station: an Architectural History* (New Haven, Conn.: Yale University Press, 1956), Christiane Scelles, *Gares: Ateliers du voyage 1837-1937* (Paris: R.E.M.P.ART., 1993).

48   For examples of the lavish furnishing of many Victorian railway carriages, see C. Hamilton Ellis, *Railway Carriages in the British Isles from 1830 to 1914* (London: George Allen & Unwin, 1965). For an analysis of nineteenth-century efforts to disguise mechanical and industrial devices and processes with padding and decoration, see John Gloag, *Victorian Comfort: a Social History of Design from 1830-1900* (Newton Abbot: David & Charles, 1973) – although Gloag overstates the Victorians' aversion to the mechanical and functional. For a more balanced view see Asa Briggs, *Victorian Things* (London: Batsford, 1988), esp. chap. 2, 'The Great Victorian Collection.'

49   Ellis, *Railway Carriages*, 44-9; Frank Ferneyhough, *Liverpool and Manchester Railway 1830-1980* (London: Robert Hale, 1980), 109; Jack Simmons, *The Railways of Britain* (1961; 4th edn., London: Macmillan, 1986), 174-6.

50   See L. T. C. Rolt, *Red for Danger: a History of Railway Accidents and Railway Safety* (1955; 3rd edn., Newton Abbot: David & Charles, 1976), 30.

51   For these innovations and other aspects of railway carriage development, see Ellis, *Railway Carriages, passim*; Simmons, *Railways of Britain*, 176-83; Simmons, *Victorian Railway*, 84-6.

52   *The Railway Times*, vol. 1 (1838), 46; quoted in Schivelbusch, *Railway Journey*, 76.

53   Ralph Waldo Emerson, *Journals*, 7 February 1843; quoted in Schivelbusch, *Railway Journey*, 52.

54   Edward Bradbury, 'Pictures in trains', *Magazine of Art*, vol. 3 (1880), 109-10.

55   Jules Verne, *Twenty Thousand Leagues Under the Seas*, trans. William Butcher (1869; Oxford: Oxford University Press, 1998), part II, chap. VII, 236.

56   James Buzard, *The Beaten Track* (Oxford: Oxford University Press, 1993), 36.

57   Raymond Williams, *The Country and the City* (London: Chatto & Windus, 1973), 240-2.

58   R. L. Stevenson, *A Child's Garden of Verses* (1885), reprinted in L. Kennedy (ed.), *A Book of Railway Journeys* (London: Collins, 1980), 9.

59   Charles Dickens, *Dombey and Son* (1848; Harmondsworth: Penguin,

1971), chap. 20, 354-5.

60   These examples are drawn from John Huntley, *Railways on the Screen* (Shepperton: Ian Allan, 1993), iv. See also Simmons, *Victorian Railway*, 151-2, and Nicholas Faith, *The World the Railways Made* (London: The Bodley Head, 1990), 253-4.

61   Anne Friedberg, *Window Shopping: Cinema and the Postmodern* (Berkeley & Los Angeles, Calif., & Oxford: University of California Press, 1993), 56. Friedberg follows Walter Benjamin in seeing in the department store, the boulevard, the shopping arcade and the railway journey 'a fitting paradigm for all modernity' (*ibid.*, 49), but – like Benjamin – fails to stress the imposed passivity of the observer which distinguishes the railway journey from the other forms of experience cited. Schivelbusch similarly elides this important distinction, despite his stress elsewhere on the passivity of the railway passenger: Schivelbusch, *Railway Journey*, 188-97.

62   *Handy Book*, 6.

63   Foxwell, *English Express Trains*, 9.

64   Sheridan Le Fanu, *Uncle Silas* (1864; Oxford: Oxford University Press, 1981), chap. LX, 390.

65   Mortimer Collins, *The Vivian Romance* (3 vols., London: Richard Bentley, 1870), vol. I, 186.

66   E. A. Duchesne, *Des chemins de fer et leur influence sur la santé des mécaniciens et des chauffeurs* (Paris, 1857). This work does not appear to have been translated into English, but seems to have been well enough known in Britain for *The Lancet* to refer to it without detailed elaboration in 1862; see 'The Influence of Railway Travelling on Public Health', *The Lancet*, 18 January 1862, 80.

67   Duchesne, *Des chemins de fer*, 183.

68   F. S. Williams, *Our Iron Roads: their History, Construction, and Administration* (1852; 7th edn., 2 vols., London: Derby, Bemrose & Sons, 1885), vol. 2, 356-7.

69   'A Trip to Paris and Belgium. II. Boulogne to Amiens and Paris', in *The Works of Dante Gabriel Rossetti*, William M. Rossetti (ed.), (revised and enlarged edn., London: Ellis, 1911), 178.

70   *The Lancet*, 11 January 1862, 51.

71   Duchesne, *Des chemins de fer*, 146.

72   *Ibid.*

73   *The Lancet*, 11 January 1862, 51.

74   'Perils of the train', *The Spectator*, 12 July 1862, 779.

75   'Effects of railways on health'. *Cornhill*, vol. VI (July-December 1862), 487-8.

76   *The Lancet*, 18 January 1862, 79-80.

77   Haviland, *Hurried to Death*, 22.
78   *Ibid.*
79   *The Lancet*, 11 January 1862, 51.
80   *Ibid,* 51-2.
81   Ruskin, *Works,* vol. V, 370.
82   Matthew E. Ward, *English Items: or, Microcosmic Views of England and Englishmen* (New York, 1853); quoted in Schivelbusch, *Railway Journey,* 60.
83   *The Lancet*, 11 January 1862, 52.
84   *Ibid.,* 50.
85   Letter from Morris to Aglaia Ionides Coronio, 24 July 1874; in Norman Kelvin (ed.), *The Collected Letters of William Morris* (3 vols., Princeton, N.J.: Princeton University Press, 1984-7), vol. I, 225.
86   *The Lancet*, 11 January 1862, 50.
87   *Ibid.,* 48-9; 8 March 1862, 259.

8

Mobility, Syphilis, and Democracy: Pathologizing the Mobile Body

Tim Cresswell

Prologue

This paper represents part of much larger project of thinking through the creation and maintenance of ideologies surrounding mobility in the American context. I am interested in those ways in which mobilities are produced within social and cultural contexts – how the raw fact of motion, the displacement of objects and people from A to B – is transformed into mobilities that are implicated in networks of meaning and power. I want to contextualise and deconstruct claims made about mobility in a number of theories ranging from poststructuralist discussions of nomadology to Harvey's time-space compression.[1] Indeed, I aim to show how the theories of academics are themselves discursive constructions of mobility that are implicated in the equation which links motion to power and meaning.

In this particular section of the work, I am seeking to provide a multi-representational framework for the production (and subsequent disappearance) of a social type – the tramp. While it is commonplace (following Foucault in particular) to speak of the production of various bodies and types in relation to discourses such as medicine, policing, the penal system or psychiatry, it is more unusual for scholars to look at the production of particular bodies through a series of different discursive nets. With this in mind, I discuss the tramp, and especially the mobility of the tramp, in terms of a number of interlinked discursive strategies which brought the tramp into being in the 1870s, and continued to act on the tramp until the Second World War. Literature, comedy, law, medicine, social reform, eugenics, the railroad, and political economy all played a role in the production of the tramp. For the purposes of brevity, I limit my discussion here to the presence of tramps in the interrelated fields of eugenics, social reform, and medicine.

The Tramp Scare 1869-1930

On May 10th 1869 a major event in the history of time-space compression occurred, as workers and officials observed the placement of the last tie, laurelwood bound in silver, and the driving of the last spike, made of gold, of the first transcontinental railroad in North America. The Union Pacific Railroad was completed, connecting the West coast to the Missouri River and thus the East coast. A nation recently divided by civil war was united by technology. In effect, Asia was connected to Europe – the Pacific rim to the Atlantic rim. The railway brought North American agricultural commodities, ore, lumber, and finished goods to the ports of the West coast, and returned to the midwest with foodstuffs and products not indigenous to the region. The landscape of the American west changed on a massive scale as wheat farms spread across the plains and irrigated fruit and vegetable plantations appeared in New Mexico and California. By 1900, the trans-Mississippi west possessed an intricate rail network connecting the United States to Canada and Mexico, and via the steamship routes of San Francisco, Los Angeles, Seattle, Portland and Galveston to Asia, Latin America and Europe. The United States entered a global economy.[2]

The technology of the railroad provided the conditions of possibility for a new social type – the tramp – to exist. Not only did it provide a form of transportation that meant that people could be on the East coast one day, and within a week turn up on the West coast, it also enabled the development of western agribusiness where fruit plantations demanded 200 workers one month and 20,000 the next. These were the jobs for migrant labourers that Steinbeck was later to make infamous.

In 1876, seven years after the completion of the transcontinental railroad, the first of many state 'Tramp Laws' was passed in New Jersey, to be followed by eighteen more in the following five years. By 1880, the whole country was in the middle of what became known as the 'tramp scare' or 'tramp evil' as people, displaced by economic downturns, took to the road in search of work. The tramp became the moral panic of the nation. Newspapers across the land prescribed radical measures for the unwanted wanderers. These ranged from poorhouses, to rural character-building labour camps to doses of arsenic. A tramp was defined by laws as an idle person without employment, a transient person who roamed from place to place, and who had no lawful occasion to wander. Making the tramp railroad connection explicit, the vagrancy law of Massachusetts made riding a freight train *prima facie* evidence of tramphood. Punishment varied from ninety days of hard labour in New Mexico to being sold into servitude for up to a year in Kentucky. In Missouri, the tramp could be hired out go the highest bidder with cash in hand.

The mobility of the tramp, then, was resisted on a number of fronts, ranging from the courtroom, to the academy, to the popular press. Here I focus on the debates over the origins of the new mobile worker and the ways which were suggested to stop this movement. In doing so, I will touch on arguments about the health of the tramp and, in a more cursory manner, his unique contribution to democracy.[3]

Theories of Origins

A great deal of intellectual labour was invested in the search for the origins of the tramp problem. In the late nineteenth century, very few people were willing to point towards economic context as a reason for taking to the road and most commentators laid the blame firmly within the individual. Eugenics was in full swing at the time, and it was explanations of heredity that held sway. Particularly influential was the analysis of a family known as the Jukes, whose family line had been studied by R.L. Dugdale. Dugdale studied six sisters and 709 of their descendants since 1750. He found the family to be thirty times more likely to be criminal than the general population. In addition, 11-25% of the sample suffered from syphilis, which, in Dugdale's view, was clearly correlated with social and behavioural conditions.[4] The social conditions of pauperism were connected to the pathology of syphilis – a connection I will return to later.

At around the same time as Dugdale's influential family history had become common knowledge, people began to notice the arrival of tramps in major cities around the country. The depression of 1873, for instance, saw the arrival for the first time of people classed as tramps in New York City. One observer, Charles Brace, warned against indiscriminate giving to the poor. Charity, he argued, would only encourage the arrival of more tramps who would lose any industrious habits they may have had and replace then with a spirit of pauperism. If not prevented, Brace warned, a community of tramps would develop transmitting pauperism to their children.

Pauperism, criminality, feeblemindedness, and alcoholism were all seen to be largely explainable as pathological conditions. In the case of tramps there was the additional pathology of wanderlust of dromomania. Wanderlust became just one of a whole series of unsavoury characteristics associated with marginal groups and believed to be the product of hereditary processes. One of the leaders of the eugenics movement, Charles Davenport, believed that tramps suffered from an inbred desire to wander which he referred to as 'nomadism'.

Davenport had studied biology at Harvard and earned a Ph.D. After serving as an instructor at Harvard, he moved to the University of Chicago in 1899, and took up the position of assistant professsor. He had already developed a passion for statistical study and had introduced Pearson's methods to the United States. Combining his interests in biology and statistics, Davenport persuaded the newly formed Carnegie Institution of Washington to establish the Station for Experimental Evolution at Cold Spring Harbour on Long Island, of which he became the first director. His work at the station initially involved extensive breeding experiments in animals ranging from snails to sheep, but soon developed into a more sinister interest in tracing 'genetic traits' in people. By 1907, he was publishing papers on the heredity of eye, skin, and hair colour in people, and his work moved towards eugenics.

As director of the Station for Experimental Evolution, Davenport became a figure of national prominence, and was able to organise a vast array of committees in everything from deaf-mutism, through feeble-mindedness and criminality, to immigration. Following a huge endowment Davenport extended his Long Island centre to incorporate a new Eugenics Record Office. Again, Davenport became its director. Beginning in 1924, the Eugenics Record Office held summer school in which young men and women were trained to be 'eugenics field workers'. The training included lectures on heredity from Davenport, methodology (the collection of family histories) and field trips to asylums, hospitals, and the homes of 'defective families'. Once trained, field workers collected endless records of family histories in prisons, asylums, and elsewhere.

One of his first forays into discussions of Mandelian rations was his book *The Feebly Inhibited* which was published in 1915. It included his work *Nomadism, or The Wandering Impulse, with Special Reference to Heredity*.[5] Davenport believed that tramps suffered from an inbred desire to wander which he referred to as Nomadism. In this work, Davenport considered a number of medico-psychological conditions related to the desire to move. Wanderlust he describes as a mild form of desire for travel which we all exhibit from time to time, but, for the most part, remains under control. At the other end of his spectrum lies the condition known as 'fugue', which he describes as an extreme and markedly pathological inability to stop moving. In addition to, and somewhere between, these two is the condition known as 'dromomania', a form of ambulatory automatism. In preference to all of these, Davenport chooses to talk about 'nomadism', which he describes as a racial or tribal tendency to wander. 'On the whole', he writes, 'I am inclined to use the word 'nomadism' just because it has a racial connotation. From a modern point of view, all hereditary characteristics are racial.'[6]

Davenport develops his thesis via a discussion of the wandering tendency as a normal characteristic of humanity and animals which sets them apart from plants. He traces nomadism through a kind of evolutionary hierarchy noting the 'wandering instinct' in anthropoid apes, in 'primitive' people, in young children, and in adolescents. By tracing these connections, Davenport sought to show how nomadism was a primitive trait exhibited most frequently in those who have not fully enjoyed the benefits of civilisation. Apes, 'primitive peoples', babies, and adolescents all suffered from an excess of primitive urges and a lack of civilised constraints and were thus likely to wander. He spends the greatest effort discussing so-called 'primitive' people in order to reveal how all of the most primitive people are nomadic. At the bottom of this hierarchy are 'Fuegians, Australians, Bushman, and Hottentots', all of whom are nomadic. He refutes the suggestion that they are nomadic because they are hunters, and instead asserts that they are forced into hunting by their nomadic traits. He continues up his hierarchy of peoples noting the nomadism of Cossacks, Turkomans, Mongols, Polynesians, and Gypsies. Indeed, his central contention is that non-nomadic lifestyles are a very recent phenomenon in human history. Nomadism, to Davenport, indicated a racial tendency to wander which, somewhat bizarrely, but in keeping with American ideology about mobility, he saw as an expression of Americanness. Quoting Lowell's *Fireside Travels*, he pointed out that: 'The American is nomadic in religion, in ideas, in morals, and leaves his faith and opinions with as much indifference as the house in which he lives.'[7] Americans, he argued, were descendants of those restless elements of other, mainly European, nations, who chose to leave their ancestral homes and so it was surely no surprise that many American families would show nomadic traits.

Like social reformers of their time, Davenport was concerned with the classification and categorisation of 'nomadism', and he looked to France for models. At the time the French were extremely concerned with vagrancy and vagabondage and a number of people in medical and pseudo-medical fields were producing explanations for and classifications of vagrancy. Of particular significance at the time was the French diagnosis of 'fugue', a diagnostic relation of hysteria which swept through psychiatric circles at the time. Fugue was identified as a pathological urge to wander restricted mainly to men. Davenport, while evidently interested in the French diagnosis of fugue as a medical condition, was concerned to show the genetic origins of 'nomadism'.

Ian Hacking has brilliantly shown how the diagnosis of fugue as a medical entity was linked in France to social concern over vagrancy.[8] Fugue (literally flight) refers to a medical disorder characterised by sudden and inexplicable travel. Someone who suffered from fugue was referred to as a fuguer. Sufferers were almost always male, could not recall their travels, and often adopted startling new identities. What interested Hacking was the observation that fugue became a medical pathology around 1887, and ceased to be a topic of much concern by 1909.

Fuguers, like tramps, were most often thought of as men. Indeed, Hacking suggests that fugue provided a diagnosis for men that closely mirrored the feminised diagnosis of multiple personality disorder:

> Fugue was commonly run alongside multiple personality. Nine out of ten people recently diagnosed as multiple personalities are women. In the past, as now, the protoypical multiple was a women. The prototypical fuguer was a man, and for good reason. It was very much more easy for a man to take off with little money and perhaps no papers than for a woman to do so. A woman who wants to lead another life better do it at home. She must dissociate and fragment. A man can become another person by hitting the road.[9]

One question raised by Hacking is why fugue never took off as a medical diagnosis in the United States. His answer revolves around the socio-historical conditions that differentiated France from other countries: 'There are some obvious reasons why fugue should not be an American preoccupation... "Go West, young man: the fuguer never came back. America was full of young men in flight, but fugue was never medicalized.'[10] The story of the 'tramp scare' makes this explanation at least a little leaky. Many migrants in the United States did follow circular paths and frequently returned to old haunts – particularly in major cities such as Chicago. On top of that all manner of diagnoses were made of tramps including Davenport's eugenic explanations which, in turn, were informed by, and a response to, French discussions of fugue and vagrancy.

In many ways the French diagnosis of fugue contrasted with Davenport's eugenicist orientation. Fugues could be caused by anything from a bump on the head to fits of epilepsy. Davenport's nomadism was a deeply ingrained family and racial trait. But, as Hacking points out, the French history of all forms of hysteria were based on a foundation of heredity and degeneracy. A weak organic stock could lead first to alcoholism, then hysteria, then epilepsy, and eventually fugue. In Davenport's discussion of 'nomadism', the urge to wander was associated with a whole litany of psychoses including suicide, temper, migraine, epilepsy, hysteria, 'sprees', and 'sexual outbreaks'. All of these could lead to a paralysis of the inhibitions that are normally relied upon to prevent nomadism in civilised people. These nomadics were, in Davenport's view, a product of their genetic make-up and thus members of a special nomadic race.

Davenport comes to the conclusion that the nomadism is the result of a simple recessive sex-linked gene associated with these psychoses. His workers discovered 168 male nomadics and only 15 female. In the extreme case of tramps and vagabonds, Davenport suggested, 'the inhibitory mechanism is so poorly developed that the nomadic tendency shows itself without waiting, as it were, for the paralysis of the inhibitions'.[11] In other words, people who led a nomadic lifestyle were in the same category as babies, 'primitive people', and others who had none of the inhibitions typical of intelligent adults and 'civilised' people.

As an appendix to his work he provides details of 100 family histories of his nomads. Some of them read as bizarre litanies of pathological traits inevitably linked to nomadic lifestyles:

> (4) Propositus is a restless visionary. He has always been shifting from one position to another. Left home some months ago saying he was going West; has not been heard from since. Sibs: 1, female, died 14 years. 2 – male, died infancy. 3, female, works in a factory; is getting divorced. 4, male, has a roving disposition; is a nurse and companion; accompanies various patients on their trips for health. 5, female, has long been lawless and violent in her actions; she ran away from home while in a commercial school; had been there only a few weeks when she got the princicpal to refund her tuition, which had been paid in advance; with this money she went to L—— and became a telephone operator, later she ran away again to marry, and since her marriage she has run away; she loses her temper.
>
> Father, unknown
> Mother, unknown. Sibs: 1, male, unknown; 2, male, drowned when 7 years old.

Mother's father. – Was a stage-driver between Salem and Boston and kept a tavern or 'roadhouse' in what is now an outskirt of L——. Some of his descendants suggest that the wanderlust and frequently erratic character of his descendants come through this ancestor.

Mother's mother unknown.[12]

(11) Propositus, born 1895 in Missouri, is (1914) a wanderer and has left home repeatedly and been away for months at a time, returning home for rest and clothes, then he goes away again; works some, but does not save or provide for the future – a disobedient boy… Smokes a pipe and cigarettes, drinks whiskey, and has used cocaine considerably… Is irregular and uncertain in his habits, does not like to stay in one place long; likes to bum and tramp around to see the world… Has flat feet, crooked toes, crooked spine, and one shoulder is higher than the other….[13]

In these family histories, anything from headaches to having crooked feet is considered evidence for the pathological nature of human wandering. The 100 entries are a remarkable routemap of the prejudices and paranoias of early twentieth-century social science.

Davenport, of course, was not a lone figure in this mapping of pathologies. Other academics in other disciplines made similar assumptions. Peter Alexander Speek roots the mobility of the tramp in psychology.[14] Tramping, he argued, is caused when 'a passion for wandering is increased almost to madness'. This passion is inevitably followed by a 'profound aversion to work', 'a liking for drink', 'a childlike perspective that he might strike rich', and a loss of 'ability to concentrate'. 'Wonderful human nature', he writes, invents other, one might say in common parlance, "artificial" substitutes for "natural" enjoyment appearing in ambition and hope. By changing environment – scenes – by constant wandering, he keeps up some sort of interest in life.'[15]

A similar logic was used by a Chicago journalist in 1917 who gives us an admirable insight into the politics of mobility in the following quotation:

> Part of hobos belongs to the class of wanderlust. They will see the world, they will learn, and it is a very strong impulse. But the world respects the rich man who turned [out] to be a globe trotter and uses first class cabins and Pullman cars, but has inclinations to look over his shoulder at the hobo who, to satisfy this so strong impulse, is compelled to use box-cars, slip the board under the Pullman or in other ways whistle on the safety of his life and the integrity of his bones.[16]

In a similar vein, the well-known tramp investigator Josiah Flynt postulated that young boys became victims of a 'railroad fever' which gripped them at a young age and doomed them to life on the rails.[17]

So wandering was described as a pathology in terms of wanderlust. This form of mobility was connected to other forms of deviance such as poverty and insanity. Every problem calls for solutions and the logic of eugenics pointed in only one direction – preventing reproduction. W.H. Brewer made the eugenics argument quite succinctly: 'This "dangerous class"', he argued:

> is a tribe. It has its origin and natural constitution of a tribe, with its own instincts, tastes, traditions, and codes. Its mental characteristics are curiously like a tribe of savages in many respects and its acts as cruel and atrocious, and like all tribes it has its foundation in heredity.[18]

Brewer cites Dugdale's work on the Jukes as evidence for his argument and suggests that the only solution to the 'tramp evil' is confinement and separation of the sexes to prevent further breeding. In addition, it was certain that tramps were either foreign or weak-willed Americans, and that their personal deficiencies and moral indulgence would lead to the eventual extinction of their family.

Similar arguments were prominent at the Fourth Annual Session of the National Conference of Charities and Corrections in 1877, where there was a special session devoted to the 'Tramp Evil'. Professor Francis Weyland of Yale gave the key address in which he drew a very negative picture of the tramp as 'a lazy, shiftless, sauntering or swaggering, ill-conditioned, irreclaimable, incorrigible, cowardly, utterly depraved savage'.[19] Such savages, he suggested were impossible to detect due to their mobility: 'He is simply a tramp.' Weyland went on: 'In other words, he belongs to that vast horde of idle and unprincipled vagrants, who, by the fatal indulgence or apathy of our criminal legislation are permitted to roam, unchecked, throughout the length and breadth of our land.'[20]

Weyland suggested that the evil could be prevented by: a) providing necessities; b) compelling them to perform work; c) preventing them committing crime; and d) rendering it impossible for them to propagate paupers. An enthusiastic participant called Mrs Dall of Boston suggested that tramps should be disenfranchised and forbidden from marriage.

It is clear, then, that the combination of the tramp's mobility with other characteristics of pauperism, alcoholism, and mental illness were considered to be pathological in the sense that they were assumed to reside within the make up of the individual, perhaps linked to family and national origin, which led to the state of tramphood. In addition to this, though, were other fears, which linked the mobility of the tramp with particular pathologies. The one I focus on here is syphilis.

Syphilis and Mobility

One way in which tramps and hobos were defined as deviant and thus a threat was the association of the tramp's mobility with syphilis and its spread. Diseases and plagues throughout history have implied a number of disturbing characteristics which combine to suggest a radical out-of-placeness. Some of the characteristics of plagues and disease that might be relevant to the association of disease and tramps include a disregard for spatial boundaries, a capacity for rapid spread, a threat to 'normal' function, and the possibility of foreign origin.

Syphilis has been explicitly connected to mobility throughout history.[21] The plagues of the pox which swept through Europe in the sixteenth century have long been thought to be the result of Christopher Columbus and his crew picking it up in the New World, and bringing it back to Spain. The success of a mercenary army headed by Charles VIII King of France in Italy in 1495 led to the eventual capture of Naples in early 1496. While in Naples, the mercenary army of Swiss, Flemish, Italians and Spaniards made merry to such a degree that they were forced to leave by Italian princes whose original enthusiasm for the invasion was transformed into hostility. Besides, a Spanish army was on its way to recapture Naples. Upon their retreat the army took with them a new and strange disease. The French called it Neapolitan disease, while the Italians called it a French sickness.[22] When the disease arrived in Bristol in 1497 it was known as the Bordeaux sickness. Everywhere the disease arrived it was named after some other place. Muscovites called it the Polish sickness, the Poles the German disease. In Holland, it was known as the Spanish disease, and the Japanese called it the Portuguese sickness. Systematic attempts to locate origins of the disease pointed towards a number of travelling groups ranging from the Moors to the Beggards – a mystic-erotic cult who roamed Europe. Later the idea that Columbus' men had imported it with their slaves became common knowledge.[23]

Early researchers into syphilis quickly made a connection between the threat of syphilis and new technologies of mobility. In Russia during the 1860s, for instance, Dr Eduard Shperk blamed the spread of syphilis on the material life of modernity. In particular, he pointed towards the deleterious effects of railroads in weakening traditional (and implicitly moral) community bonds. Syphilis, he argued, was least rampant in agricultural peasant villages where traditional ties remained strong between people and between people and land. 'As the railroad enters a given locality', wrote Shperk, 'it increases the number of rented apartments, rented carriages ... and rented women.'[24]

Syphilis was also explicitly connnected to migrant workers in the United States and played an important role in the tramp scares that haunted the nation after the completion of the Union Pacific. Clearly, the address 'of no fixed abode' insinuated a looseness of morals and disconnection from normality. It was mobile people, such as sailors, soldiers, and tramps that were seen as the spreaders and even the causes of the disease. Of these, it was hobos and tramps who were believed to have the highest incidence. Nels Anderson, for instance, claimed that hobos in Chicago exhibited a 10% infection rate, twice that of servicemen.[25] Radical Chicago reformer Ben Reitman was keen to have hobos tested for the disease. He pointed out that 'the majority of them are between 18 and 45. They are unmarried and they take on all kinds of sex partners. Outside of the South side groups, they have more syphylis and gonorrhea than any other group in the city.'[26] In another letter to the Chicago medical authorities, Reitman made his case for a VD clinic in the hobo district by suggesting that 'transients are coming and going, bringing syphilis to Chicago and carrying gonorrhea to some other state. And nothing has been done about it.'[27] In Connecticut, another, less radical but still liberal social reformer James McCook was also dealing with the connectin between the mobility of tramps and the spread of syphilis.

McCook wrote to doctors all over the country to assess the prevalence of syphilis amongst tramp populations. He reported his findings in his paper 'Some New Phases of the Tramp Problem'.[28] He noted that 9.8% of 1,200 tramps surveyed had syphilis, and explicitly asks if there is a connection between physical health and political health. He recounts a letter from R.W. Taylor, MD, Professor of Veneral Diseases at the College of Physicians and Surgeons, New York, which reads:

> I think you are under the mark in assuming a 9.8% of these revolvers, as we call them, who are infected with some loathsome disease ... I think a large number certainly are diseased. I have no doubt that the widespread existence of itch in this county – it was a

rare disease here twenty years ago – is largely due to tramps. As to
their spreading syphilis, there can be no doubt and I am sure
gonorrhea is spread [and] broadcast by these wretches.[29]

Another letter from Dr C.I. Fisher, the Superintendant of the State
Almshouse in Tewkesbury, Massachusetts, reads:

> During the year ending March 1890, there were admitted to the
> hospital 1,058 men. Of these, 551, or more than 52%, were
> syphilites.… . Next to intemperance I hold that syphilis is the most
> important factor in the development and perpetuation of the
> dependent classes. It is everpresent as a factor of depression,
> weakening the will, lessening the vigour and lowering the sense of
> responsibility.[30]

Again connecting syphilis with wider political and social health,
McCook relates a meeting with a tramp in Worcester, Massachusetts,
who had voted in California within the year. Using his extensive
notes on tramps he had met, he picks out another example:

> #2 is a labourer; last worked at anything 'a long time ago', 'doesn't
> know when he is going to work again'; health 'good', 'but has had
> syphilis'; has been in the almshouse; generally sleeps 'anywhere';
> secures his food by 'begging', is intemperate and has been convicted
> of drunkenness … He … votes in Hartford. And what type of votes
> are they apt to be? Men who pass nearly half their time in jail, and
> never draw a sober breath when thay can help it, would hardly have
> much intelligence or conscience to go by; but such as it is would they
> use it? Or would they sell themselves readily to the highest bidder?[31]

James McCook was in many ways sympathetic to tramps and their
way of life. He kept in constant touch with one tramp, Roving Rob
Aspinwell, and obviously slipped into romantic notions of the life on
the open road. Here, though, McCook makes quite clear the litany
of pathologies associated with trampdom. In #2, we have a body
which refuses to be disciplined.

A few months later, McCook published another paper in the
popular magazine *Forum*. In this paper, he discussed the alarming
proportion of venal voters, suggesting that as many as 25,000 out of
166,000 votes in a recent election had been bought and paid for. Of
this 25,000, he suggested, the majority were tramps who often voted
more than once.[32]

McCook was certainly not the only person to note the threat to
democracy posed by the tramp. Reitman in Chicago noted how

whole electoral wards were easily fixed by buying hobo votes. 'The vote buyers', he said, 'can always be depended upon to buy the hobo ward.' 'Election day in Hoboland', he went on:

> is always a gay day. The men look forward to it with great pleasure. They are always sure of a fee for voting and around election time drinks are plentiful, panhandling is profitable and it is comparatively easy to get a drink or a night's lodging on the cuff. Probably no other form of social behaviour is so demoralizing to the individual and the community as this nefarious business of buying and selling votes.33

Nels Anderson too noted that hobos travelled as far as a thousand miles to cast a vote and would occasionally accept money for it. During the tramp scare, the equation mobility = democracy that is central to mainstream American historiography was reversed, and the mobility of the tramp became a codeword for corruptions of democracy. The solution that was demanded was disenfranchisement and confinement.

Syphilis and venal voting both played a part in the labelling of the nomadic tramp as a threatening other and both helped lay the ground for repressive actions by the medical establishment and the state. The mobile body of the tramp was inscribed with signifiers of pathological deviance from an inbred disposition to take to the road, to an economically driven desire to sell votes. In using disease in the description of transgressive people and actions, society is often compared to the human body. In the tramp example, hegemonic society is the social body that is threatened by the actions of the mobile workers. Professor Francis Weyland, in the address mentioned earlier, concluded that: 'The evil, as we have seen, is one of enormous magnitude, and unless speedily arrested, threatens the very life of society.'34 The idea of society having a life is, of course, one that goes back to Hobbes' *Leviathan* and beyond – the idea of the social body. I would like to suggest here that the connection of tramps with the disease of syphilis simultaneously drew correlations between the physical body of the infected tramp and the metaphorical body of the American democracy. In the notes of social reformers and others, tramps are blamed for the spread of syphilis and for the practice of multiple voting for money. In some cases, the two are connected and it is suggested that mobile people suffering from syphilis are a threat to democracy and the social body – the tramp becomes the equivalent of a disease.

I find Susan Sontag's discussion of *AIDS and its Metaphors* particularly useful here.35 She describes a variety of metaphors used to

273

construct discursively the human body and AIDS, of which the most powerful is the analogy to the military. She decribes the ways diseases, and particularly sexually transmitted ones, have been used to denote gult and irresponsibility. Military metaphors of disease, she argues:

> implement the way particularly dread diseases are envisaged as an
> alien 'other', as enemies are in modern war; and the move from the
> demonization of the illness to the attribution of fault to the patient
> is an inevitable one, no matter if patients are thought of as victims.
> Victims suggest innocence. And innocence, by the inexorable logic
> that governs all relational terms, suggests guilt.[36]

Sontag's argument, in its simplest terms, is that metaphors (e.g. military metaphors of illness) directly intervene in the perception and treatment of the people to which the metaphor is applied; that is, disease and treatment are thought of and acted upon as war. In war situations, extreme measures are called for, and normal legal process is suspended. The use of military metaphors in the description of AIDS is inevitably linked to the treatment of AIDS. The military metaphor, Sontag insists, 'overmobilizes, it overdescribes, and it powerfully contributes to the excommunicating and stigmatizing of the ill'.[37]

The conceptual metaphor *society as human body* makes possible the metaphor of transgression as disease and legitimates the (military) remedy. Returning to the nexus which links the mobile body of the tramp, the disease of syphilis, and the threat to the social and political body, we can see how the idea of tramps as diseased and as a disease was metaphorically linked to treatments, which, in line with Sontag's logic, were often expressed in military terms. The various methods of dealing with tramps from the Tramp Laws to hard labour, to imprisonment or to the whipping post, were all metaphorically justified by the threat – both literal and metaphorical – of disease.

Conclusion

I have shown a number of ways in which the figure of the tramp and the hobo were pathologized in turn-of-the-century America. The mobility exhibited by these migrants was clearly found to be distasteful by contemporary observers. In order to combat the perceived 'tramp evil', new laws were brought into being, draconian measures were suggested in the popular press, and social scientists proposed a number of disciplinary measures. But in addition to this, the tramp was associated with a number of pathologies. He was alleged to be pathologically disposed to roving due to the pseudoscientific phenomenon of wanderlust or dromomania. In addition, the threat posed by the mobility of these migrants included the spread of syphilis, as indicated by the observations of social reformers over a fifty year period. And it did not stop there: the fact of syphilis among hobos pointed towards a lack of moral character and an inability to make reasonable decisions. Reitman, McCook and others indicated the threat to democracy posed by venal voting on the part of these migrants. So not only was the human body threatened but also the body-politic – the social body. The tramps became, as it were, the syphilis germs circulating within the social body and threatening to undo it. Tramps, then, not only suffered from particular pathologies, but were also represented as pathologies themselves – pathologies which demanded draconian treatments.

The pathologization of the hobo points to the differential mobility effects of new technologies of mobility. Doreen Massey has suggested that generalised and generalising theories of time-space compression – the effective conquest of space and time said to result from new technologies of communication and transportation – mask the differential effects of these ·technologies on different social groups.[38] She argues instead for a politics of mobility grounded in the material conditions of people's lives as they move or are prevented from moving. If we look closely at the effects of the railroad in North America, we see that whole new experiences became possible – from the tourism of the leisured classes to the less comfortable travel of the tramp. New technologies of travel produce new transgressions and new pathologies such as the tramp scare. Mobility is too often generalized. Whether it is the traditional liberal formulation of mobility as freedom, the postmodern use of mobility as a form of anti-foundationalism, the use of mobility as a central pivot of American historiography, or the generalized claims of time-space compression, mobility has been subject to too many a grand narrative, and little in the way of grounded analysis. Mobility is a geographical phenomenon laden with power and meaning. The question is, how does mobility get its meaning, and how is it positioned in relation to power? To answer such questions, we need to ask more questions. Who moves? How do they move? How do people react to this movement? What boundaries and categories get disturbed via movement through space? Which get reinforced? In short, what is the spatiality of mobility?

Notes

1. For discussions of these issues, see David Harvey, *The Condition of Postmodernity* (Oxford: Blackwell, 1989); Doreen Massey, 'Power-Geometry and Progressive Sense of Place', *Mapping the Futures: local cultures, global change*, J. Bird *et al.* (eds), (London: Routledge, 1993), and C. Kaplan, *Questions of Travel: postmodern discourses of displacement* (Durham, NC: Duke University Press, 1996).
2. On railroads in American culture and political economy, see John Agnew, *The United States in the World Economy* (Cambridge: Cambridge University Press, 1987); George Douglas, *All Aboard! The Railroad in American Life* (New York: Paragon House, 1992).
3. For a lively discussion of media coverage of the tramp scare, see Kenneth Allsop, *Hard Travellin': the story of the migrant worker* (Pimlico: London, 1993).
4. R. Dugdale, *Hereditary Pauperism as illustrated by the Juke Family*, Conference of Charities (Saratoga: A. Williams & Co, 1877). For a history of eugenics in the United States. see M. Haller, *Eugenics: hereditarian attitudes in American thought* (New Brunswick: Rutgers University Press, 1963).
5. Charles Davenport, *The Feebly Inhibited: Nomadism, or the Wandering Impulse, with Special Reference to Heredity* (Washington DC: Carnegie Institution, 1915).
6. *Ibid.*, 7.
7. *Ibid.*, 7.
8. Ian Hacking, 'Les aliénés voyageurs: how fugue became a medical entity', *History of Psychiatry*, vii (1996), 425-49.
9. *Ibid.*, 429.
10. *Ibid.*, 426.
11. Davenport, *The Feebly Inhibited*, 25.
12. *Ibid.*, 28-9.
13. *Ibid.*, 31.
14. Alexander Speek, 'The Psychology of the Floating Worker', *Annals of the American Academy of Political and Social Sciences*, 6 (1917), 72-8.
15. *Ibid.*, 78.
16. Harvey M. Beardsley, 'Along the Main Stem with Red', *Chicago News*, 29 March 1917, 13.
17. J. Flynt, 'The Tramp and the Railroad', *Century Magazine*, lviii (1899), 258-66.
18. W.H. Brewer, 'What shall we do with the Tramps?', *New Englander*, xxxvii (1878), 522.
19. F. Weyland, *The Tramp Question*, National Conference on Charities

19. F. Weyland, *The Tramp Question*, National Conference on Charities and Corrections (St Paul: 1877), 112.

20. *Ibid.*, 114.

21. For social histories of syphilis, see Allan Brandt, *No Magic Bullet* (Oxford: Oxford University Press, 1985); Claude Quetel, *History of Syphilis* (Cambridge: Polity, 1990).

22. Quetel, *History of Syphilis*, 10.

23. A. Brandt, *No Magic Bullet*.

24. Laura Engelstein, 'Morality and the Wooden Spoon: Russian doctors view syphilis, social class, and sexual behaviour, 1890-1905', in
C. Gallagher and T.W. Laqueur (eds), *The Making of the Modern Body* (Berkeley, CA: University of California Press, 1987), 171.

25. Nels Anderson, *The Hobo* (Chicago: University of Chicago Press, 1925).

26. Reitman's papers are kept at the University of Illinois, Chicago Circle Library in the Special Collections division. This quotation is from Supplement II, VD Reports #104, 21/8/38.

27. Reitman Papers, Supplement II, VD Report #17, 1938.

28. James McCook, 'Some New Phases of the Tramp Problem', *Charities Review*, i: 8 (1892), 355-64.

29. *Ibid.*, 355-6.

30. *Ibid.*, 357-8.

31. *Ibid.*, 361.

32. J. McCook, 'The Alarming Proportion of Venal Voters', *Forum*, xiv: 1 (1892), 1-13.

33. Reitman Papers, 'Vote Selling and the Criminal Hobo', Supplement II.

34. Weyland, *op. cit.*, 120.

35. Susan Sontag, *AIDS and its Metaphors* (New York: Farrar, Strauss and Giroux, 1988).

36. *Ibid.*, 11.

37. *Ibid.*, 95.

38. Massey, 'Power-Geometry and Progressive Sense of Space'.

9

The Politics of Medical Topography: Seeking healthiness at the Cape during the nineteenth century

Harriet Deacon

Introduction

In the nineteenth century there were, it was said, three reasons for travel, 'infirmity of the body, imbecility of mind, or inevitable necessity'.[1] In his 'Introductory lecture on climate', delivered at Edinburgh Medical School in 1857, A.W. Pulteney Pinkerton M.D. advised students that convalescence abroad could be an important part of a cure, especially for the chronically insane, rheumatic or tuberculous patient.[2] As a contemporary cartoon suggested, doctors (and the families of patients) may have used the foreign health resort or the sea voyage to shift responsibility for a difficult cure away from themselves. In choosing a health resort, doctors had to consider both temperature and humidity. Pinkerton counselled that the combination of heat and moisture (such as on islands or at the seaside) produced a relaxing effect, while dry heat and cold were stimulating.

One of the health resorts considered by British doctors in the nineteenth century was the temperate Cape Colony (now part of South Africa), under varying degrees of British control from 1795 to 1961. A visit to the Cape offered European invalids a sea voyage and a choice of coastal verdure or a dry arid interior. The Cape had always been depicted as a healthy place for Europeans to visit, but its popularity as a health resort fluctuated and, within the colony, the locus of healthiness moved inland during the course of the nineteenth century. By analyzing these shifts, we can begin to understand more fully the economic, political and moral undertones influencing the European invalid's choice of a health resort abroad.

The selection of a health resort did not rest on a simple measurement of climate or ease of access: it was closely related to what theorists of tourism call the symbolic value of place.[3] Descriptions of climate were themselves also evaluations of the social or political status of a place and its inhabitants. As Livingstone suggests:

> Geographical discussions of climatic matters throughout the nineteenth, and well into the twentieth century were profoundly implicated in the imperial drama and were frequently cast in the diagnostic language of ethnic judgement.[4]

Dane Kennedy's work on colonial Kenya and Rhodesia in the twentieth century, for example, implies that contemporary theories about climate (the dangerousness of exposing Europeans to the tropical sun) were influenced by differing programs for white settlement and expressed European settler anxiety about their new home. Steps taken against overexposure to tropical heat shaped the defensive way in which European settlers responded to the colonial environment and the people in it.[5] Colonial health resorts thus benefited from their association with the healing countryside, but they also carried a potential threat of moral and social degeneracy for European invalids.

Medical Topography and Imperialism

As a restocking point for ships on the East Indian trade route, the Cape was associated with health and recuperation from the very beginning of the colonial encounter. It was considered a particularly healthy place for ships to stop because of the 'temperate' climate and easy access to fresh food and water. A British chaplain travelling along the East Indies route in 1693 described the Cape as 'this Paradise of the World', where

> '[t]he Air ... is ... temperate and sweet, healthful and pleasant, and very agreeable to the constitution of the Dutch, as well as the Natives, to whom it gives great activity and vigour'.[6]

Travel accounts of the eighteenth and nineteenth centuries were increasingly specific in their details of the Cape climate, the quality of water and food, altitude and prevalent diseases. Such accounts were part of the genre of medical topography, which arose out of an increasing interest in documenting and measuring the relationship between disease and the environment in seventeenth- and eighteenth-century Europe.

Medical topography emerged out of a revival of classical humoral aetiological theory and a new interest in classification and

280

measurement of the natural world.[7] The classical writers had interpreted disease as an imbalance of the four humours: blood, bile, black bile and phlegm. The humours were linked to the four seasons and the four elements, binding man, nature and the universe tightly together.[8] 'Airs, waters and places' influenced disease patterns. After the early modern period and the discovery of new parts of the world, environmental influence on human health and culture was considered even more important than before, an idea which was taken up and extended in the seventeenth and eighteenth centuries by writers like Sydenham, Montesquieu and Buffon.[9] They employed new methods of meteorological measurement. These did not provide scientific proof of their theories, as measuring disease and statistical analysis remained in their infancy, but lent them a new scientific credibility.[10] As Europeans became more confident about their role as stewards of nature,[11] they sought to control disease by adjusting the micro-environment – the 'non-naturals' such as air, diet, sleep, exercise, evacuations and passions of the mind – to counter broader climatic and topographical effects.[12] The greater prominence of social and hygienic factors in these evaluations of the environment – the inclusion of people in the environmental equation – was part of a trend towards more specific disease aetiologies in the nineteenth century.[13]

The genre of medical topography reveals a relationship between environment and disease deeply inscribed with moral and political overtones and profoundly influenced by social and economic trends. In analyzing accounts of the medical topography of 'temperate' colonies like the Cape we cannot dismiss them simply as medical mumbo-jumbo, cynical imperialist justification, or marketing hype, although they performed all these functions too.[14] Environmental disease aetiologies, in both meteorological and sanitary forms, were so powerful that they were able at first to incorporate, and later exist alongside, germ theories of disease, especially in popular culture (we still feel 'under the weather' when unwell).[15] Imperial expansion was at the very origin of the revival in environmental disease aetiology in the seventeenth century; it provided new ground for scientific investigation and demanded better medical care for sailors, soldiers and settlers on long voyages and in different environments.[16] Travel accounts aimed at the medical and emigrant markets drew extensively on the attractions of a healthy climate to attract tourists and settlers to temperate colonies. To be healthy, however, a new environment had to be domesticated and conquered first. The image of the garden thus played an important function in asserting human

281

control over nature and place.

Descriptions of climate, an essential element in any nineteenth-century explanation for disease patterns and the identification of healthy places, were thus profoundly affected by the political, economic and moral economy of imperialism. European adaptation to colonial climates was morally important as a mark of their rationality and politically important as a sign of their fitness to rule other nations.[17] It was also a necessity where they planned to exploit the natural resources of their colonies, and to civilize and evangelize the 'natives'.[18] While there was some doubt about the ability of Europeans to settle in tropical regions, their physical fitness to settle (and by extension their moral fitness to rule) was less questionable in temperate colonies. There, European settlement was not as threatened by new diseases as in the tropics. Indeed, the introduction of European diseases to temperate regions actually reduced indigenous resistance to colonization.[19]

The definition as 'temperate' of the major settler colonies in the nineteenth century (the Cape, parts of America and Canada, New Zealand and Australia) carried broader political connotations too. By the eighteenth century older ideas about the relative virtues of hot, cold and temperate climates[20] had been used to explain the relative civilization of temperate regions in Europe compared to the tropical world.[21] Temperate climates were thought to endow their inhabitants with special ability to rule and trade,[22] and connoted areas of highest civilization and democracy.[23] The political and moral healthiness of the colonies was also tagged to their climate. The healthy climate and abundant landscape of opportunity thus became a central part of colonial identity in the temperate colonies.[24]

The Colonial Health Resort: *rus in urbe*

To be popular with wealthy medical tourists, the colonial health resort had to be both physically rural and socially cosmopolitan. The European spa town was physically separate from the city, but modelled on it socially: while characterized by its healthy natural environment, it had to be domesticated and socialized – Eden was always a garden rather than a jungle. In the spa, conspicuous consumption replaced the crass acquisitiveness of the city, while its frenetic social life made up for the loneliness of the landed gentry on their rural estates.[25] In the colonial context the establishment of a health resort therefore relied on the prior conquest of territory and people, but this relationship with conquest had to be hidden. This was done in the same way that natural history 'asserted an urban, lettered, male authority over the whole of the planet', a 'passive innocence of hegemony' which Pratt calls 'anti-conquest'.[26] This helps to explain why the Cape health resort followed the boundary of conquest, just far enough inside it to be secure in its 'innocent hegemony', yet still at a healthy distance from urban squalor.

In the first half of the nineteenth century, Cape Town, situated conveniently on the sea route to the East, was popular with 'travellers in pursuit of sport, health or science'[27] as a health resort for Anglo-Indian officials and British emigrants *en route* to Australasia or the East. From 1816 to 1846 the Cape, alongside New South Wales, recorded the lowest mortality rate among white troops and was proclaimed 'eminently healthy'.[28] Because of the idea that they could not adapt easily to a tropical climate, ailing British officers in India (and sometimes also those whose conduct was unsatisfactory) were allowed the option of convalescence 'upon the sea coast, or in any other healthy situation, or to go to sea, to China, to St Helena, or even to Europe for their recovery'.[29] From soon after the British captured the Cape in 1795[30] until the 1850s, a considerable number of these men – called Indians or Hindoos locally[31] – went to Cape Town and neighbouring villages.

As the colonial frontier moved outwards and conditions in the growing town began to evoke comparisons with unhealthy urban environments in Europe, Cape Town's leafy suburbs and domesticated hinterland became more attractive than the town itself. At the end of the century a local newspaper commented:

> [Life in the Cape Town suburbs has] that particular rus in urbe – that happy blend of sylvan beauty with access to all the social stimuli of a capital. [The climate is good], if without the peculiar snap and tingling dryness of the characteristic upcountry air.[32]

Cape Town's pernicious urban influence was by this time distinguished from the gentle healthiness of the suburbs. Significantly, however, by mid-century most of the praises of the Cape countryside were being sung by and for Cape Town residents rather than visitors from abroad. The Cape suburbs and country town retreats were cast in the same terms as the English countryside, drawing on settler desires for acceptance in Europe rather than a colonial identity of their own.[33] For those seeking particular climatic conditions for rheumatism or tuberculosis, the Cape interior offered something different – new and exciting, and close to the growing wealth of the gold and diamond fields.

The temperate colonies stood in the same symbolic relation to the imperial metropole as the 'countryside' did to the 'city'. As Raymond Williams has said, Empire was the countryside writ large: an idyllic retreat, an escape and an opportunity to make a fortune.[34] This made the temperate colonies ideal health resorts, but at the same time underlined their subordinate position in relation to the metropole. As colonies expanded, new urban-rural gradations of power and healthiness emerged and health resorts shifted accordingly. But although the Cape was always considered healthy in some part, its continued political and economic weakness meant that residence there continued to be associated more with degeneracy and provincialism than with regeneration. This hampered the development of a 'new world' image for the colony and the establishment of high-status health resorts there.

Colonial Degeneracy and Urban Decay

British settlers and travellers to colonial territories in the nineteenth century were worried about maintaining their standards of civilization, preventing any physical and moral degeneracy in hot climates. Inventiveness and hard labour were considered to be at the very origin of the civilizing impulse.[35] Natural abundance was thus welcomed for the economic growth it promised many colonies, but at the same time a climate which made growing and hunting food a relatively easy task was not thought to be as stimulatin283g to human creativity and civilization as was the colder European climate.[36] In spite of greater confidence about European ability to control new disease environments during the nineteenth century,[37] a growing polygenist conviction that races were physiologically and mentally attuned to their ancestral racial environment,[38] fuelled the fear that Europeans who stayed in hotter countries too long could degenerate.[39] Leaving the climate of one's birthplace could produce negative physical and moral effects.[40] British writers in the 1830s suggested that the Hindu in India had become racially degenerate because the hot climate enabled them 'to live heedless and slothful'.[41] While the Cape was classified as 'temperate', the summers were hotter than British ones and living off the land was considered to be easier.

British commentaries on the Cape in the late eighteenth century began to point out the moral and physical degeneracy of the Cape Dutch settlers and indigenes, in marked contrast to descriptions of their 'activity and vigour' in the late seventeenth century.[42] Some visitors argued that the moral degeneration of Cape Dutch settlers – excessive eating, drinking and indolence – caused ill-health,[43] which would explain the presence of disease in spite of the excellent climate.[44] British visitors extended these criticisms to Dutch town planning, suggesting that the Dutch-built canals beside the Cape Town streets exerted a 'noxious influence on the health of the inhabitants'.[45] This negative attitude formed part of a general British attack on Dutch rule of the Cape, the idleness encouraged by slave-owning and the immorality and unhealthiness of Dutch culture. This critique stemmed partly from the fact that the British were at war with the Netherlands from 1795 until 1815, a war in which they annexed the Cape. But expansionist imperialism and the incorporation of conquered indigenous societies had also intensified the identification of indigenous culture with immorality and idleness by this time.[46] Medical commentators had shifted greater responsibility for disease onto the poor and indigenes.[47] It is not altogether surprising therefore that, by the late eighteenth century, British visitors to the Cape were eager to point to the moral degeneracy of Cape Dutch settlers and indigenes.

Once the British began to send their own settlers to the Cape after 1795, British commentators tried to draw a contrast between Cape Dutch 'boors' and British settlers. They were sensitive to critical comments about their own settlers, and more eager to explain illness with reference to climatic location or urban decay rather than a creeping moral degeneracy. The critics' attention was focussed on Cape Town, which was at this time the main destination for British settlers and visitors. Although never overwhelming enough to discourage immigration, the unhealthy effects of the 'strong winds' and sudden variations in temperature in Cape Town now became more prominent in accounts of the Cape than before.[48] Moodie noted in the 1830s that while the colony as a whole was healthy, 'Cape Town and the country skirting the base of the mountains are, notwithstanding their proximity to the sea, very warm, and less healthy than the other districts of the colony'.[49] There was general praise of the 'dryness of the atmospheric air' and the bracing influence of its 'brisk circulation' by the prevailing winds,[50] but the South East wind was represented as a healthy influence mainly because of its ability to reduce the oppressive heat or remove the noxious fumes of urban decay from slums and Dutch canals.[51]

Although the problems of urbanization and the need to find a suitable scapegoat for settler illness clearly influenced the trend towards more measured accounts of the Cape Town climate, the discourse about the unhealthiness of Cape Town was closely related to a deliberate redefinition of the role the town played in relation to the rest of the colony and to the metropole. The town's unhealthiness was a symptom of its progress towards urban maturity. Between the third and the fifth decades of the nineteenth century, middle-class English settlers in Cape Town scrambled to establish morally- and culturally-protective social institutions to preserve their moral status and enhance their political power in the colony. Public health improvements were part of this effort to assert power through mimicry of British models and they were associated with the reconstruction of public and political space in the urban area. Through the establishment of commercial and public institutions, urban sanitation, street cleaning and better policing, Cape Town could be redefined as a British urban environment with a controlled underclass in the sanitized or partitioned slums, a central, modern, civilized public sphere and a healthy residential environment in the middle-class suburbs.

In the town, a Commercial Exchange (built in the 1820s) became the centre of male society and high-status streets were gradually dominated by business premises rather than houses with shops in the front rooms.[52] By conquering the unhealthy influences of some of its inhabitants and becoming a public space, Cape Town became the masculine, powerful 'city' centred on trade and institutionally-driven progress in relation to the feminine, domesticated 'countryside' and suburbs. By providing the institutions and structure of a British urban space Cape Town could now represent the attainment of civilized modernity in the colony. This meant that the symbolism of Cape Town had to move away from the imagery of the healthy countryside which had served to boost its reputation as a health resort in the past. The suburban villages around Cape Town now became the focus for visitors seeking health resorts and for wealthy settler residents.

The Cape Town suburbs, once described by a visitor as 'a desert' compared to the industry of the town,[53] were gradually recast as a garden-like region with a markedly more healthy climate than the town. They included the green and traditionally picturesque[54] villages of Wynberg, Newlands and Rondebosch on the cooler, wetter side of Table Mountain and the more distant towns of Stellenbosch, Paarl and Somerset West.[55] In 1818 a British woman visiting the Cape commented that 'behind the mountain, the air is much cooler' than in the Town during summer, and that in Simonstown, 'the air is considered cooler, purer and more healthy than that of Cape Town'.[56] Many wealthier Capetonians moved permanently into these suburbs during the 1840s. The Cape 'countryside' became a more appropriate site than the town in which to seek health and residential bliss. Thirty years later one of the Cape Town doctors still acknowledged that in the leafy suburbs there was 'more exposure to healthy winds and cooler climates' while the old town was 'saturated by exhalations from squalid tenants and pythogenic [sic] diseases'.[57]

From the very beginning of the century, invalids had gone to visit the 'country' towns for their health.[58] As early as 1806, Stellenbosch had become, at least in the summer, 'a fashionable resort for parties of pleasure [to which] many ... who are in a bad state of health, [go] to avoid the heat and violent south-east winds of Cape Town.'[59] In 1858 the Professor of Classics and English at the South African College, Langham Dale, while suffering from a 'nervous headache', was prescribed a 'change of air' by his doctor in Cape Town, and was sent to Somerset West, 'then very popular as a health resort', where the doctor's son and professional partner was, conveniently, resident.[60] Although there were several hot springs in the colony,[61] they did not become popular health resorts during the nineteenth century, perhaps because of the lack of high-status facilities. The Caledon Baths, the oldest and closest to Cape Town, were criticized in 1822 as lacking 'amusement' or 'society',[62] although up to 200 visitors per annum had visited them in the late eighteenth century.[63]

The Lack of Society at the Cape

Provincialism was a persistent problem which reduced the appeal of Cape Town and its suburbs to medical tourists. Even in the heyday of its popularity as a health resort in the early nineteenth century, the Cape had to defend itself against suggestions in the London and Indian press that its inhabitants were 'in the lowest possible state of moral degradation', and that it was wanting in 'civility' and proper facilities.[64] Like the English countryside, the colonies lacked the protective institutions of civilization and the instruments of commercial and industrial progress which characterized the metropole and symbolized its power. Institutions were considered important because theories of climatic influence on human physical and mental characteristics had opened up the possibility during the Renaissance that vice and virtue was partly out of human control. Only by overcoming climatic control over human society through industry, culture and innovation, were people able to progress beyond the limitations of their environmental heritage, a consequence of the Fall from Grace. Any laxness in the institutions of civilization and the gathering of knowledge about nature would reassert climatic control and thus encourage degeneration.[65]

These ideas were articulated differently by metropolitan and local commentators and formulated in various ways among the colonies. In America, early Virginians saw their country as a paradise where they would be made regenerate by a new relationship with the abundant earth, improving on nature by making plantations (although their vision was disrupted by the presence of the black slave as gardener).[66] Metropolitan commentators on New Zealand and Australia got around the lack of institutions by describing the colonies as Arcadia, an egalitarian land of plenty in which a people of moderation and contented simplicity did not require formal institutions.[67] By contrast, during the early nineteenth century the Cape was represented by British commentators and settlers more in the style of the 'Land of Cockaygne',[68] where the environmental cornucopia was abused by the Dutch and the 'Hottentots' because of their innately gross and insatiable appetites. The relative absence of the trappings of civilization was thus particularly severely felt at the Cape, where Dutch settlers were considered to be country bumpkins who not only lacked modern institutions (like theatres and a Commercial Exchange) but patronized old-fashioned ones (like fairs and shops in houses).

Especially before middle-class institutions like theatres, museums and literary societies were established in the 1820s and 1830s, Cape Society was an unwelcome contrast to that in contemporary resorts such as Bath or Brighton in England where royal patronage was ideally combined with organized high-status activities (such as balls and recitals) for large groups of better-class visitors during the Season.[69] In the absence of an aristocracy, military and naval officers were considered to be among the upper echelon of Cape society.[70] As one visitor complained after a visit in 1820, the Anglo-Indian invalids 'may be said to comprise nearly all there is of gentility' in Cape Town:[71]

> A society ... dependent upon such moveable gentry for its tone and brilliancy, must be subject to incessant changes ... There is, at present, little or no visiting going on at the Cape; and few amusements ... What is wanting to their festivities ... in 'pomp and circumstance' – is made up for in solid feeding.[72]

Port Elizabeth, an arid town on the Eastern frontier, tried to attract Anglo-Indians from Cape Town, but with little success.[73] An Anglo-Indian traveller commented in the 1850s that Port Elizabeth was a place 'where ladies are not, and where gentlemen are scarce' (after a complaint he was forced to add a comma before 'scarce').[74] These Anglo-Indian visitors abandoned the Cape when changes in their leave and pecuniary allowances in the late 1840s[75] and the opening of the Suez canal in the 1860s[76] made it easier for them to go to Europe for medical leave instead.[77]

The Waning Popularity of the Cape as a Health Resort

Ideas about the Cape's natural healthiness were thus intertwined with the threat of physical and moral degeneracy and cultural provincialism. This was to have some effect on its 'symbolic value' as a health resort. Pinkerton suggested in 1857 that the temperate colonies, Canada, New Zealand or the Cape, were best chosen as health resorts for 'men of energy and perseverance', and not suitable for weaker invalids (including women) and the higher classes, who should go to the Mediterranean instead.[78] It was often difficult to persuade even those living in the temperate colonies and ex-colonies to eschew Mediterranean resorts for their own.[79] Colonial resorts in general were of a lower status than European ones and were, like the colonies themselves, brash and possibly dangerous for the weak. Within this skewed market, the Cape competed rather ineffectually against the other temperate colonies for those strong enough to brave the colonial health resorts. It was unable to attract many medical tourists when the general traffic around the tip of Africa decreased after 1850 and military confidence about protecting troop health in tropical climates through sanitary measures increased.

When the 'Hindoos' departed, temperate colonies like the Cape turned towards the private health-resort trade. After mid-century some Karoo towns and Bloemfontein, close to the diamond fields of Kimberley and *en route* to the gold fields of the Transvaal, attracted a small number of tuberculosis sufferers who were prepared to endure a social wilderness there. Emma Murray (*née* Rutherford), the wife of a missionary in Bloemfontein and the daughter of a Cape merchant, suggested at this time that

> The cold up here [in Bloemfontein] is far more bracing than in Cape Town, we have snow and ice and in winter a dry cold considered most bracing, in summer our rain.[80]

In the quest for tourist numbers, the temperate colonies competed with each other and the wealthy and fashionable Mediterranean resorts. Cape and Australasian resorts suffered particularly as a result of this competition – they did not feature at all in Bradshaw's *Bathing*

Places and Climatic Health Resorts at the end of the century, although California, Jamaica and Tunis did.[81] After the 1860s the popularity of the curative sea voyage had waned and high-altitude or seaside resorts closer to Europe boomed.[82] As one Cape supporter commented wanly in 1869:

> Without attempting to compete with foreign watering-places in mere gaiety and public amusements, we are only a month behind the larger towns of England in commercial, political and social intelligence [i.e. news] ... at all events, we can supply abundance of fresh air and water and ... out-of-door enjoyment.[83]

The fashion for oriental furnishings in the late nineteenth century created another competing exotic focus in the East, which the Cape could not match. In attracting medical tourists in the latter half of the nineteenth century, therefore, the Cape competed for a very small slice of the market, mainly with Australia.[84] In 1885 Dr Atherstone, a prominent practitioner in the Eastern Cape, said on providing a report on the Cape for the Colonial and Indian Exhibition that:

> We must not let the matter of our sanatory superiority to other colonies fall through. Our health resorts as such are superior in every way to the Australian colonies, and easier of access.[85]

The Cape Medical Board sought, on the request of the Cape Government, to collect information from local doctors on 'the salubrity of our Climate and its beneficial effect in many complaints'.[86] Attracting invalids was a serious matter, both economically and in terms of status and identity. As one British commentator pointed out:

> Invalids bring money with them, and for that reason, if for no other, I think it would be a very good thing if doctors would discover that our British Colonies are good health resorts.[87]

Atherstone was told that through his submission he would 'be able to show at least that the old settlers have lost nothing, physically and mentally by being transposed to an African Climate'.[88] As British experience of tropical Africa grew, so too did their fear of its dangers, fears which were transposed onto the temperate South; there was also greater publicity about the poor white problem in South Africa by the 1880s, which symbolized degeneracy. The Exhibition publicity was not just intended to attract medical customers, but simultaneously to allay European concerns about degeneracy and by extension, bolster the image of Cape settlers.

290

Conclusions

A number of medical tourists visited the Cape Colony during the early nineteenth century, a time when British employees in India sought relief from their tropical surroundings and many travellers passed the tip of Africa on their way to the East. By the second half of the century, however, the Cape was competing less successfully with other countries for European medical tourists. Promoters of health resorts within the colony gradually shifted their attention out of urban Cape Town during the 1830s, and looked towards the sylvan beauty of the suburbs. After the 1860s, their focus was on the dry and arid hinterland as a cure for the ailing consumptive. Altitude and dry air tuberculosis cures became increasingly important in attracting health tourists to the Cape. These shifts were consistent with a search for new health resorts in established settlements which were safely inside the moving colonial frontier, but not yet sullied by the foulness of a city.

The Cape's popularity as a resort was partly a function of its changing position on trade and emigration routes from Europe to the East, but it was also related to the colony's symbolic positioning within an Imperial 'countryside' and the moral desirability of its 'temperate' climate. In general, however, the Cape failed to provide a strong symbolic association with high-status health and pleasure to counterbalance the growing disadvantage of its distance from Europe and the threat of provincialism and degeneracy which colonial resorts – and the Cape in particular – posed to their European visitors. High-status resorts had to offer visitors both sophisticated social stimulation and natural beauty, a combination which the Cape was hard-pressed to offer.

It is only during the twentieth century that the symbolic value of Cape healthiness has been cemented as part of the broader appeal of the controlled natural environment of South Africa for European and white South African tourists when the natural (but safe) attractions of game parks in the Transvaal and Natal were juxtaposed against the restful leafy beauty of the Western Cape. This view was encapsulated in the advertising jingle 'Braaivleis Biltong, Sunny Skies and Chevrolet' in the 1970s. The South African natural environment was there to be eaten ('braai-ed' or barbecued), enjoyed (in healthy sunshine) and traversed (by car) – (white) culture had triumphed over nature. This has metamorphosed into a vision of the country as one giant safari, shared by rich (white and black) South Africans and tourists alike.

Notes

1 Laurence Sterne quoted in J. Spillane, *Medical travellers: narratives from the seventeenth, eighteenth and nineteenth centuries* (Oxford: Oxford University Press, 1984), 1.

2 A.W.P. Pinkerton, 'Introductory lecture on climate' (Edinburgh: Sutherland & Knox, 1857), 10, 21-23.

3 K. Meethan, 'Place, image and power: Brighton as a resort', in T. Selwyn (ed.), *The Tourist Image: myths and myth-making in tourism* (Chichester: Wiley, 1996), 179-96.

4 D.N. Livingstone, 'Climate's Moral Economy: Science, Race and Place in Post-Darwinian British and American Geography', in A. Godlewska and N. Smith (eds), *Geography and Empire* (Oxford: Blackwell, 1994), 137.

5 D. Kennedy, 'Climatic theories and culture in colonial Kenya and Rhodesia', *Journal of Imperial and Commonwealth Studies*, X(1) (1981), 50-66.

6 J. Ovington, *A voyage to Suratt in the year 1689 ... Likewise a description of ... the Cape of Good Hope* (London: Tonsen, 1696), 486.

7 C. Hannaway, 'Environment and Miasmata', in W.F. Bynum and R. Porter (eds), *Companion Encyclopedia of the History of Medicine* (London: Routledge, 1993), 292-308, 300. See also C.J. Glacken, *Traces on the Rhodian Shore: Nature and Culture in Western Thought from Ancient Times to the end of the Eighteenth Century* (Los Angeles: University of California Press, 1967).

8 V. Nutton, 'Humoralism' in W.F. Bynum and R. Porter (eds), *Companion Encyclopedia of the History of Medicine* (London: Routledge, 1993), 281-91, 288.

9 C.J. Glacken, *Traces on the Rhodian Shore*, 429, 502, 566, 620-22. See also M. Harrison, *Public Health in British India* (Cambridge: Cambridge University Press, 1994), 38.

10 C. Hannaway, 'Environment and Miasmata', 299.

11 C.J. Glacken, *Traces on the Rhodian Shore*, 480-84, 661.

12 V. Nutton, 'Humoralism', 289; C. Hannaway, 'Environment and Miasmata', 293.

13 C. Hannaway, 'Environment and Miasmata', 302.

14 D. Kennedy, 'Climatic theories and culture', 50, 55 makes the same point.

15 This was generally true in Europe, but is particularly noticeable in tropical medicine. See M. Harrison, *Public Health in British India*, 53-57. D. Kennedy shows that climatic theories were still prevalent

in psychiatry during the 1930s ('Climatic theories and culture', 58).

16 C. Hannaway, 'Environment and Miasmata', 302; see also R. Grove, *Green Imperialism*, 42-45.

17 M. Harrison, *Public Health in British India*, 39, 43-44. See also M. Worboys, 'Tropical Diseases', in W.F. Bynum and R. Porter (eds), *Companion Encyclopedia of the History of Medicine* (London: Routledge, 1993), 511-535.

18 Sir Harry Johnston, Commissioner for the British Central African Protectorate, made this point explicitly in his introduction to Dr Kerr Cross, *Health in Africa: a medical handbook for European travellers and residents* (London: J. Nisbet, 1897), vii.

19 A.W. Crosby, *Ecological Imperialism: the biological expansion of Europe, 900-1900* (Cambridge: Cambridge University Press, 1986).

20 C.J. Glacken, *Traces on the Rhodian Shore*, 440-41.

21 On British experiences in tropical environments, see articles by M. Harrison and W. Anderson in a special issue of the *Bulletin for the History of Medicine*, 70 (Spring 1996).

22 C.J. Glacken, *Traces on the Rhodian Shore*, 440-41.

23 *Ibid.*, 539, 547, 592-93.

24 One example would be the construction of the high-altitude Andean superman M. Cueto, 'Andean biology in Peru: Scientific Styles on the Periphery', *Isis*, 80(304) (Dec. 1989), 646).

25 J. Urry, *The Tourist Gaze: Leisure and Travel in Contemporary Societies* (London: Sage, 1990), 5.

26 M.L. Pratt, *Imperial Eyes: Travel writing and transculturation* (London: Routledge, 1992), 7, 38-39.

27 A. Gilchrist, *The Cape of Good Hope: a Review of its Present Position as a Colony* (London: Hamilton, Adams and co., 1844), v.

28 A.K. Johnstone, 'Essay on the geographical distribution of health and disease', 1856, National Library of Scotland, Acc. 5811, box.13. A similar opinion had been advanced in Great Britain, Army Medical Department and War-Office, 'Statistical Reports on the sickness, mortality, and invaliding among the troops in Western Africa, St Helena, the Cape of Good Hope and Mauritius' (London: n.p., 1840), introduction.

29 Wellesley to Pole, 12 Nov. 1805, UCT Manuscripts, BCS 274.

30 R. Percival, *An account*, 133, 138-39.

31 N. Polson, *A subaltern's sick leave*, 78.

32 'How girls live', *Cape Times*, 4 Sept. 1897.

33 This is in interesting contrast to America in the nineteenth century, where A. Miller suggests landscape representations there 'carried a new weight of national meaning' and helped to form a distinctive

cultural identity for the American middle class (*The Empire of the Eye: Landscape Representation and American Cultural Politics 1825-1875* (Ithaca: Cornell University Press, 1993), 1-2).

34   R. Williams, *The country and the city* (St Albans: Paladin, 1975), 337. See also S. Pugh, 'Introduction' in S. Pugh (ed.), *Reading Landscape: country – city – capital* (Manchester: Manchester University Press, 1990), 5.

35   The idea that Europeans could not work in the hot sun, which justified the employment of black slaves and workers in America (G. Puckrein, 'Climate, health and black labor in the English Americas', *Journal of American Studies*, XIII (1979), 179-93, 180) and tropical parts of Africa (D. Kennedy, 'Climatic theories and culture', 53), was said by one visitor to be the (indefensible) reason why the Dutch had imported slaves to the Cape (E. Blount, *Notes on the Cape of Good Hope ... 1820* (London: J. Murray, 1821), 20.) Manual labour continued to be seen as *kaffirwerk* into the 20th century.

36   C.J. Glacken, *Traces on the Rhodian Shore*, 539, 547.

37   M. Harrison, 'Disease and Climate in India and the West Indies', *Bulletin for the History of Medicine*, 70 (Spring 1996), 68-93, 73. See F. Nightingale, *How people may live and not die in India* (London: E. Faithfull, 1863).

38   W. Anderson, 'Disease, race and empire', *Bulletin for the History of Medicine*, 70 (Spring 1996), 62-67, 64.

39   J.W. Tripe, 'On some relations of meteorological phenomena to health', International Health Exhibition: 'Meteorology in relation to Health', conference hosted by the Royal Meteorological Society, July 17-18 (London: IHE, 1884). See also D. Kennedy, 'Climatic theories and culture', 53-54.

40   C. Hannaway, 'Environment and Miasmata', 302-4; C.J. Glacken, *Traces on the Rhodian Shore*, 558-61. See also D. Kennedy, 'Climatic theories and culture'.

41   M. Harrison, *Public Health in British India*, 48.

42   J. Ovington, *A voyage to Suratt in the year 1689*, 486.

43   R. Percival, *An account of the Cape of Good Hope* (London: Baldwin, 1804), 224-30.

44   J. Barrow, *Travels into the interior of South Africa*, 2 vols. (London: Cadell and Davies, 1806), vol.2, 13.

45   G. Forster, *A voyage around the world* (London: White, 1777), 58-59, 78-79.

46   J.M. Coetzee, *White writing: on the culture of letters in South Africa* (London and New Haven: Yale University Press, 1988), chapter 1.

47   R. Viljoen, 'Disease and society: VOC Cape Town, its people and

the smallpox epidemics of 1713, 1755 and 1767', *Kleio* XXVII
(1995), 22-45, 42; J.W.D. Moodie, *Ten years in South Africa* 2 vols.
(London: Richard Bentley, 1835), i, 41.

48   G. Forster, *A voyage around the world*, 58-59, 78-79. See also J.A
Backhouse, *Narrative of a visit to the Mauritius and South Africa*
(London, 1844), 84.

49   J.W.D. Moodie, *Ten years in South Africa*, i, 39.

50   S. Henderson, *An inquiry into the causes which produce disease among
the troops at the Cape of Good Hope* (?, 1795) [copy in South African
Library, Cape Town AZP 1993-1], 457; J.W.D. Moodie, *Ten years in
South Africa*, i, 40.

51   Anon., *Gleanings in Africa: exhibiting a faithful and correct view of the
manners and customs of the inhabitants of the Cape of Good Hope*
(London: Cundee, 1806), 46. See also N. Polson, *A subaltern's sick
leave* (Calcutta: ?, 1837), 80.

52   See for example M. Marshall, 'The growth and development of Cape
Town' (unpublished UCT M.A. thesis, 1940); W.W. Bird, *The state
of the Cape of Good Hope in 1822* (London: John Murray, 1823),
140.

53   Sir G.M. Keith, *A voyage to South America and the Cape of Good
Hope* (London: Vogel, 1819), 58.

54   J.M. Coetzee, *White writing*, chapter 2.

55   On Paarl as a resort see Letters to the Editor, *South African
Commercial Advertiser*, 23 Dec. 1826.

56   S.N. Eaton, *Journal by Sarah Norman Eaton ... of a voyage to the
Cape ...* (Mimeograph, Pretoria, 1953), 66, 68.

57   W.J. Black, 'On the sanitary state of Cape Town', *The Sanitary
Record*, 17 Aug. 1877.

58   A.M.L.R., 'An American Girl at the Cape in 1834', *Quarterly
Bulletin of the South African Library*, XXIII (3) (March 1969), 84.

59   Anon., *Gleanings in Africa*, 222.

60   J. Murray (ed.), *Mrs Dale's Diary 1857-1872* (Cape Town: Balkema,
1966), 4.

61   On this see B. Booyens, *Bronwaters van genesing: die tradisionele
warmbron-waterkuur in ons volksgeneeskunde* (Cape Town: Tafelberg
Press, 1981).

62   W.J. Burchell, *Travels in the interior of Southern Africa* (London:
Longman, 1822), 98.

63   A. Sparrman, *A voyage to the Cape of Good Hope, towards the
Antarctic Polar circle, and around the world: but chiefly into the
country of the Hottentots and Caffers from the year 1772 to 1776*,
trans. from the Swedish (London: Robinson, 1786), 137.

64 See for example, refutations of these claims in 'Critical Notices', *Cape of Good Hope Literary Gazette*, 1(5) (Oct. 1830), 63-65 and in 'Introductory Sketch', *The Cape of Good Hope Almanac and Annual Register for 1847* (Cape Town: Van der Sandt, 1847).

65 C.J. Glacken, *Traces on the Rhodian Shore*, 439, 472.

66 L.P. Simpson, *The dispossessed garden: pastoral and history in Southern Literature* (Athens (Georgia): University of Georgia Press, 1975), 15-16.

67 M. Fairbairn, *The ideal society and its enemies* (Auckland: Auckland University Press, 1989), and C. Lansbury, *Arcady in Australia: the evocation of Australia in nineteenth-century English literature* (Melbourne: Melbourne University Press, 1970).

68 See M. Fairbairn, *The ideal society and its enemies*, 26, for a discussion of this idea.

69 P. Hembry, *The English Spa, 1560-1815: a social history* (London: Athlone, 1990), 309 and K. Meethan, 'Place, image and power: Brighton as a resort'.

70 J.W.D. Moodie, *Ten years in South Africa*, i, 31-32.

71 E. Blount, *Notes on the Cape of Good Hope*, 97.

72 E. Blount, *Notes on the Cape of Good Hope*, 98.

73 P.W. Laidler, and M. Gelfand, *South Africa: its medical history 1652-1898: a medical and social study* (Cape Town: Struik, 1971), 262.

74 A.W. Cole, *The Cape and the Kaffirs* (London: Bentley, 1852), 65.

75 Nealds to Editor, 15 Sept. 1847, *Cape Town Medical Gazette*, 1(4) (Oct. 1847), 82.

76 E. Burrows, *A History of Medicine in South Africa up to the End of the Nineteenth Century* (Cape Town: Balkema, 1958), 139.

77 J. Noble (ed.), *The Cape and its people, and other essays* (Cape Town: Juta, 1869), 38, 40.

78 A.W.P. Pinkerton, 'Introductory lecture on climate', 22, 29.

79 For example, see B.W. James, *American resorts, with notes upon their climate* (London: F.A. Davis, 1889), 7.; J. Murray, *Young Mrs Murray goes to Bloemfontein* (Cape Town: Balkema, 1954), 8, and 'Our Thermal Springs', *Cape Illustrated Magazine*, IV(6) (Feb. 1894), 185-88.

80 J. Murray, *Young Mrs Murray goes to Bloemfontein*, 41.

81 B. Bradshaw, *Bathing Places and Climatic Health Resorts* (London: Kegan Paul, 1903).

82 C.T. Williams, 'Aero-therapeutics in lung disease', *Journal of British and Foreign Health Resorts*, IV(3) (July 1893), 95.

83 Prof. Noble, *The Cape and its people*, 25.

84 See for example, the way in which J.A. Ross, 'Consumption and its

treatment by Climate: with reference especially to the health resorts of the South African colonies' (London: Henry Renshaw, 1876), compares South Africa with Australia and no other colony.

85 Atherstone to Herman, 17 March 1885, Dr W.G. Atherstone Collection, UCT Manuscripts, BCS 139.

86 Herman to Atherstone, 3 May 1885, Dr C.L. Herman Collection, UCT Manuscripts, BCS 138.

87 Lt.-Col. Sir Charles Mitchell, commenting on a paper by E.S. Thompson, 'South Africa as a health resort', read before the Royal Colonial Institute, 13 Dec 1888 in *Proceedings of the Royal Colonial Institute* (London: 1888).

88 Herman to Atherstone, 25 Nov. 1885, Dr C.L. Herman Collection, UCT Manuscripts, BCS 138.

10

Sleepers Wake:
André Gide and Disease in *Travels in the Congo*

Russell West

The future Nobel Prize winner André Gide left Paris in July 1925, accompanied by his young friend and apprentice film-maker Marc Allégret, on a journey which would take him into the heart of the African continent, lasting until May of the following year. Gide had been an inveterate traveller all his life and it was thus no surprise to see the fifty-five year-old setting off on what would become a physical and moral test of endurance. The ageing writer left in search of an exotic Africa which had formed part of his personal mythology since of his youth. More than thirty years previously, in Tunisia, the young Puritan had fallen ill with tuberculosis, had recovered, and at the same time shaken off the shackles of a Protestant upbringing and discovered his homosexuality. Early experiences as a 'delicate child' and the subsequent experiences in North Africa moulded Gide's personal philosophy, to the extent that he could claim in his autobiography that he 'wouldn't mention the question of health had it not been so important in [his] life'.[1] Such questions of health and disease dominated almost all of his writing from the early novels including the modernist *Marshlands*, via the famous *Immoralist* and *The Counterfeiters*, through to his last novel *Theseus*. It is this constant preoccupation with disease in Gide's literary production which justifies a reading of his 1925-26 travel narrative foregrounding the language of health and sickness. Indeed, it would have been difficult to avoid mention of matters of health and disease when reporting on a journey in colonial Africa in the mid-1920s, as European presence in Africa was from the very beginning, as Alfred Cosby has demonstrated, accompanied by the ravaging effects of new and destructive diseases.[2] Gide's account of the African journey, *Travels in the Congo*, is the story of a journey through a panorama of diseases, which in turn became the catalyst of the traveller's changing attitude to Africa.

299

Gide's highly personalised narrative needs to be placed in the specific context of French imperial presence in Africa and the colonial rhetoric of illness. From the 1860s onward, through to 1900, increasing military expansion secured French control of large expanses of Equatorial and West Africa. After this date, large trading companies were able to expand their activities in the region, developing from trade and export firms of modest proportions to immense undertakings making substantial profits on the basis of forced labour from the middle of the first decade of the century onwards. The companies increasingly relied upon the labour of the African people, who were extensively exploited for the production of crops such as rubber and coffee; the French administration was in general powerless to control the activities of the trading companies, and if anything, tended to facilitate their operation, and the concomitant destruction of the native primary economy, by introducing taxes on imported commodities to the exclusion of locally produced goods. Through the first two decades of the century, despite scandals and attempts at reform, colonialism literally devastated the cultural, social and geographic fabric of indigenous life. Natives fled from the threat of forced labour, entire regions were laid waste in reprisal for inadequate productivity, and the conditions of exploitation caused famine and disease to spread. Census figures for French Equatorial Africa recorded a drop in population from 15 million at the turn of the century to a little under 3 million in 1921, shortly before Gide's journey through Africa.[3] Malnutrition resulting from the conditions of forced labour, the destruction of indigenous agriculture, infant mortality, newly introduced diseases and military reprisals were some of the causes of the drastic reduction of the population. Clearly the colonial economy took a heavy toll on the lives of the indigenous inhabitants.

Colonisation, however, was not without its costs for the colonisers themselves. The European soldiers and administrators who undertook the task of conquering and occupying large parts of the African and Asian world suffered heavy losses upon contact with a climate hitherto unknown to them and diseases against which they had no resistance. An issue of *The Lancet* pointed out, for instance, that service on the West Coast of Africa was so dangerous to British military officers' health that a year's service there counted for two elsewhere, with equivalent promotion.[4] The ravages of such diseases among colonial personnel, the very real threat they posed for the continued viability of the European expansionist project, and the development of tropical medicine that grew out of the great concern on the part of the colonial authorities, have been extensively documented by Philip Curtin.[5] Despite the emphasis laid upon indigenous health by some colonial regimes, such as the Belgians, the attention of colonial medical authorities, both in policy and in cultural representations of the colonial enterprise, was almost exclusively directed towards the well-being of Western military and civilian personnel in the tropics. It was only in 1905 that a government decree established a General Medical Service including what was known as 'Native Medical Care' in French West Africa – initially equipping this huge colony with twenty-one doctors, a figure that rose to nearly a hundred fifteen years later.[6] The scarcity of resources made available for native health facilities becomes clear when one realises that this handful of doctors covered an area which is today made up of fifteen African nations.

This imbalance in the distribution of medical resources between Western and indigenous populations is reflected in the cultural representations of disease in Africa. As Pierre Halen has remarked, colonial literature was overwhelmingly preoccupied with the health of colonial settlers rather than that of the native population, despite the avowed colonial commitment to native health on the part of an administration such as that of the Belgian colonies.[7] The realities of indigenous disease were elided by Western stereotyping and essentialising. Rather than accurately representing the nature and causes of illnesses among colonisers and colonised, colonial literature, whether French or English, tended to operate with a set of binary oppositions governed by images of a vulnerable (European) Self and a threatening (African) Other capable of dissolving the identity of the Self. 'It is the fear of collapse, the sense of dissolution, which contaminates the Western image of all diseases', claims Sander Gilman: 'How we see the diseased, the mad, the polluting is a reflex of our own sense of control and the limits inherent in that sense of control'.[8] A brief glimpse of several writers of the early colonial period demonstrates to what extent Gilman's remarks aptly describe stereotyping in the representation of Africa and its diseases.

The French colonial novelist Pierre Loti referred to the 'accursed climate' of Africa, where 'great stinking swamps, stagnant waters, [were] saturated with miasmas of fever'.[9] Joseph Conrad depicted 'rivers, streams of death in life, whose banks were rotting into mud, whose waters, thickened into slime, invaded the contorted mangroves, that seemed to writhe at us in the extremity of an impotent despair'.[10] Such lurid personifications of a vague and generalised menace from the environment were replicated in medical

301

textbooks: the German doctor Hirsch and his British informant Annesley were in agreement regarding the nefarious character of particular types of soil in the African countries, which emit 'terrestrial emanations'; such notions were echoed by a Professor Mahé at the Brest Naval Medical School who told his students that in Africa 'the earth and waters exhale a poisonous breath'.[11] Sir James Ranald Martin analysed in great detail the nature of air, soil and water as sources of disease in his textbook of tropical medicine in 1861.[12] Such opinions should have been overhauled by advances in the rapidly changing field of medical sciences at the end of the nineteenth century. However, the tendency to identify Africa and Africans themselves with the causes of disease, persisted well into the twentieth century. Women in particular were singled out as symbols of contamination. Loti's hero contracts his first illness, the classical colonial 'fever', when he cedes to the sexual temptations of a half-caste woman. Loti draws a parellel between the 'black blood' boiling in the natives' veins and the poisonous sap rising in the vegetation, excluding venom-like perfumes in the tropical spring, and Jean's later black mistress, a 'fruit' hastily ripened in the tropical climate, 'bloated with toxic juices, filled with unhealthy, feverish and strange desires' to which the defenceless young man succumbs.[13] The demise of Conrad's Kurtz comes about as a result of his ceding to the 'heavy mute spell of the wilderness', which had 'taken him, loved him, embraced him, got into his veins, consumed his flesh'; this wilderness is embodied in a savage African woman.[14] These literary images of contamination by indigenous women were not taken for mere fictions: the *Lancet* could express great concern over the proliferation of brothels in India, for example; prostitution represented a dangerous loss of control over gender and race boundaries, symbolised by a rhetoric of contamination.[15]

These colonial images of disease as pollution constituted a significant component of the literary tradition inherited by Gide as a *fin-de-siècle* novelist. In an early novella, *Urien's Voyage* (1893), Gide had described the threat posed to Urien and his chivalric travelling companions by the seductions of the exotic but diseased women of Queen Haïtalnefus' realm. This depiction of gender and geographical otherness as potential dangers for the Western traveller immediately preceded Gide's departure for Tunisia, where he fell ill with tuberculosis, triggering a reappraisal of himself and his attitudes, and the consequent acceptance of his homosexuality. Gide's view of exoticism thus altered radically, becoming one at odds with the reigning colonialist view of Africa as a domain of contagion. This crucial early experience of illness and recovery in Africa endowed him with a mythical image of a *healthy* Africa which would determine his later attitude towards disease there.

It is significant that Gide's *Travels in the Congo* opens with a dedication to Joseph Conrad. This is a reflection of Gide's indebtedness to Conrad as a colonial author – but also reveals the extent to which Gide's attitude to disease in Africa was soon to question the hegemonic perception of Africa as a source of contagion.[16] It is by no means unimportant that Conrad's *Heart of Darkness* moves away from the exclusive preoccupation with the health of the colonisers, to include that of the natives: 'They were dying very slowly – it was very clear ... Brought from all the recesses of the coast ... lost in uncongenial surroundings, fed on unfamiliar food, they sickened, became 'inefficient, and were allowed to crawl away and rest.' When Conrad does utilise the reigning topoi of contagion, his language turns against its culture of origin. Marlow ruminates upon 'disease, exile, and death, – death skulking in the air, in the water, in the bush. They must have been dying like flies here.' Ironically, he is referring not to Africa here, but to a Britain colonised by the Romans, abruptly reading the centre of the civilised world through the same filter of conceptions of periphery and darkness as were habitually applied to Africa. Most significantly, Conrad portrays mercantile European expansion as a contagious plague, whose epicentre is London, proximity to which causes the evening sun to lose its brilliance, 'as if stricken to death by the touch of that gloom brooding over a crowd of men'.[17] Colonialism, he suggests, causes death by its very operation, a perception that Gide would gradually come to share as he travelled through French Equatorial Africa.

Conrad's narrative probably contributed to some extent to Gide's limited awareness, even before he left for Africa in 1925, to the darker side of colonialism. But what he was to find in Africa would make much more of an immediate impact upon him than the vague reports of abuses heard in far-away Paris. Travelling through the French colonies in Africa, partly as a private tourist and partly as a representative of the French government, Gide was confronted with a colonial administration whose exploitative character became more and more evident. Upon his return to Paris in 1926, he set about issuing a series of attacks, mainly upon the conduct of the Western trade companies in the French colonies, but whose force would lend fuel to the growing groundswell of anticolonial agitation.

A year later, he published *Travels in the Congo*. This travel narrative is little more than the annotated and edited version of his daily diary entries; Gide stressed that he was not working as a novelist, in his time in Africa, but simply as an eye-witness reporter of facts observed on the ground. Nonetheless, Gide's narrative *is* a narrative; it is structured by an interplay of themes and images, and by a teleogical drive which increasingly demystifies the private mythology of health which Gide had initially imposed upon Africa. Such a mythology and the tropes which replace it help the traveller to make sense of his journey, to construct a coherent set of meanings out of a wealth of confusing impressions. Moreover, both the mythology of health and the subsequent reversal of such images of 'natural Africa' to some extent participated in, but often contested, the customary topoi of exoticism, particularly those of disease. In what follows, I wish to demonstrate to what extent illness is a preoccupation of Gide the tourist in *Travels in the Congo*. Two 'diseases' in particular underpin Gide's narrative: on the one hand, sleeping sickness, epidemics of which decimated the native population; and on the other hand, sleeplessness, Gide's own insomnia, which regularly punctuates the traveller's narrative of native illness. These two 'diseases' exist in a dialectical relationship, contributing to the development of Gide's nascent critique of Western expansion in Africa.

Sleeping sickness and other diseases of colonialism

In 1925, Gide discovered a French Equatorial Africa which resurrected his earlier ecstatic experiences in North Africa. The older Gide saw West Africa as a continuation of those earlier experiences, a place where perfect bodily harmony and equilibrium was attainable. 'Beauty of the trees', he wrote, 'of bare-chested, laughing children with a languid gaze. The sky is low. Extraordinary peace and softness of the air. Everything here seems to promise happiness, sensuality, forgetfulness' (685). Gide observed that 'people are smiling and happy, yes, even the feeble and the sick' (816). But these perceptions of Africa as a paradise would not endure for long, and soon gave way to a more ambiguous version of the continent he was traversing, comparable to a description of an epileptic child he met in Fort-Archambault. During a fit, the child had fallen into a fire, so that 'one side of his face is hideously burned; the other side smiles, quite angelic' (816). Gide's Africa had two faces, like the burnt child; one side was that of a preconceived mythical health and harmony, the other was that of disease and death. Little by little, the destruction of African bodies, rather than their mythological beauty, would come to occupy the foreground of Gide's narrative.

But it took him some time to discover this second face of Africa in all its reality. It is perhaps Gide's observations regarding sleeping sickness (African trypanosomiasis), a disease of mental deterioration caused by a tsetse-fly-borne parasite, and resulting in a somnolent condition and eventual death, which best characterise the gradual change of his attitude to disease in Africa. At the very beginning of the tour, Gide noted that he and his companions were 'crossing regions being decimated by sleeping sickness' (707). Further on he noted: 'Last night, in the villages, a large number of sick natives, terribly thin – sleeping sickness. And are those tsetse flies, these horse-flies that have covered our sedan-chairs for the last two days and wait for every chance to bite?' (805). In the last stages of the journey, sleeping sickness was still a danger: 'We will have to send the horses back to N'Gaoundéré once we get beyond Tibati because of the tsetse flies, and consequently, because of sleeping sickness' (989). Of course, other diseases are mentioned in Gide's narrative: recurrent fever, tuberculosis (930), one unidentified epidemic (939), not to mention the thousand small complaints, sunburn, adenitis, pneumonia, vomiting and so on, which were scribbled down by Gide in his daily notebook. But sleeping sickness constitutes a thread running through the account, making disease into one of the narrative's ordering principles. This was perhaps, in part, because it was one of the few diseases which colonial administrations made real efforts to combat (albeit often with barbaric methods[18]), as it directly threatened the availability of cheap African labour. It attained considerable media prominence among the European public, as a new and romantic field of scientific endeavour with its own glorious rhetoric.[19] Despite the fact that the very availability of this disease as part of the Western perception of Africa was heavily overlaid with ideological meanings, it is in conjunction with images of sleeping sickness that Gide's narrative records his rapidly changing view of Africa and the shocking facts which obliged him to modify an originary mythology.

Gide appears initially as the impartial Western observer, recording the attempts of the colonial administration to deal with the ravages of sleeping sickness. He noted the departure for the Grimari region of a team of doctors to test the effectiveness against the disease of a new preventative medicine called 309 Fourneau (717). Elsewhere he met a sergeant who claimed to give his patients six hundred injections a day against sleeping sickness, and a hospital team who thought they could cure sleeping sickness even in the third [sic] phase (850, 872). Here Gide's discourse follows the rhetoric of

305

medical care as an integral part of the *mission civiliatrice* which would be invoked, in French colonialist circles, well into the '30s and even later.[20] Gide appears not to contest this enlightened Western medical discourse, whose hallmarks are its triumphalism and its claims to neutrality and universal validity, but also its elision of the social and political context of disease. It is, however, the socio-political aspect of illness that the reader increasingly detects coming to the fore in Gide's travel narrative.

Initially Gide draws attention to the limits of colonial medical campaigns, pinpointing the lack of resources available in contrast to the extent of the problems to be dealt with. 'We need more doctors, and we need to pay them better. And we lack medication. Everywhere one can see a lamentable penury which allows the most easily conquerable diseases to spread triumphantly' (710). Too little, too late, declares, but apparently without scrutinising the role that European expansion might play in the causes of disease. Little by little, however, the text reveals, for instance, that the natives do not have access to adequate food supplies, which are usually sold to the whites, leaving only the barest necessities to the indigenous population (796). It is only later on that Gide, having identified these economic inequalities, then links such injustices to the spread of diseases which Western medical resources are inadequate to control. Gide recognises, at an even later stage, that: 'Three quarters of the diseases from which the natives suffer (apart from epidemics) are diseases linked to malnutrition' (810, n. 1). He also begins to identify the links between the absence of accommodation provided for native labourers and the proportion of respiratory diseases among them (811-12, n. 1). But Gide's commentaries in *Travels in the Congo* are largely restricted to demands for improvement of conditions of native health, rather than a recognition of the essential link between colonialism itself and the existence of disease. The text espouses a reform of a badly managed colonial enterprise, rather than radical change to the colonial system. Such reforms, Gide appears to believe, would cause disease to disappear from the face of Africa.

Evidently such a point of view ignores what is increasingly accepted today, the fact that colonialism itself was responsible for the emergence of hitherto non-existent or little known diseases. Gide's inability to recognise the essentially destructive nature of colonialism and the direct physical consequences of Western expansion for the bodies of Africans was radically modified, however, when he was confronted with the evidence of torture: the most extreme point on a continuum whose less acute graduations were malnutrition and disease. Gide describes an ex-prisoner from the Boda gaol showing the scars left by whippings and beatings (74). In the Lake Chad region, Gide receives a native who 'bends down to show a large and evident scar from recent injuries above the neck; he pulls aside his bou-bou to show another scar between the shoulders'; and the same process of exhibition of scars is repeated a day later with other victims (841, 842). At this point, Gide's text displays the naked violence of a colonial regime, which it has until now slid over with well-meaning goodwill or simple non-recognition of the connections between bodily suffering and the European invasion of Africa.

Gide's gradual perception of the intimate links between colonisation and the spread of disease also held good for sleeping sickness, the disease which we have already identified as the most prominent in his narrative. The disruption of indigenous society, demographic mobility, widespread malnutrition and inhuman work conditions all contributed to produce the spread of this disease in the colonies. Gide came close to reaching such a conclusion in his comments on the treatment of the native workers by the concessionaire companies:

> The doctor speaks to us at some length about the 'compagnie forestière', which finds ways and means, he says, to get around health regulations, avoiding medical check-ups and ignoring medical certificates for the natives which it recruits from village to village to constitute the troops of Bakongos in its employment – which leads to the uncontrollable spread of sleeping-sickness. (757)

Gide perceives here that colonialism aids the spread of such epidemic diseases. What is recognised as the aggravation of a problem already in existence can be seen, however, as typical of the *emergence* of such diseases. John Ford has demonstrated that before the arrival of the white colonisers, stable populations and agricultural methods insured that sleeping sickness only ever occurred endemically, if at all. Western expansion destroyed the natural social and demographic barriers which minimised the impact of such diseases. What the Europeans assumed to be the cause of such diseases, the mobility of the native peoples, was in reality a direct result of the disruptive presence of the invaders. Ford quotes natives in Uganda saying that: 'Tsetses, Glossina morsitants, had been advancing in Ankole from the south since 1907, and the local people asserted that until the Europeans arrived in that part of the continent, just west of Lake Victoria, there had been no tsetstes in their country'.[21] Gide too increasingly noticed this association of geographic mobility, an index of dislocated social structures, and the presence of disease: 'We learn that the gloomy village is losing its population little by little. Recurrent fever and emigration' (824). Occasionally Gide gives glimpses of this on-going process of social destruction at work. He cites the example of the missionary priest at Lingara who leaves the mission station to receive medical care at Brazzaville, taking with him particularly ill children from the mission school. Gide comments that the area is ravaged by sleeping sickness: ironically, the priest perpetuates the massive geographical disruption caused by colonisation, which triggered the epidemics of sleeping sickness, in the very attempt to fight disease (707).

Travels in the Congo gives, at most, partial glimpses of the colonial system in its essentially pathological functioning. For Gide himself was part of that system, caught up in the very process he increasingly singled out for criticism, in no way a distanced observer. But this very same involvement with a pathological system informing his own writing would in turn produce the most trenchant critique of that system manifest in Gide's travel narrative. Illness and physical abuse of the natives would become the site of a conversion in Gide's account of his journey, from complicity to resistance to colonial power structures.

Gide and Marc Allégret were increasingly called upon as part-time doctors as they followed their chosen route into the heart of Africa and back towards the coast. Their teams of porters and guides were constantly falling ill, and Gide's text reads at times like a doctor's case-book, filled with lists and attempted cures: 'Patient's heart beating as if fit to burst. 39°. Gave quinine and stovarsol' (952). Sometimes the journal entries include notes on up to five or six ailing porters, not to mention the tourists' own ills. As the group moved forward with their journey, the mentions of illness and of therapeutic measures become more frequent. During some phases of the journey it was evidently Gide's major preoccupation, giving him first-hand experience of the health problems of natives in colonial Africa.

Ironically, he often played the role of coloniser in these scenarios, despite his frequently critical stance towards the colonial empire and his benevolent role of doctor for his little group of natives. For Gide came to Africa as a 'Chargé de mission', as an official representative of the French government. Indeed, his links with government officials, among others Marcel de Coppet, who was a colonial administrator, were instrumental in making such a journey possible. Yet these links, while indispensable for Gide's African sojourn, forced him to remain silent on certain issues. For fear of prejudicing the position of friends such as Marcel de Coppet, Gide refrained from criticising the colonial administration itself, reserving his attacks for the concessionaire companies. Gide thus became an accomplice of the colonial regime whose abuses he could not help but see, but was unable to report. His position of connivance with the government is elided in the text of *Travels in the Congo*, but curiously laid bare by the appellation of the native carriers. Gide reports that: 'Since Fort-Lamy the boy, then the whole group of carriers, have promoted me. "Commandant" didn't satisfy them. Later, "Governor" wasn't enough either. Nothing stops them. Soon, out of pure enthusiasm they'll be calling me "Government"' (892, n. 1). The main benefit conveyed by his honorary status as a government representative was that it allowed Gide to obtain carriers from local French government administrators, considerably facilitating the journey through the African interior. Gide tried as much as possible to avoid having recourse to the sedan-chairs with which the carriers were equipped – as often as not it was the sick porters themselves who were carried by their compatriots. Nonetheless, these carriers *were* requisitioned, and though Gide (unlike the majority of colonial personnel) paid them for their labours, they were co-opted as part of the standard colonial policy of forced labour imposed upon the native population. Disturbingly, he condoned the system of 'porterage', by which natives were forced to carry heavy load for colonial officers – himself included. Porterage, Gide claimed, was a necessary evil, essential in order to establish other means of transport which would then supersede it: 'It's not the porterage system one should condemn', he wrote, 'but the excessively long distance of each leg of the journey, and the excessive distance between administrative posts, a problem easily remedied' (859, note). Gide's reluctance to condemn a system of forced labour, from which he benefited as a representative of the French colonial government, makes him appear a less that wholehearted critic of colonialism, and a sinister doctor for his carriers – for he directly supported and perpetuated the system causing the ills from which they suffered and which he in turn looked after.

Gide's ambiguous position as a critic of colonialism simultaneously participating in the regime he condemned is particularly evident in some of the episodes of illness he reported. In such episodes, his own text lays bare the contradictory position he occupied in colonial Africa. During the middle phase of Gide's journey, along the Logone river close to Lake Chad, the rowers were frequently ill. On one occasion, Gide treated two Sara native rowers with cupping glasses; the next day another paddler fell ill; several days later, four others were sick (907, 910, 913). 'Every day', he reported in his diary, 'new invalids' (915). Among the invalids was the 'capita', the head-rower and pilot, who fell ill and died after three days of suffering (910, 915). It is the death of this rower which makes particularly clear the delicacy of Gide's position. The capita had caught pneumonia; Gide prescribed medication, not without recording his anxiety whether the sedative wouldn't be too strong a medicine for the weakened patient – who was indeed found dead the next morning: 'I rather suspect that the small dose of sédebrol – and it was a very small dose indeed – that we gave the patient, might put him, in his weakened state, to sleep forever. But at least he will have had a more peaceful death' (917). At the same time, Gide, incapable of sleep, exhausted by the events of the day and forced to bed down in the filthy, stinking river-boat, had himself taken a dose of sleeping draught: 'I resign myself to the way things are; at least I can take some sonéryl which will procure me salutary oblivion' (917). There is a strange phonetic and functional similarity between the two sedatives taken by Gide and his head-rower, sédobrol and sonéry. But their simultaneous effects are also linked by a kind of perverse causality. Gide is exhausted by the difficult conditions surrounding him, and takes a sedative to block out the noise, the filth, the chaos; part of this chaos is the sick capita, disposed of by Gide's amateur medical skills. Gide's approximate attempt at bush medicine becomes, in this episode, as much a symbol of his part in a colonial enterprise which annihilates the black Africa subject, as of his concern for the indigenous population with whom he comes in contact.

Gide's insomnia

But Gide's response to the natives' suffering was not always to seek oblivion in putting them or himself to sleep. When the rowers camped out in the open air, rapidly developing pneumonia and other related illnesses in the freezing nights that followed the heat of the day, Gide made no secret of his acute awareness of his moral dilemma. 'I'm very pleased with myself to have bought an extra woollen blanket for each of our boys', he commented. 'But these poor people close by, are naked, their backs chilled by the wind, their chests roasted by the fire, unable to let themselves fall asleep for fear of waking up half cooked (one of them showed us the skin on his chest singed and covered with blisters) after labouring the whole day – this is completely monstrous' (890). Gide's consciousness of this terrible dilemma keep him too from sleep: 'The rowers... hardly stopped coughing all night. The sense of their discomfort, for which I am indirectly responsible, keeps me awake' (890). Here Gide recognises his ambiguous position to an extent nowhere else evident in his narrative. His comments reveal the manner in which his employment of the native rowers, essential to the journey and the subsequent public criticism which it will allow, encourages the very respiratory illness which he elsewhere attacks as an exemplary of the negligence of the concessionaire companies (811-12, n. 1).

Insomnia is the motif that constantly reoccurs in the text to mark Gide's awareness, however involuntary, of the suffering for which he is in some way responsible. 'The Sara natives coughed, spat, hawked, cleared their throats well into the night. Even with ear plugs in, I heard the wheezing and gurgling of their breathing' (904). The worried traveller, unable to sleep, is vigilant, in the literal sense of the word: 'In the middle of the night, I get dressed to see why those whose coughing prevents me sleeping have preferred to sleep on the river bank' (913). Insomnia summons Gide to a vigil over his natives, taking responsibility, to some small extent, for the illnesses of which he cannot help but be in part the cause.

The appearance of insomnia in the text is highly significant, for sleeplessness is one of the most constant and present features in Gide's fiction, diaries and letters. Éric Marty rightly calls it a 'fundamental theme in Gide', present from the beginning to the end of his literary enterprise, as the author himself noted in the meditations written shortly before his death, *So be it.*[22] Gide's African journey may have been a journey to a land of mythological health, but the author's own private malady remains no less present in the pages of *Travels in the Congo*. Frequent mentions confirm this:

> Very mediocre night's sleep. Incessant bleating of goats around our hut. Got up at five-thirty. (766)

> Too tired, could hardly sleep. (780)

> A touch of fever towards evening. The nights have been pretty bad. (820)

> [The noise of the river-boat] completely prevented me from sleeping. (845)

> Strange queasiness at the beginning of the night. It wasn't too hot, almost fresh, but it was impossible to breathe. A sort of extreme discomfort which sleep couldn't overcome without help. I tried, for the first time, sonéryl ('talc and starch', Marc reads in the brochure)

whose effect I was not long in experiencing. (849)

Night almost without sleep. (874)

This accumulation of quotations – and it is far from complete – shows just how constant an anxiety this private and relatively trivial illness is in Gide's travel narrative. Sleeplessness becomes a thread running through the whole narrative in the same way that sleeping sickness also represents a thematic constant in *Travels in the Congo*. These are the two faces, individual and collective, occidental and indigenous, of disease in Gide's text. In my concluding remarks I will make a more audacious claim: namely, that insomnia responds to the implicit question of sleeping sickness as representative disease of colonial oppression.

Gide's mentions of insomnia become more and more frequent as the journey progresses into its second half. This was partly due to the increasing fatigue of the elderly traveller, but also because each new discovery made the tourists a little more aware of the atrocities committed in the name of Western expansion. The sight of colonial oppression became less and less tolerable, and Gide was more and more preoccupied, during his sleepless nights, by cruelties which he could no longer pass over in silence. Literary critics have drawn attention to the links between abnormal psychological states and intensified perception;[23] Gide had, in his *Immoralist*, illustrated this in the person of the tuberculosis-patient Michel, whose somatic consciousness is so acute that it precludes the oblivion of sleep. In *Travels in the Congo* a similar state of sleeplessness accompanied by heightened perception is transmuted into ethical and political awareness. Sleeplessness becomes the very site, in the Gidean travel narrative, where real solidarity comes into being, where moral *responsibility*, understood in the sense of responding *to* and *for* an Other, is born.

In a crucial episode, at Bangui, Gide is woken in the night by a native desperate to obtain the tourists' intervention in an intolerable situation of colonial abuse:

> Having retired early, we were both fast asleep under the mosquito nets, in the passengers' huts. About two in the morning, the sound of steps and voices woke us. Someone wanted to enter the hut. We shouted in Sango: 'Zo niè?', 'Who is there?' It was a prominent native chief – distraught to see his hopes of speaking with us dashed, he had resolved to come to find us at this ungodly hour. (736-37)

The important chieftain, Sanba N'Goto, had come to report the brutal practices of a certain M. Pacha: in particular the Bambio 'Ball' a torture festival perpetrated by the colonial administrator, where a group of natives were punished for inadequate productivity as slave labourers by carrying heavy weights in the midday sun until they collapsed, dying from exhaustion and beatings. Gide immediately responded to Samba N'Goto by promising to take responsibility for the man's potentially fatal confession, assuring him there would be no retributions, and asking him to come back in the morning to give a more detailed account. The interruption of sleep becomes, in Gide's narrative, the topos par excellence of an ethical response to the evidence of oppression. Éric Marty claims that insomnia in Gide's writing is the site of a loss of self, confirming Lévinas's contention that ethical responsibility displaces the claims of egoism, indeed, displaces the primacy of selfhood to place it under the mastery of a suffering Other.[24] This is the type of ethical confrontation which emerges when Samba N'Goto disturbs Gide's sleep to make him aware of the atrocities committed against Africans. From now on, insomnia remains the site of moral concern for the natives in Gide's text:

> Impossible to sleep. The Bambio 'Ball' haunts my nights. One can no longer be content to say, as one often hears it said, that the natives were unhappier before the French occupation. We have taken on responsibilities towards the natives that we do not have the right to shirk. From now on, an immense lamentation fills me: I know things that I cannot accept. What demon drove me to Africa? What was I looking for in this land? Now I know: I must speak out. (745)

This statement is justly perhaps the most famous passage from *Travels in the Congo*, and marks the apex of Gide's moral outrage, which would result in a campaign against the abuses of the concessionaire companies upon returning to Paris. Gide's apparently private and insignificant sleeplessness is a sort of moral watchfulness which replies to the shocking evidence of colonial oppression to be seen in Pacha's brutal repression and, in a chronic form, in the widespread sleeping sickness which Gide met all through his journey in French colonial Africa.

The vigilance of insomnia remains the key term in the last lines of *Travels in the Congo*. Gide, back on board the ship that would carry him home to France, commented on the other passengers returning from the colonies. He described them as 'not reflecting, not reading, not praying, and sleeping like a log. Nothing disturbs them' (1008). Such people, Gide implies, 'sleeping the sleep of a brute', to translate literally his turn of phrase, are not worthy of the name of human beings – precisely because they are unconcerned by the plight of others, because they can sleep, despite all that is happening in colonial Africa. Sleep symbolises the absence of an ethical relationship with others; insomnia, it seems, is the malady that marks out moral sensibility from egoism.

Sleeping sickness is representative, in Gide's narrative, of disease which the traveller gradually came to recognise, albeit only incompletely, as the result of European expansion. As Gide gradually realised that disease was not a neutral fact, but in some way associated with the worst excesses of French colonialism, he also began to notice his own participation in a colonial regime responsible for the deterioration of the health of the indigenous population. This uncomfortable realisation translated itself, in the text, as insomnia, which in turn became the place of an acceptance of responsibility in the face of the unacceptable atrocities of colonial regimes. Together, sleeping sickness and sleeplessness are the textual indices of a gradually developing critical understanding of European expansion in the non-European world. To this extent, Gide's double panorama of private and collective illnesses offers the first glimpse of a critique which would eventually culminate in the progressive collapse of the colonial empires thirty years after his journey.

Four years after his return from the Congo, Gide wrote in his diary, 'I believe that illnesses are keys which can open certain doors for us. I believe that there are some doors that illness alone can open. There is a state of health which allows us not to understand everything… health cuts us off from some truths, or shields us from those truths such that we are not disturbed by them.' The alert reader might be forgiven for detecting an oblique reference here to the author's own 'malady' of insomnia in Africa and the manner in which it opened his own eyes to the suffering of the native population. But a subsequent observation is even more revealing, in which he recalls a witty quip about: 'illnesses [as] the travels of the poor'.[25] This comment nicely describes the inner crossing of boundaries which experiences of illness provoked in Gide. But at the same time, he also inverts, in this slick proverb, the relationships between travel, illness and poverty which had structured his own recent experience. For this now renowned novelist and polemicist, travel had become a means of escaping from his own privileges as an upper class writer with private means, living in the capital city of one of the two major colonial empires of the day, to discover aspects of human existence in Africa that his aestheticist ethos had never allowed him to suspect. For Gide in Africa, travel was his means of discovering the illnesses of the empire's poor.

Notes

1 Gide, *If it die* (*Si le grain ne meurt*) in *Journal 1939-1949, Souvenirs* (Paris: Gallimard/Pléiade, 1954), 552-53. Also included in this volume is *Travels in the Congo* (*Voyage au Congo* and *Retour du Tchad*); references to this work will be indicated in the text. Unless stated otherwise, all translations from the French are my own.

2 Alfred W. Cosby, *Ecological Imperialism: The Biological Expansion of Europe 900-1900* (Cambridge: Cambridge University Press/Canto, 1993).

3 Jean Suret-Canale, *French Colonialism in Tropical Africa 1900-1945*, trans. Till Gottheiner (London: C. Hurst, 1971), 36.

4 *The Lancet*, 19 March 1870, 424.

5 Philip D. Curtin, *Death by Migration: Europe's Encounter with the Tropical World in the Nineteenth Century* (Cambridge: Cambridge University Press, 1989).

6 Suret-Canale, *French Colonialism*, 406.

7 Pierre Halen, 'Notes de lecture sur la maladie, la fièvre et la folie dans la littérature coloniale belge', in *Littérature et maladie en Afrique: Image et fonction de la maladie dans la production littéraire*, (ed.) Jaqueline Bardolph (Paris: L'Harmattan, 1994), 57.

8 Sander L. Gilman, *Disease and Representation: Images of Illness from Madness to AIDS* (Ithaca: Cornell University Press, 1988), 1, 3.

9 Pierre Loti, *Le Roman d'un spahi* (1881) (Paris: Gallimard/Folio, 1992), 53, 109.

10 Joseph Conrad, *Heart of Darkness* (1901) (London: Dent, 1946), 63.

11 August Hirsch, *Handbuch der historisch-geographischen Pathologie* (Stuttgart: Verlag Ferdinand Enke, 1886), Vol. 3, 238, 249; Suret-Canale, *French Colonialism*, 404.

12 Sir James Ranald Martin, *Influence of Tropical Climates in Producing the Endemic Diseases of Europeans* (London: John Churchill, 1861), 16ff.

13 Loti, *Le Roman d'un spahi*, 83, 110, 111.

14 Conrad, *Heart of Darkness*, 144, 115.

15 *The Lancet*, 19 February 1870, 274.

16 See my *Conrad and Gide: Translation, Transference and Intertextuality* (Amsterdam/Atlanta GA: Rodopi, 1996), esp. Ch. 5.

17 Conrad, *Heart of Darkness*, 66, 49, 46.

18 See Suret-Canale, *French Colonialism*, 408-11, on Dr Jamot's campaign against sleeping sickness in Africa in the 1920s.

19 See Maryinez Lyons, 'Sleeping Sickness, Colonial Medicine and Imperialism: some connections in the Belgian Congo', in *Disease,*

Medicine and Empire: Perspectives on Western Medicine and the Experience of European Expansion, Roy McLeod and Milton Lewis (eds), (London: Routledge, 1988), 242-56.

20 Raoul Girardet, *L'Idée coloniale en France 1871-1962* (Paris: Éditions de la table ronde, 1972), 183.

21 John Ford, *The Role of the Trypanosomiases in Africa Ecology: A Study of the Tsetse Fly Problem* (Oxford: Clarendon Press, 1979), 419-20, 7.

22 Éric Marty, *L'Écriture du jour: Le Journal d'André Gide* (Paris: Seuil, 1985), 161, 165-68; *Ainsi soit-il*, in *Journal 1939-1949, Souvenirs*, 1213.

23 Clemens Heselhaus, 'Die Metaphorik der Krankheit', in *Die nicht mehr schönen Künste: Grenzphänomene des Ästhetischen (Poetik und Hermeneutik III)*, H.-R. Jauß (ed.), (Munich: Wilhelm Fink Verlag, 1968), 423.

24 Marty, *L'Écriture du jour*, 167; Emmanuel Lévinas, *Autrement qu'être ou au-delà de l'essence* (Paris: Livre de poche, 1990), 15-16, 84.

25 Gide, *Journal 1889-1939* (Paris: Gallimard/Pléiade, 1948), 998.

INDEX

A

accidents, during travel *53–54*
   railway travel *229*
acclimatisation failure *50*
Addington, Anthony *164*
Addison, *Spectator* essays *143–144*
adventure *157, 188*
Africa
   carriers for travellers *308, 309, 310–311*
   climate *301*
   colonialism *see* colonialism
   diseases *299*
   Gide's travels *see* Gide, André
   Gide's two faces of *304–305*
   medical resources/care *301, 306*
   social destruction *308*
   see also Cape Colony; French Equatorial Africa
African trypanosomiasis *see* sleeping sickness
After-Care Association *39*
ageing, railway season-ticket holders *250*
agitation, travel causing *184–185*
agoraphobia *12*
AIDS, metaphors *273–274*
air
   benefits in mental disease *36–37*
   fresh, 'gospel of' *36, 37*
   Rome *208*
airing yards *37*
Akenside, Mark *136, 142, 151*
Albani, Cardinal *189*
albatrosses *158, 169*
   sooty *160*
Allégret, Marc *299, 308*
Allen, Hannah *32–34, 58*
Alps *185–186*
   destabilizing effect *193*
America
   neurasthenia and *56*
   tramps *262*
   see also United States
anatomy, education on *92, 95*
Anatomy of Melancholy (Burton) *28*
Ancient Mariner *see The Rime of the Ancient Mariner*
Anderson, Nels *271, 273*
animal spirits *30*
Annals of Medicine *105*
Anson, Lord *160–161, 165, 166, 167*
Antarctic waters *158*
Antarctica *158, 159*

317

anxiety
about nervous illness *64*
murders on trains and *235–236*
archaeologists *215*
Archer, John *47, 50*
Archer, Lord, estates *126–127, 131*
'aria cattiva' *207*
see also 'mal' aria'
aristocracy, unpopularity of railways
231
Arnold, Matthew *236*
art
as reviving experience *200*
Roman peasants and *217*
science interrelation *209*
viewing *199–200*
artists, travel *53*
Aspinwell, Roving Rob *272*
Association Medical Journal 241
railway stations *233–234*
asylum doctors *35*
asylums *30*
payment for *38*
poor reputation of care *34*
private patients *27*
public's lack of faith *71*
'reformed' *37*
seasonal excursions from *37–41*
siting *37*
stigma *34*
temperature changes effect
49–50
travel as adjunct/alternative
71–72
Atherstone, Dr W. G. *290*
Autun, France *179*
Avon, River *130*
Azores, islands *160*

B
bad airs *36*
in Rome *208*

see also 'mal' aria'
Baedeker, ... *219*
Baillie, Matthew *92*
Bakewell, Thomas *54–55, 66*
Bambio 'Ball' *313*
Bangui, Congo *312*
banishment, in mental illness *26*
Banks, Joseph *92, 93, 166, 171*
Barbault, Mrs *169, 172*
Barclay, Mr *91–92*
Barrell, John *6–7*
Barzellotti, Giacomo *219*
Bath *42, 137*
resort for mentally afflicted *41,
42*
Battie, William *31, 48, 59*
Battle of Edge Hill *123, 125, 133,
134*
battlefields
landscaping *123–124*
publicity on gardens *124*
Beddoes, Thomas *159, 162*
Beireis, Professor *95*
Berlioz, Hector *219*
Bethlem Hospital *26, 30, 31, 37,
50*
birdsong *168*
Birmingham (UK) *141*
Blackmore, Richard *32, 48*
Blaine, Gilbert *92*
Bligh, William *167–168*
Bloemfontein (South Africa) *289*
blood, scurvy and *161, 162*
body-politic, landscape as
expression *15*
Bologna, Italy *100, 179*
Bordeaux sickness *270*
Boughton, Northamptonshire *147*
Bounty 167–168
bourgeois society *5, 6, 7, 9*
Bouverie, Augustus *181, 197, 198*
Brace, Charles *263*

bracing effects of sublime *183–186*
Bradbury, Edward *243*
Bray, William *147*
Brest Naval Medical School *302*
Brewer, John *123*
Brewer, W. H. *269*
Briggs, Thomas *235–236*
British Medical Journal (BMJ) 70
  see also *Association Medical Journal*
bromides *55*
brothels *302*
Browne, W. A. F. *34, 40, 60*
Brugnatelli, Professor *99*
Brunswick, Andrew Duncân in *94–95*
Burgess, T. H. *214*
Burke, Edmund *171, 184, 186, 195, 197*
  Philosophical Enquiry 186, 195
Burns, Robert *91*
Burton, Robert *28, 35, 65, 73*
Bury Pomeroy, gothic ruins at *138*
Bute, Lady *60*
Buzard, James *244*

C

Cagnati, Marsilio *210*
Caledon Baths *287*
Campbell, John *127*
Cape Colony *280*
  climate *280, 282, 285*
  fears of dangers *290*
  as health resort *18, 279–280*
  medical therapeutic effects *18*
  waning popularity as health resort *289–290, 291*
  see also Cape Town
Cape Dutch settlers *284–285*
Cape Medical Board *290*
Cape Town *18, 283*
  Ango-Indian invalids *283, 288*

Cape Dutch comparison with British settlers *285*
  climate *285*
  degeneracy and *284–287*
  lack of society *284, 287–289*
  popularity as health resort *283–284*
  public health *286*
  suburbs *283, 286–287*
  unhealthiness *285–286*
  urban decay *283, 284–287*
  waning popularity as health resort *289–290*
Carlsbad, spa resort *43, 44*
Carnegie Institution, Washington *264*
Caroline, Queen *130*
carriers, in Africa *308, 309, 310–311*
Carter, Paul *169*
Catcott, Alexander *125*
Caygill, Howard *170*
Centurion 161, 165, 167, 170
Chad, Lake *307, 309*
chalybeat preparations *41, 42*
Charlecote, George Lucy of *130*
Charles VIII, King of France *270*
Cheyne, George *41*
Chicago, hobos and syphilis *271*
chlorals *55*
chlorosis *42*
cinema, sensory experience of travel and *245*
circulation of travellers, health and *146–147*
civilisation, organic cycle *134*
Clark, James *212*
  dangers of cultural tourism *214*
Clark, John *161, 166*
Clark, Michael *31*
cleanliness, concepts *5*
Clerke, Mrs *58*

Cleves, spa resort *42*
Clifford, James *2*
climate
  advice on specific travel types
    67
  Africa *301*
  Cape Colony *280, 282, 285*
  descriptions *280*
  hot, degeneracy in *284–287*
  mental disorders caused by
    47–53
  Naples *180, 183*
  Rome *16, 183, 210, 211, 213*
  seasonal/topographical variations
    211, 212, 214
  temperate, for mentally afflicted
    46
  warm, receptiveness to pleasure
    186–187
climatology *70, 220*
  literature *61, 213*
clinical teaching *109*
  in Italy *99*
Clouston, Thomas *36–37, 44, 50,*
  56, 59, 63
  advice on types of travel *62*
  travel as rest cure *66–67*
  travel prescription *62–64*
Cobham, Lord *124, 126, 145*
Cohen, Patricia Cline *239*
Cold Spring Harbour *264*
Coleman, Deirdre *162*
Coleridge, Samual Taylor *15, 157*
  knowledge of scurvy *157, 159*
  The Rime of the Ancient Mariner
    157–178
  The Watchman 162
College of Physicians, Edinburgh
  105
College of Physicians, London *48*
College of Physicians and Surgeons,
  New York *271*

Collins, Mortimer *247*
Collins, Wilkie *233*
Cologne *108*
colonial health resorts *280,*
  282–284
  degeneracy *284–287*
  social status *289*
  urban decay *283, 284–287*
  waning popularity *289–290*
  see also Cape Town
colonial settlers
  health and disease *301*
  image of disease as pollution
    302–303
  physical abuse of natives *307,*
    308, 312
colonialism *18, 308–309*
  adverse effect on natives *300*
  dark side to *303–304*
  death due to *303*
  demand for improved
    conditions for natives *306*
  Gide as accomplice *308–309*
  ill-health of natives *303*
  physical abuse of natives *307,*
    308, 312
  responsibility for diseases and
    spread *306–307*
  sleeping sickness as
    representative disease of
    oppression *312*
  violence *307, 308, 312*
  see also imperialism
colonisation *282*
  costs to colonisers *300–301*
  costs to natives *300*
colours, sensitivity to *167, 168*
Columbus, Christopher *270*
Commercial Exchange, Cape Town
  286
communications technology *3–4*
commuters, railway *249–250*

confinement *30, 31*
  concept *5*
  of insane *26*
Congo *see* Gide, André; *Travels in the Congo*
Conrad, Joseph *303*
Continental Tour *90, 91*
  see also Grand Tour
convalescence, abroad *279*
  see also Grand Tour; health resorts
convalescent homes, seasonal excursions to *37–41*
Cony, Carlos *59*
Cook, Captain James *159, 160, 171*
Cooper's Hill *128*
coping strategies *8*
Coppet, Marcel de *308*
Cosby, Alfred *299*
country, trips to for mentally afflicted *63*
Cox, Joseph Mason *66*
Cox, Thomas *123*
Crell, Professor *111*
Creuzé de Lesser, Auguste *208*
crime
  railway compartments *234–236*
  vulnerability in trains *236*
Cromwell, Oliver *128, 129*
Crowther, A. *4*
Cullen, William *29, 32*
cultural tourism *208, 214*
culture, travel meanings *28*
curiosity *195*
  scorbutic symptom comparison *169–170*
'curious inspector' *151*
Curtin, Philip *301*

D

Daer, Lord *103*

Dale, Langham *287*
Dall, Mrs, of Boston *269*
Dampier, William *157*
Dancel, Jean-François *214*
Daniels, Steve *9–10*
Davenport, Charles *264, 265–268*
Davidson, John *232, 233*
de Coppet, Marcel *308*
De Mowbray, Lord *231*
De Quincey, Thomas *6–7*
De Quiros *162, 167, 168*
Deacon, Harriet *67*
death
  abroad *179, 181*
  amid delights of Warm South *189–190*
  due to colonialism *303*
  'mal'aria' *189*
  scurvy causing *161*
Decaisne, Emile *214*
Defoe, Daniel *54, 140, 161, 166*
delusional insanity *63*
delusions *47*
  of suspicions *62*
Denham, Sir John *128*
Derbyshire, Allen H.'s travel from *33*
destabilization by travel *187–190*
  aim to avoid *190–191*
  Alpine sublime *193*
  excitement of travel and *197*
Devon County Asylum *40*
Diary of an Ennuyée (A. Jameson) *179–180*
Dickens, Charles *245*
Diderot, D. *164*
Dinas Bran, hilltop fort *139*
disasters, travel *53–54*
  railroad *8*
disease
  Africa *299*
  cycle of health and *134*

environmental influence *281*
Hippocratic theory *210*
as imbalance of four humours
281
interpretation *121*
landscape *126, 132, 134*
mental *see* mental disorders
see also specific diseases
disorientation *28*
Disraeli, Benjamin *231*
distemper *47*
diversion, principle *28, 29, 30*
'dromomania' *265, 275*
Drysdale, Mr *38–39*
Duchesne, E. A. *247*
Dugdale, R. L. *263*
Duncan, Andrew Jr *15, 89–119*
aims of travel *90, 93, 100*
apologies to father *101*
appointments after travels
105–106
birth and parents *89*
comparison with Charles Este
106–108
comparison with medical
student travellers *106–111*
consolidation of father's interests
in Europe *98, 111*
financial arrangements for travel
94
in Germany *94–98*
in Italy (*1795*) *98–102*
knowledge of Continental
medical practice *99, 101, 102,*
109
in London (*1794-1795*) *91–94*
as medical attendant *102–103*
medical education *90*
network of personal contacts *93*
non-medical interests *95–96*
purchase of books *98*
second trip to Italy (*1796-1798*)

102–106
Duncan, Andrew Sr *89, 109*
apologies of A. Duncan Jr *101*
in London *91–92, 93*
medical jurisprudence *96, 106*
Dupaty, Charles *187*
Dusky Bay *160, 169*
Dyer, John *10*
Dyke, Sir Thomas *148*

E

Eaton, Charlotte *198*
Ebel, Hoffrath *95*
Edge Hill *15, 145*
Battle of *123, 125, 133, 134*
battlefield *123*
flowers and meaning *136*
gothic tower *123–124, 129,*
135, 145
landscape viewed *129, 131*
landscaping *123–124*
owner *see* Miller, Sanderson
view from *125*
Edge-Hill (Jago, R.) *121–152*
battle description *131*
book *1* and book *2 126, 133*
book *3 141*
book *4* (final) *126, 132*
friendliness of landscape *131*
historical background *128*
hospitality *146, 147*
indigenous *vs* foreign travel
135–136
key concepts *126*
land management *126–127,*
130, 146–147
national progress *140, 141*
political issues and *127, 134,*
136
praise of 'local' *129–130, 131*
prevailing themes *126,*
151–152

publication *122*
revisited *121–152*
spatial *vs* historical prospect
125–126
state of health/disease of
landscape *126, 132*
Edinburgh
Charles Este's visit *107*
Royal Medical Society *89, 98*
*Edinburgh Medical and Surgical
Journal 105*
Edinburgh Medical School *279*
Edinburgh New Dispensatory 105
Edinburgh Royal Asylum *36, 89*
Edinburgh Royal Public Dispensary
89
Edinburgh University *89, 90*
comparison with other medical
institutions *92*
Medical Jurisprudence and
Medical Police, chair *106*
Medical Jurisprudence chair
105
Emerson, Ralph Waldo *243*
Empson, William *157, 160*
enclosure schemes *131, 147*
The English in Italy (Normanby,
Marquis) *181*
English landscapes *135, 136*
ENO's Fruit Salts *11*
environmental influence, disease
281
Ernst, Waltraud *52*
Eschenburg, Professor J. J. *95*
Esquirol, Jean Etienne Dominique
49
Este, Charles *94, 106–108*
comparison with Andrew
Duncan *106–108*
travel book *94, 107*
Este, Charles Sn. *107, 109*
Ettrick, Henry *165*

eugenics *263, 264, 269*
eugenics field workers *264*
Eugenics Record Office *264*
euphoria *15–16*
excitement, travel *195–201, 215*
excursions
from asylums *37–41, 71–72*
to form 'idea of England' *123*
exercise
bracing effects of travel
184–185
for mental illness *66–67*
travel as form *65*
exhaustion, from travel *199,
246–247*
eyes
effect of railway travel *250–251*
liberty of *143*
eyewitnesses *171*

F
false association *29–30*
false judgement *29*
family
influence on medical care *37, 39*
travel on advice of *32–34, 39, 58*
see also Duncan, Andrew
family history, nomads and tramps
263, 267–268
fatigue *199, 246–247*
fears, of travel *12*
of dangers in Cape Colony *290*
over technological modernity of
railways *231–232*
railway tunnels *236–237*
on social mixing, railway travel
232
Ferrier, David *54*
fetishised commodity *11*
Fisher, Dr C. I. *272*
fixed ideas *29*
Fletcher, Ralph *65–66*

flowers, smell *167*
Floyer, John *42*
Flynt, Josiah *269*
follies *144–145*
Ford, John *307*
forensic medicine *109*
Forster, E. M. *238*
Forster, George *159, 163, 167, 168*
Forster, Johann Reinhold *158, 309*
Fourneau (medicine) *305*
Foxwell, E. *231, 246*
France, models of nomadism *265–266*
Frank, Johann Peter *96, 97, 99, 102*
translation of *System 96, 100, 106*
Frank, Joseph *99*
freedom, sense of *193*
French Equatorial Africa
Gide's perceptions/experiences *304–310*
population drop *300*
see also colonialism
French imperialism *300*
French sickness *270*
French West Africa *301*
Freud, Sigmund *8, 236*
Friedberg, Anne *245*
Frings, P. *36, 49*
fugue *28, 264, 265–266*
French diagnosis *266*
social concern over vagrancy and *266*

G
Gairdner, Meredith *42–44*
gardens
Andrew Duncan's interest *95*
battlefield sites *123, 124*
flow of water *126*

Gastein, spa waters *43*
General Medical Service *301*
Genoa, Anna Jameson's visit *179*
geographical advantages *127*
geographical space *9*
George III, King *35, 58*
Germaine de Staël, Anne Louise *189–190, 196*
Germany
Andrew Duncan in *94–98*
spa resorts *42–44*
Gibbon, Edward *134*
Gide, André *18, 299–316*
as accomplice of colonial regime *308–309*
ambiguous position as critic and participant *309, 310–311*
autobiography *299*
demand for improved conditions for natives *306*
illness of carriers *308, 309, 310–311*
insomnia *310–314*
insomnia as vigil over natives *311*
in North Africa *299*
as 'part-time' doctor (to carriers) *308, 310*
social destruction in Africa *308*
travel for discovery of illness of empire's poor *314*
two faces of Africa *304–305*
Urien's Voyage 302–303
see also Travels in the Congo
Gilchrist, Ebeneezer *45–46*
Gilman, Sander *301*
Gilpin, William *126, 143*
Giraud, Pierre François Eugène *217, 219*
Glasgow Royal Asylum *38, 39, 40, 51*
gloom, Antarctic sea travel *158*
Gloucester 161

Gloucester Lunatic Asylum *65–66*
'gospel of fresh air' *36, 37*
gothic buildings, follies *144–145*
gothic designs *150*
gothic hospitality *145–146*
gothic ruins *134, 138*
gothic towers *123–124, 129, 135, 145*
Göttingen, Germany *96–97, 111*
Grand Tour *14, 182, 200–201*
  Anna Jameson *179–180*
  change of air *180–183*
  English landscape *vs 135, 136*
  excitement *198*
  invalid version *60*
  Italy *100*
  as leisure *191*
  for melancholia *69*
  for young physicians *110–111*
Granet, François Marius *215, 216*
Grant, Mr *101, 104*
Granville, Sir Bevile *137*
Granville, Augustus Bozi *42, 43*
Great Eastern Railway *236*
Great Windmill Street School *92*
Greenblatt, Stephen *172, 198*
Guildford, Lady *60*
Gulliver's Travels 47
Gunn, Ben *54*

H

Hacking, Ian *266*
Halen, Pierre *301*
Hales, Dr Stephen *141*
Hall, Marshall *54*
Halsam, John *30, 47*
Hamilton, Duke *110*
Hardman, Sir William *238–239*
Harrington, Ralph *54*
Harriot, John *52, 57*
Harte, Sir Percyvall *148, 150*
Hatley, Simon *158, 172*

Hawkins, Sir Richard *160, 163, 167, 168*
hazards to health, of travel *52, 61–62, 74*
  cultural tourism *214*
  James Johnson and *188, 199, 215*
  railway travel *see* railway travel
Hazlitt, William *190, 191, 213*
health
  circulation of travellers and *146–147*
  travel as detrimental *see* hazards to health
  travel connected *10*
  see also public health
health resorts *279*
  Cape Town *see* Cape Town
  colonial *280, 282–284*
  Mediterranean *289*
  see also spa resorts
hearing, railway travel effect *252*
heat
  adverse effect *182–183*
  extremes in Italy *182*
  railway travel *252*
Hébert, Ernest *217*
hill tops
  constitutional walking *151*
  as places of transcendent vision *122*
Hippocratic principles *210, 213*
Hippocratic theory of disease *210*
Hirsch, Auguste *302*
historical progress, of nation *140*
historical vision *125*
  as cycle *134*
history, obsessive preocupation *197–198*
hobos *17, 268–269*
  syphilis and *271*
  vote fixing and *273*

see also nomadism; tramps
Hobsbawm, Eric *4*
home, removal from *31*
homesickness *166*
horse riding *65*
horses, mechanical *66*
hospitality *151*
  Gothic *145–146*
  'old English' *146, 147*
hostility, to travellers *147*
Hulme, Peter *172*
Hunt, S. Leigh *52*
Hunter, William *90–91*
'hurrygraphs' *243, 244*
hydrotherapy *42*
hypochondriasis *32, 63, 65, 185*
hysteria *266, 267*
  treatment *66*

I

icebergs *158, 159*
identity, escape by travel *191*
illnesses
  as metaphors *10*
  of travel *48*
imagination *142*
imperialism
  environmental disease aetiology
    and *281*
  French, in Africa *300*
  medical topography and
    280–282
  temperate regions *282*
  see also colonialism
India
  British in *50, 51, 52, 283*
  concern over brothels *302*
  sunstroke *50*
industrialisation *8, 17, 253*
insanity, medical *vs* lay views *51*
insomnia *18, 69*
  André Gide's *310–314*

Institutes of Medicine, Edinburgh
    University *89, 106*
Ireland, Mr *93*
Ireland, visits by asylum patients
    39
iron industry *141*
Islington Waters *41*
Italy *16*
  adverse effects of travel
    182–183
  Andrew Duncan in *98–102*
  benefits of travel *183–187*
  danger and destabilization of
    travel *188–190*
  relaxing effects of travel
    186–187
  therapeutic effects *182*
  see also Rome; Warm South

J

Jacobite Rebellion (*1745*) *129*
Jacobitism *128, 148*
Jacyna, Stephen *109*
Jago, Richard *121–152*
  education and background *123*
  see also Edge Hill
Jamaican trading ship case *47*
James, Henry *214*
Jameson, Anna *179–180, 187, 192*
  Alpine travels *185–186, 193*
  Bay of Naples *193*
  fatigue *199*
  'Song of the Syren Parthenope'
    193, 196
  travel as novelty and excitement
    195–196
Jean, James *231*
Jebb, John *59*
Jewish Ghetto, Rome *212*
Jewson, N. *64*
Johnson, James *182, 183*
  benefits of travel *184–185*

dangers of travel *188, 199, 215*
　Rome as filthy city *212*
　warning of fatigue *199*
Joyce, James *245*
Juan Fernandez *167, 168*
Jukes family *263, 269*

K

Keats *190*
Keene, Henry *148*
Kennedy, Dane *280*
Kenny, Alexander S. *52*
King, Dr William *128, 139*

L

Lake Chad *307, 309*
The Lancet 70
　anxiety over railway
　compartments *232–233*
　concern over brothels in India
　302
　dangers of service in West Africa
　300
　effect of railway travel on eye
　and brain *250–251*
　effect of railway travel on
　hearing *252*
　harmful effects of railway *234,
　248, 249*
　railway commuting *249–250*
Lancisi, Giovanni Maria *210*
land management *126–127, 130,
　146–147*
landscape
　Andrew Duncan's interest *95*
　cycle of health and disease *134*
　disease *126, 132*
　English *135, 136*
　enjoyment of railway travel
　251–252
　friendliness *131*
　guarantors of health of *151*

　as indicator of health/prosperity
　140
　mapping, concepts *125*
　openness *131, 151*
　pathologising *15*
　political implications *127, 134,
　136*
　prone to general state of
　health/disease *126*
　from trains *243, 244*
　travellers' observations on health
　of *121–152*
landscaping, battlefields *123–124*
Lansdowne, Lord *137*
Lansdowne Hill *137*
Lapi, Giovanni Girolamo *220*
Lassel, Richard *191*
Laycock, Thomas *54*
Le Fanu, Sheridan *246*
Leghorn *101, 104*
leisure, travel as *191*
leisure travel *121*
Lettsom, John Coakely *92*
liberty *131, 134*
　of eye *143*
'liberty' of vision *143*
Lind, James *161, 165, 169–170*
Lingara, Congo *308*
Lipscombe, George *138, 140*
literature
　climatology *61, 213*
　medical *100, 209*
　of travel *see* travel literature
Livingstone, D. N. *280*
local image *129–130*
　vs expansive vision *130–131*
Locatelli, Dr *99, 111*
London, Andrew Duncan in
　91–94
Lorenzetti, Ambrogio *140*
Loti, Pierre *301*
love melancholy *28*

Lowes, John Livingston *159*
Lucy, George, of Charlecote *130*
Lullingstone Castle, Kent
  147–148, 150, 151
Lunacy law *27*
Lyceum Medicum *92*
Lyndhurst House *40*
Lyttleton, George *145*

M

MacCulloch, John *188, 189,
  207–208, 220*
MacKenzie, John *241*
mad-doctors *35, 73*
madness *13*
  models of theories of causes *29*
  sunstroke causing *48*
  see also mentally afflicted
Magellan, F. *167*
Mahé, Professor *302*
'mal'aria' (malaria) *17, 188,
  207–228, 208*
  advice on avoidance *208*
  changes in location and *213*
  local advice *218–220*
  location *212–213*
  mapping in Rome *209, 210*
  misery and death *189*
  'nest of' *214*
  role of winds *210, 212, 213*
  in Rome *210–211*
malarial fever *212–213*
malnutrition, French Equatorial
  Africa *300*
mania *133*
manic hyperactivity *28*
mapping *125*
  landscape *125*
  mal'aria in Rome *209, 210*
Marienbad waters *43*
Martin, Sir James Ranald *302*
Marty, Éric *311*

Massey, Doreen *275*
Materia Medica *106*
Matthews, Henry *54, 61, 64, 67,
  182, 183, 208*
McClintock, Anne *11, 12*
McCook, James *271, 272–273*
Mead, Richard *29–30, 48, 65, 167*
mechanical horses *66*
medical advice
  on travel *52–53, 57*
  whilst travelling *52*
medical attendant *102–103*
Medical Commentaries *90*
medical education *90, 97*
medical journals *105–106*
  see also Association Medical
  Journal; The Lancet
medical jurisprudence *96, 105,
  106*
medical knowledge, uncertainties
  about travel *62*
medical literature *100, 209*
medical police *96, 106*
medical resources, in Africa *301,
  306*
Medical Society *92*
medical students *90, 106*
  in Germany *96–97*
  travel by *106–111*
medical topography
  imperialism and *280–282*
  'mal'aria' in Rome *210–211*
medical travellers *89*
medico-legal aspects of travel *54*
Medico-Psychological Association
  (MPA) *67, 69–70*
melancholia *28, 32*
  risks of travel *69*
  scurvy causing *159*
  travel advice *62, 73*
Melville, Herman *167*
mental disorders *13–14, 25–88*

caused by travel *47–53*
models of theories of causes *29*
travel pathologised as *47–57*
mental health, travel as detrimental
52, 61–62
mentally afflicted
activities/exercise *66–67*
criticisms of travel for *67–68*
late Victorian travel guidance
60–70
reasons for travel *25*
sea voyages *45–46*
seasonal excursions to
convalescent homes *37–41*
travel as therapy *27–35*
travel for airing mental
problems *35–37*
travel to spa resorts *41–45*
metaphors
military, of travel *273–274*
society as human body *274*
of travel *1–2*
Metropolitan Railway Company
240
Michel, Jean-Baptiste *211, 219*
migrant workers, syphilis *271*
Milan *99*
military surgery *93–94*
Miller, Sanderson *123, 128*
enclosure schemes *131*
gothic tower *123–124, 129*
pro-Stuart sympathies *128–129*
publicity on battlefield garden
124
Shenstone's views *135*
mind and body interactions
scurvy *162, 163*
travel *197*
mining *141*
Mitchell, Silas Weir *41, 68*
mobility *9, 10–11, 261–277, 275*
politics *268*

sleeping sickness spread
307–308
syphilis and *270–274*
tramps *see* nomadism; tramps
see also railway travel
monomania *29, 63*
Monro, Dr Alexander *92*
Monro, John *26, 30, 31, 36*
Mont Blanc *185*
Montagu, Lord *147*
Montesquieu, Charles Louis de
Secondat, Baron de *184*
Montpellier *61*
Montrose Royal Lunatic Asylum *60*
monuments, English *137*
Moore, John *110*
Moorfields hospital *37*
moral responsibility, colonialism
and *312*
moral therapy *34–35, 38, 71*
morbid introspection *31–32*
Mordaunt, Charles *131*
Morgan, Charles, Sir T. *182*
Morgan, Sydney *182, 189*
Morison, Alexander *31, 44, 60*
Morris, William *252*
Morton, Richard *41*
motion, continual *183–184, 196*
mountain regions *67*
Munro, John *47, 59*
murders, railway trains *234–236*
Murray, Emma *289*
mutiny *167–168*
A Mystery of the Underground (J.
Oxenham) *235–236*

N

Naples
Anna Jameson's visit *179*
climate *180, 183*
Naples Bay *193*
Nasmyth, James *240*

National Conference of Charities
and Corrections (*1877*) 269
natives, colonialism and *see*
colonialism
Neapolitan disease 270
nervous disorders/illness 32
anxiety about 64
sea voyages for 45
nervous strain, due to travel
55–56, 246–247
neurasthenia 53–57
criticisms 56
diagnosis 55
popularisation 56
N'Goto, Sanba 312–313
Nirvana principle 180
nomadism 264
family history 267–268
French models 265–266
genetic origins 266, 267
origins 265–266
see also tramps
Normanby, Marquis 181, 183,
187, 197
North, W. 213
North Africa, André Gide in 299
nostalgia 166
'old English hospitality' 146,
147
nourishment, mentally afflicted 63
novelty, travel as 195–201, 215

O

obsessive disorders 29
ocean, putrefying 163
opium 163
Oppenheim, J. 31, 62, 64
on treatment of Virginia Woolf
69
Orford, Lord 27
overwork 65
Oxenham, John 235–236

P

Pacha, M. 313
Pacific Ocean
albatrosses 158
scurvy 160–161
Padua, Italy 101
paintings, of Gothic ruins 139
paranoia 62
paranoid psychoses 29
Pargeter, Reverend William 49
Paris, France 104
'pathology,' definition and reason
for use 2–3
patriotic tourists/travellers 123,
151
pauperism, tramps and 263
paupers 38, 39
Pavia, Italy 99, 108
Pearson, Dr 93
Pemble, John 221
peripatetic, walking and 6
personality disorder, multiple 266
phosphorescence 159, 163
pilgrimages 27–28
Pils, Isidore 214
Pincio hill 213
Pinkerton, A. W. Pulteney 279
Playfair, W.S. 41
pneumonia 310
poetic realism 217
Poinsot, Chief Justice 234–235
political aspects
art in Rome and 218
landscape implications 127,
134, 136
mobility 268
Poole, Thomas 168
poor whites, South Africa 290
Pope, Alexander 127, 133
Port Elizabeth, South Africa
288–289

Porter, Roy *70, 90*
porterage, in Africa *308, 309,*
  310–311
postgraduate medical education
  90, 97
post-traumatic stress disorder *54*
Prague *102*
Pratt, Mary Louise *172*
prescriptions of travel *16*
private patients, in asylums *27*
provincialism, Cape Town *287*
psychic forms, travel *5, 6*
psychological effects, sea voyages
  46
psycho-social benefits of travel *44*
psychosomatic benefits of travel *44*
public health
  Cape Town *286*
  railway issues *233, 246*
Purcell, John *41–42, 44, 57*

R

Radcliffe Camera *128*
Radway, Warwickshire *123*
railroad disasters *8*
'railroad fever' *269*
railway
  as symbol of human encounter
    with technology *234*
  as symbol of progress *229*
  as symbol of society *233*
railway carriages
  fatigue from and vibrations
    247–248
  open (American) *237*
  purpose-built *242–243*
  sexual assault *238–239*
railway compartments *242–243*
  anxiety over social mixing
    232–233
  crime and dangers *234–236*
  as prison and as protection *236*

'railway fatigue' *247*
'railway spine' *8, 54*
railway stations
  clocks *241–242*
  public health issues *233–234*
  as symbol of human encounter
    with technology *234*
  violence *233*
railway trains
  anxiety over social mixing in
    compartments *232–233*
  class system *230, 242*
  crime *234–236*
  'intruders' *233*
  road carriages on *242*
  see also railway carriages; railway
    compartments
railway travel *7–8, 229–259*
  accidents *229*
  as alarming and threatening *229*
  boredom and monotomy *243*
  classes of passengers *242*
  as collective social experience *230*
  commuters and season-ticket
    holders *249–250*
  criticisms for melancholics *69*
  degenerative assault on
    body/mind *229*
  degenerative threat *246*
  effect of regulation on mind *241*
  enjoyment of landscape
    251–252
  exhaustion from *246–247*
  fears on social mixing *232*
  fears over technological
    modernity *231–232*
  on footplate *247–248, 253*
  harmful effects on health *234*
  heat and ventilation problems
    252
  levelling effect on society *231*
  middle classes *236*

nervous strain due to *55–56,*
246–247
opportunities for women
travellers *237–238*
passenger numbers *240*
perceptual experience *244–245*
public health issues *233–234,*
246
regulation and rigidity of
239–241
relationship of view and viewer
244
responses to *17*
sensory experience connection
to cinema *245*
tramps *262–263*
trauma of *230*
views from windows *243–244*
visual stimuli and damage
250–251
vulnerability to crime *235, 236*
The Railway Traveller's Handy Book
237, 241, 246
railway tunnels, fears *236–237*
railway workers *247*
Ratisbon *98*
Raynal, *164*
recreational activity, for asylum
patients *39–40*
Reitman, Ben *271, 272–273*
relaxation, effect of travel *186–187*
reputation, safeguarding in mental
illness *25, 26, 27*
Resolution 159
rest cures *41, 65, 66–67, 68*
Restoration *128*
Richards, Jeffrey *241*
The Rime of the Ancient Mariner
157–178
absurd and unintelligible
165–166
aesthetic complexity *164*

Death's Partner *162, 163*
eras in reception/understanding
157
moral regeneration of mariners
167
scurvy and *see* scurvy
spectre ship *162, 163, 164*
starvation and scurvy effects *161*
road carriage, on trains *242*
Robert, Léopold *217*
Robertson, George *166*
Robinson Crusoe (D. Defoe) *161,*
169
Rogers, Samuel *191–192, 195*
Rogers, Woodes *157, 160*
'Roman fever' *213*
Roman ruins *134*
Romantic Travel 188
romanticism *53*
Rome *101*
bad air *208*
change of air *182*
climate *16, 183, 210, 211, 213*
contemporary neglect *218*
cultural and therapeutic
contradiction *208, 214, 221*
cultural tourism *208*
fatigue in *199*
as filthy city *212*
insalubrity and disease *212*
mal'aria *see* 'mal'aria'
as museum city *208*
opinion of doctors in *219*
pathological topography *211*
peasants *217, 220*
pursuit of culture *214*
ruins as wonder *198*
seasons and risks/benefits *209,*
213
Villa Albani *189*
Rossetti, Dante Gabriel *248*
roundworm *160*

Rowley, William *42*
Royal College of Physicians,
  Edinburgh *89*
Royal Medical Society *89, 98*
Royal Public Dispensary *105*
Royal Society *92*
Runymede *128, 151*
Ruskin, John *240, 251*
Rymer, James *164*

S
sailors, ballad for *157, 159*
St Luke's Hospital *31*
San Martino ai Monti *215–216*
Santa Croce *199*
Saumarez, Philip *170*
Savage, George Henry *26, 46, 59,
  71*
  advice on specific travel types *67*
  advice on travelling for mental
    illness *64*
  career *72*
  criticisms of travel *67–68*
  Medico-Psychological
    Association *67, 69–70*
  travel as exercise *66–67*
  treatment of Virginia Woolf
    68–69
Scarpa, Antonio *99*
Schivelbusch, Wolfgang *7–8, 17*
science
  art interrelation *209*
  impact on writing *221*
scurvy *16*
  alternation between horror and
    pleasure *15–16, 163, 166–167,
    169–170*
  ballad about *see The Rime of the
    Ancient Mariner*
  causes *162, 164, 165*
  Coleridge's knowledge *157, 159*
  effect on mind *164, 166*

melancholy due to *159*
mortality *160–161*
preventive measures *160*
sense perception alterations
  167–168
South Seas *159–160*
sugar for *171*
symptoms *158, 161, 163,
  164–166*
theory on *162*
sea voyages *45–46, 68, 279*
  for mentally afflicted *45–46*
  risks to melancholics *69*
  scurvy *see* scurvy
  South Seas *160*
  waning popularity *290*
sea-sickness *45–46*
seaside, trips to for mentally
  afflicted *63*
seasonal excursions, to convalescent
  homes *37–41*
sedatives *310*
Sekora, John *146*
self-help guides *52–53*
Selkirk, Earl *103*
sexual assault, in railway carriages
  238–239
shapes, pleasure from *167*
Shelley, Mary *194*
Shelley, Percy Bysshe *190*
Shelvocke, George *157–158*
Shenstone, William *123, 135*
'Ship of Fools' *26*
shipwrecks *54*
shock *53–57*
shock therapy *66*
Shorthouse, John *33*
Shperk, Dr Eduard *270–271*
sightseeing mania *215*
Simmons, Jack *241*
Simonstown, Cape Colony *286*
Simplex, Sir John *232*

Sirocco *183*
Skae, Francis *50*
slave trade *162, 171*
sleep, as symbol of absence ethical
    relationship *314*
sleeping sickness *304–310, 314*
    as representative disease of
    colonial oppression *312*
    spread *307–308*
sleeplessness *69*
    see also insomnia
slums *5*
Smith, Bernard *159, 169*
Smollett, Tobias *183–184*
soap, development *11*
social classes
    mixing, fears in railway travel
    232
    railway travel *230, 231*
    therapeutic travel *73*
social demarcation, therapeutic
    travel *64*
social progress *140*
social spaces, contested, railways as
    232
social stigma *26*
society
    lacking in Cape Town *287–289*
    levelling effect of railways *231*
    metaphor, as human body *274*
    railways as symbol *233*
soil, mal'aria location and *210*
sojurns, mentally afflicted *38–39,
    71–72*
Somerset West, Cape Colony *287*
Sontag, Susan *10, 273–274*
South Africa *291*
    see also Cape Colony; Cape
    Town
South Seas *15, 168*
    collectors *170–171*
    scurvy *160*

sea voyages *160*
Southey, Robert *165, 171*
spa, endorsement of value *43–44*
spa resorts *282*
    European/foreign *42, 43*
    travel to *41–45*
    see also health resorts
Sparrman, Anders *169, 172*
spectre ship *162, 163, 164*
Speedwell 159
Speek, Peter Alexander *268*
stage-coaches *54, 65*
Stainborough Castle *147*
Stallybrass, P. *5*
starvation
    scurvy effects with *161*
    at sea *166*
State Almshouse, Tewkesbury
    (Massachusetts) *272*
Station for Experimental Evolution
    264
steam boats *55*
Steiglitz, Dr *111*
Stellenbosch, Cape Colony *287*
Stendhal, [Henri Beyle] *192, 199*
Stevenson, Christine *37*
Stevenson, Robert Louis *245*
stigma, asylums *34*
Stock Exchange *56*
Stowe *124, 126, 143*
Strafford, Lord *145*
streams *127*
stress *53–57*
    of journeys *33, 55–56,
    246–247*
Stuart reign *127, 128, 129, 133,
    137*
Success 159
sugar *171*
suicide *183, 184*
Sumatra *52*
'summer quarters' *39*

sunstroke *47–53, 74*
  case numbers *51*
  as cause of madness *49, 50*
Swift, Jonathan *47*
Sydenham, Thomas *41*
symbolic domains, of travel *5–6*
Syme, James *54*
syphilis *263, 275*
  migrant workers *271*
  mobility and *270–274*
  origins and historical
    background *270*
  transmission *17*

T

taste, practice *170–171*
Tayleur, Dr *106*
Taylor, R. W. *271*
technological modernity, fears
  about railways *231–232*
telescopes *142, 143*
temperate regions, imperialism and
  282
temperature extremes, madness due
  to *48–49*
Temple of Ancestral Liberty *124,
144, 145*
Temple of Saxon Liberty *124, 143*
Thomas, Nicholas *170*
Thomas, Pascoe *165*
Thompson, Joseph *11*
Thompson, Dr Symes *70*
Tilt, E. J. *55*
Toeplitz *43*
Toryism *136, 139, 148*
tourism *190–192*
  cultural in Rome *208, 214*
  rise *3*
  symbolic value of place *280*
  wonders /sights *198*
tourists
  patriotic *123*

travellers *vs 4*
trade *220*
train travel *see* railway travel
trains *see entries beginning railway*
'tramp evil' *269*
'Tramp Laws' *262*
tramps *4–5, 18, 261–277*
  definition/description *263–263,
263,
269*
  as pathologies *274, 275*
  psychological origin *268*
  scare over (*1869-1930*)
    262–263
  syphilis association *270–274*
  theories of origins *263–270*
  threat to democracy *272–273*
transport revolution *3, 13*
'traumatic insanity' *50*
'traumatic neurosis' *8*
travel
  adverse effect of heat/cold
    182–183
  on advice of family/friends
    32–34, 39
  aims/role *5–6, 190*
  bracing effects of sublime
    183–186
  danger and destabilization by
    187–190
  as diversion *28, 29, 30*
  escape from depressing effects of
    north *194*
  escape from identity *191*
  excitement and novelty
    195–201, 215
  exhaustion/fatigue from *199,
246–247*
  fears *see* fears
  as form of exercise *65*
  hazards to health *52, 61–62,
74, 214*
  indigenous *vs* foreign *135*

industrialization *240–241*
as leisure *191*
metaphors *1–2*
psychic form *5, 6*
railway *see* railway travel
reasons for *279*
recommendation by physicians
181
relaxing effects *186–187*
resistance to *33–34*
romantic view *188*
as stabilising and destabilising
force *4, 5*
symbolic domain of body *5–6*
symbolic domain of
geographical space *9*
therapeutic effects *187*
as threat to medical practitioners
71
as 'translation term' *2*
warnings about threats of *55*
travel books *192*
travel guidance, lay *vs* medical
57–60
travel industry, Victorian era
61–62
travel literature *13, 14, 60*
demands *94*
medical literature interchange
209
for mentally afflicted *60–61*
travel writings
therapeutic effect of Italy *182*
therapeutic effects of travel *187*
travellers
historical progress of nation
140
hostility to *147*
tourists *vs* *4*
travelling doctors *60*
Travels in the Congo *299–316*
insomnia as moral concern for

natives *310–314*
insomnia mentions *311–312*
publication *303–304*
sleeping sickness *304–310*
see also Gide, André
tropical medicine, development
300
Trotter, Thomas *162, 166,*
169–170
trypanosomiasis, African *see*
sleeping sickness
tsetse flies *305*
tuberculosis *289*
Tunbridge Wells, resort for
mentally afflicted *41*
Tunisia, André Gide in *299*
tunnels, fears *236–237*
Turner, Brian *12*
Turner, J. M. W. *9–10*
tyranny *134*

U

Uganda, sleeping sickness spread
307
Understade *127*
Union Pacific Railroad *262*
United States
syphilis and migrant workers
271
see also America
University of Pavia *97, 99*
urbanism *12*

V

vagrancy *265–266, 266*
'vapours' *36, 45*
venal voting *272, 273*
Venice *101*
Anna Jameson's visit *179*
ventilation machines *141–142*
ventilation problems, railway travel
252

Verne, Jules *244*
vibrations, railway travel *247–248*
Vienna *102*
views, quest for *121–122*
Vigor's Horse-Action Saddle *66*
violence, railways and *233*
'violent motion' *66*
Virilio, Paul *4*
visions, historical *see* historical
   vision

W
Wales, William *159, 160, 171*
walking
   attitudes to *6*
   constitutional *151*
Wallace, Anne *6*
Wallis, Samuel *166*
Walpole, George *58*
Walpole, Horace *27, 58*
Walpole, Sir Robert *36*
Walter, Richard *164, 165, 166*
wanderlust *263, 264, 269, 275*
Ward, Matthew E. *251–252*
Warm South *179–205*
   aquatic sublime *192–195*
   bracing and relaxing travel
   183–187
   change of air and *180–183*
   danger and destabilization
   187–190
   death amid delights *189–190*
   excitement and novelty
   195–201
   'indolent delicious reverie' *179,*
   180
   myth *214, 220*
   relaxing effects of travel
   186–187
   as therapeutic *192*
   tourism and *190–192*
   see also Italy

Warnke, Martin *129–130*
The Watchman (Coleridge) *162*
water *126*
Watt, Sir James *160*
Weatherly, (General Practioner) *72*
Weber, Sir Hermann *70*
Weisser Stein, Germany *95*
Wells, H. G. *230*
Wentworth Castle *147*
Weyland, Professor Francis, of Yale
   269, 273
White, A. *5*
White's Town (America) *57*
Wiesbaden *43*
Williams, Frederick *248*
Williams, Raymond *244, 284*
Williams Wynn family *139*
Willis, Dr *166*
Willis, Francis *35*
Wilson, Richard *139*
Wilson, William, S. *46*
winds
   Cape Town *285*
   role in mal'aria *210, 212, 213*
winter, in *Edge Hill* *126, 132*
women, as symbols of
   contamination *302*
women travellers
   opportunities from railways
   237–238
   risks *239*
Woodall, John *165*
Woodward, Dr John *125*
Woolf, Virginia *68–69, 245*
Wordsworth, William *4, 6, 158*
Wrigley, Richard *53*
Wynn, Watkin Williams *139*
Wynn, Williams *139*

Y
Yellowlees *54*
York railway station *233*

Young, Arthur *140–141, 147*

Z

zymotic theory *37*

DIEGO SAGLIA

Poetic Castles in Spain
British Romanticism and
Figurations of Iberia

Amsterdam/Atlanta, GA 1999. 355 pp.
(Internationale Forschungen zur Allgemeinen und
Vergleichenden Literaturwissenschaft 39)
ISBN: 90-420-0428-2   Hfl. 120,-/US-$ 66.50

British culture of the Romantic period is distinguished by a protracted and
varied interest in things Spanish. The climax in the publication of fictional, and
especially poetical, narratives on Spain corresponds with the intense phase of
Anglo-Iberian exchanges delimited by the Peninsular War (1808-14), on the one
hand, and the Spanish experiment of a constitutional monarchy that lasted from
1820 until 1823, on the other. Although current scholarship has uncovered and
reconstructed several foreign maps of British Romanticism - from the Orient to
the South Seas - exotic European geographies have not received much attention.
Spain, in particular, is one of the most neglected of these 'imaginary' Romantic
geographies, even if between the 1800s and the 1820s, and beyond, it was a site
of wars and invasions, the object of foreign economic interests relating to its
American colonies, and a geopolitical area crucial to the European balance
designed by the post-Waterloo Vienna settlement. This study considers the
various ways in which Spain figured in Romantic narrative verse, recovering
the discursive materials employed in fictional representation, and assessing the
relevance of this activity in the context of the dominant themes and
preoccupations in contemporary British culture. The texts examined here
include medievalizing and chivalric fictions, Orientalist adventures set in
Islamic Granada, and modern-day tales of the anti-Napoleonic campaign in the
Peninsula. Recovering some of the outstanding works and issues elaborated by
British Romanticism through the cultural geography of Spain, this study shows
that the Iberian country was an inexhaustible source of imaginative materials
for British culture at a time when its imperial boundaries were expanding and
its geopolitical influence was increasing in Europe and overseas.

------------------------------   *Editions Rodopi B.V.*
USA/Canada: 2015 South Park Place, Atlanta, GA 30339, Tel. (770)
933-0027, *Call toll-free* (U.S.only) 1-800-225-3998, Fax (770) 933-9644

All Other Countries: Tijnmuiden 7, 1046 AK Amsterdam, The Netherlands.
Tel. + + 31 (0)20 6114821, Fax + + 31 (0)20 4472979
             orders-queries@rodopi.nl —— http://www.rodopi.nl

MEDICINE AND MODERN WARFARE

Ed. by Roger Cooter, Mark Harrison & Steve Sturdy

Amsterdam/Atlanta, GA 1999. X,286 pp.
(Clio Medica 55/The Wellcome Institute Series in the History of Medicine)
ISBN: 90-420-0546-7   Bound Hfl. 150,-/US-$ 83.-
ISBN: 90-420-0536-X   Paper Hfl. 45,-/US-$ 25.50

After years at the margins of medical history, the relationship between war and medicine is at last beginning to move centre-stage. The essays in this volume focus on one important aspect of that relationship: the practice and development of medicine within the armed forces from the late nineteenth century through to the end of the Second World War. During this crucial period, medicine came to occupy an important position in military life, especially during the two world wars when manpower was at a premium. Good medical provisions were vital to the conservation of manpower, protecting servicemen from disease and returning the sick and wounded to duty in the shortest possible time. A detailed knowledge of the serviceman's mind and body enabled the authorities to calculate and standardise rations, training and disciplinary procedures.

Spanning the laboratory and the battlefield, and covering a range of national contexts, the essays in this volume provide valuable insights into different national styles and priorities. They also examine the relationship between medical personnel and the armed forces as a whole, by looking at such matters as the prevention of disease, the treatment of psychiatric casualties and the development of medical science. The volume as a whole demonstrates that medicine became an increasingly important part of military life in the era of modern warfare, and suggests new avenues and approaches for future study.

-------------------------------   *Editions Rodopi B.V.*

USA/Canada: 2015 South Park Place, Atlanta, GA 30339, Tel. (770) 933-0027, *Call toll-free* (U.S.only) 1-800-225-3998, Fax (770) 933-9644

All Other Countries: Tijnmuiden 7, 1046 AK Amsterdam, The Netherlands. Tel. ++ 31 (0)20 6114821, Fax ++ 31 (0)20 4472979
orders-queries@rodopi.nl — http://www.rodopi.nl